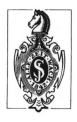

Functional Partial Laryngectomy

Conservation Surgery for Carcinoma
of the Larynx

Edited by M. E. Wigand, W. Steiner, and P. M. Stell

With 211 Figures and 88 Tables

Springer-Verlag
Berlin Heidelberg New York Tokyo 1984

Proceedings of the Third Course for Head and Neck Surgery, Erlangen 1982

Editors

Professor Dr. MALTE ERIK WIGAND
Direktor der Klinik und Poliklinik für Hals-Nasen-Ohrenkranke
Universität Erlangen-Nürnberg
Waldstraße 1, D-8520 Erlangen

Priv.-Doz. Dr. med. WOLFGANG STEINER
Klinik und Poliklinik für Hals-Nasen-Ohrenkranke
Universität Erlangen-Nürnberg
Waldstraße 1, D-8520 Erlangen

P. M. STELL, M.D., F.R.C.S.
Professor and Chairman of the Department of Oto-Rhino-Laryngology
Royal Liverpool Hospital
Prescot Street, Liverpool L69 3BX, Great Britain

ISBN-13:978-3-642-69579-7   e-ISBN-13:978-3-642-69577-3
DOI: 10.1007/978-3-642-69577-3

Library of Congress Cataloging in Publication Data. Course for Head and Neck Surgery (3rd : 1982 : Erlangen, Germany). Functional partial laryngectomy. "Proceedings of the Third Course for Head and Neck Surgery, Erlangen, 1982"—T.p. verso. Includes bibliographies and index. 1. Larynx—Cancer—Surgery—Congresses. 2. Laryngectomy—Congresses. I. Wigan , M. E. II. Steiner, W. (Wolfgang), 1942– . III. Stell, P. M. (Philip Michael) IV. Title. [DNLM: 1. Laryngeal Neoplasms—surgery–congresses. 2. Laryngectomy—congresses. W3 C09998B 3rd 1982f / WV 520 C861 1982f] RF516.C68 1982   616.99'422059   84-5592
ISBN-13:978-3-642-69579-7 (U.S.)

This work is subject to copyright. All rights are reserved, whether the whole or part of the material is concerned, specifically those of translation, reprinting, re-use of illustrations, broadcasting, reproduction by photocopying machine or similar means, and storage in data banks. Under § 54 of the German Copyright Law where copies are made for other than private use, a fee is payable to "Verwertungsgesellschaft Wort", Munich.

© by Springer-Verlag Berlin Heidelberg 1984.
Softcover reprint of the hardcover 1st edition 1984

The use of registered names, trademarks, etc. in this publication does not imply, even in the absence of a specific statement, that such names are exempt from the relevant protective laws and regulations and therefore free for general use.

Product Liability: The publisher can give no guarantee for information about drug dosage and application thereof contained in this book. In every individual case the respective user must check its accuracy by consulting other pharmaceutical literature.

2122/3130-543210

List of Contributors

ALONSO REGULES, J. E., Professor and Director del Centro de Estudios des Càncer laringeo, Br. Artigas 1659/303, Montevideo, Uruguay

BRADLEY, P. J., M.D., Department of Oto-Rhino-Laryngology, University of Liverpool, Royal Liverpool Hospital, PO Box 147, Liverpool L69 3BX, Great Britain

BRYAN NEEL III, H., Professor and Chairman, Department of Otolaryngology, Mayo Clinic, Rochester, Minn. 55905, USA

CALEARO, C., Professore e Direttore della Clinica Otorinolaringoiatrica, Università Cattolica, Largo Gemelli, Via Ubaldi 136, Rome, Italy

CATALA, M., M.D., Instituto Oncologico, Servicio O.R.L., Hospital Provincial de Madrid, Carbonero Y Sol, 42-B, Madrid 6, Spain

COLLO, D., Professor Dr. med., Oberarzt der HNO-Klinik im Klinikum der Johannes-Gutenberg-Universität, Langenbeckstr. 1, 6500 Mainz, FRG

CZIGNER, J., Dozent Dr. med. habil., Weil Emil Krankenhaus, Uzsoki u. 29, 1145 Budapest, Hungary

DALBY, J. E., M.D., Mersey Regional Centre for Radiotherapie & Oncology, Clatterbridge Hospital, Wirral, Merseyside, Great Britain

DENECKE, H.-J., Professor Dr. med., Hals-Nasen-Ohrenarzt, Moltkestraße 20, 6900 Heidelberg, FRG

DEV, R., M.D., Sir Harkisandas Hospital & Tata Memorial Hospital, Ben-Nevis, B, Desai Road, Bombay 400 036, India

FARAGO, L., Dr. med., GÖD, SOMOGYI U 3, 2131 Hungary

FEDERSPIL, P., Professor Dr. med., Leitender Oberarzt der Hals-Nasen-Ohrenklinik der Universität, im Landeskrankenhaus, 6650 Homburg/Saar, FRG

FLOOD, L. M., M.D., University College Hospital, London WCIE 6AU, Great Britain

FRASER, J. G., M.D., University College Hospital, London WCIE 6AU, Great Britain

GRUNDMANN, E., Professor Dr. med., Direktor des Pathologischen Instituts der Universität, Domagkstraße 17, 4400 Münster, FRG

GUERRIER, Y., Professeur et Chef de Clinique Oto-Rhino-Laryngologique et Chirurgie Cervico-Faciale, 75, Avenue de Lodève, 34000 Montpellier, France

HARRISON, D. F. N., M.D., F.R.C.S., Professor of Laryngology and Otology, University of London, 330/332 Gray's Inn Road, London WC1X 8EE, Great Britain

HOMMERICH, K. W., Professor Dr. med., Reichsstraße 84 a, 1000 Berlin 19, FRG

JACH, K., M.D., Klinika Otolaryngologii ul Unii Lubelskiej Nr. 1, 71-344 Szcecin. Poland

JAZOULI, N., M.D., Clinique Oto-Rhino-Laryngologique et Chirurgie Cervico-Faciale, 75, Avenue de Lodève, 34000 Montpellier, France

KIRCHNER, J. A., M.D., Professor and Head of the Department of Otolaryngology, Yale University, School of Medicine, 333 Cedar Street, New Haven, Conn. 06510, USA

KITTEL, G., Professor Dr. med., Leiter der Abteilung für Phoniatrie und Pädaudiologie, HNO-Universitätsklinik, Waldstraße 1, 8520 Erlangen, FRG

KOSOKOVIC, F., M.D., Full Professor of I ENI-Department of Medicine Faculty Zagreb, Salata 4, Zagreb, Yugoslavia

KOTHARY, Pramod M., M.S., D.L.O.R.C.S. (Lon.), Hon. E.N.T. Surgeon, Sir Harkisandas Hospital & Tata Memorial Hospital, Ben-Nevis, B, Desai Road, Bombay 400 036, India

KRAJINA, Z., Dr., Professor and Head, Klinika Za Bolesti Uha, Nosa I Grla, Medicinskog Fakulteta Sveučilista, Salata 4, Zagreb, Yugoslavia

LABAYLE, J., Docteur, Professeur au Collège de Médecine, Hopitaux Oto-Rhino-Laryngologiste Honoraire, Hopitaux de Paris, 51, Boulevard Murat – XVI E, 75016 Paris, France

MAJ, P., M.D., Klinika Otolaryngologii ul Unii Lubelskiej Nr. 1, 71-344 Szcecin, Poland

MEYER-BREITING, E., Priv.-Doz. Dr. med., Oberarzt der Universitäts-HNO-Klinik, Theodor-Stern-Kai 7, 6000 Frankfurt/Main 70, FRG

MONNIER, Ph., Docteur, Service d'Oto-Rhino-Laryngologie, Centre Hospitalier, Universitaire Vaudois, 1011 Lausanne, Switzerland

MORTON, R. P., M.D., Department of Oto-Rhino-Laryngology, Royal Liverpool Hospital, Prescot Street, P.O. Box 147, Liverpool L69 3BX, Great Britain

MOZOLEWSKI, E., Professor Dr. med., Director, Klinika Otolaryngologii ul Unii Lubelskiej Nr. 1, 71-344 Szcecin, Poland

NAUMANN, C., Priv.-Doz. Dr. med., Oberarzt der Universitäts-HNO-Klinik, Kopf-Klinikum, Josef-Schneider-Straße 2, 8700 Würzburg, FRG

OLOFSSON, J., Associate Professor, Linköping University, University Hospital, Department of Otolaryngology, 581 85 Linköping, Sweden

PASCHE, R., Docteur, Service d'Oto-Rhino-Laryngologie, Centre Hospitalier, Universitaire Vaudois, 1011 Lausanne, Switzerland

PIQUET, J.-J., Docteur, Professeur et Chef de Clinique Oto-Rhino-Larnygologie, Hôpital Régional, Place de Verdun, 59037 Lille Cedex, France

SAUER, R., Professor Dr. med., Direktor der Strahlentherapeutischen Universitätsklinik, Krankenhausstraße 12, 8520 Erlangen, FRG

SAVARY, M., Docteur, Professeur et Chef de Service d'Oto-Rhino-Laryngologie, Centre Hospitalier, Universitaire Vaudois, 1011 Lausanne, Switzerland

SCOLA, B., M.D., Instituto Oncologico Servicio O.R.L., Hospital Provincial de Madrid, Carbonero Y Sol, 42-B, Madrid 6, Spain

SERAFINI, I., Professore e Direttore della Divisione O.R.L., Ente Ospedaliero di Vittorio Veneto, Via Forlanini, 31029 Vittorio Veneto, Italy

SINGH, S. D., M.D., Department of Oto-Rhino-Laryngology, Royal Liverpool Hospital, Prescot Street, Liverpool L69 3BX, Great Britain

STAFFIERI, A., Professore della Clinica Otorinolaringoiatrica, Universitá di Ferrara, Arcispedale S. Anna, 44100 Ferrara, Italy

STEINER, W., Priv.-Doz. Dr. med., Universitäts-HNO-Klinik, Waldstraße 1, 8520 Erlangen, FRG

STELL, P. M., M.D., F.R.C.S., Professor and Chairman of the Department of Oto-Rhino-Laryngology, Royal Liverpool Hospital, Prescot Street, P.O. Box 147, Liverpool L69 3BX, Great Britain

STRICKLAND, P., M.D., Regional Radiotherapie Centre Mount Vernon Hospital, Northwood, Middlesex HA 6 2RN, Great Britain

List of Contributors

STRUPLER, W., Professor Dr. med., Chefarzt der Klinik für HNO-Kranke, Kantonsspital St. Gallen, 9007 St. Gallen, Switzerland

SULIKOWSKI, M., M.D., Klinika Otolaryngologii ul Unii Lubelskiej Nr. 1, 71-344 Szcecin, Poland

TARNOWSKA, C., M.D., Klinika Otolaryngologii ul Unii Lubelskiej Nr. 1, 71-344 Szcecin, Poland

TEATINI, G. P., Professore e Direttore della Clinica Otorinolaringoiatrica, Università di Sassary, Sassary/Sardinien, Italy

THEISSING, J., Professor Dr. med., Direktor der HNO-Klinik der Städtischen Krankenanstalten, Flurstraße 17, 8500 Nürnberg, FRG

TRAISSAC, L., Professeur Agrégé et Chirurgien des Hôpitaux, Chef de Service O.R.L., Centre des Spécialités, Hôpital des Enfants, 33077 Bordeaux Cedex, France

VECERINA, S., M.D., Klinika Za Bolesti Uha, Nosa I Grla, Medicinskog Fakulteta Sveučilista, Salata 4, Zagreb, Yugoslavia

VEGA, M. F., M.D., Insituto Oncologico, Servicio O.R. L., Hospital Provisial de Madrid, Carbonero Y Xol, 42-B, Madrid 6, Spain

WASILEWSKA, M., M.D., Klinika Otolaryngologii ul Unii Lubelskiej Nr. 1, 71-344 Szcecin, Poland

WDOWIAK, P., M.D., Klinika Otolaryngologii ul Unii Lubelskiej Nr. 1, 71-344 Szcecin, Poland

WEILAND, L. H., M.D., Professor and Chairman of the Department of Surgical Pathology, St. Mary's Hospital, Mayo Clinic, Rochester, Minnesota 55905, USA

WIGAND, M. E., Professor Dr. med., Direktor der Universitäts-HNO-Klinik, Waldstraße 1, 8520 Erlangen, FRG

WILKE, J., Professor Dr. med., Direktor der HNO-Universitätsklinik, Hamburger Berg 21, 5032 Erfurt-Bischleben, GDR

WYSOCKI, R., M.D., Klinika Otolaryngologii ul Unii Lubelskiej Nr. 1, 71-344 Szcecin, Poland

Preface

Cancer of the head and neck continues to be a challenge. Increasing incidence has pushed malignancy of the upper aerodigestive tract into the first rank of cancer. In some countries it follows bronchial carcinoma in frequency and is more common than gastro-intestinal and gynaecological cancer. This increasing incidence makes it difficult to train enough highly specialised staff who are also responsible for the care of many other patients, requiring sophisticated microsurgery of the ear and nose.

The question of quality is even more difficult. Oncological success in the treatment of head and neck cancer is bought at the price of crippling of vital functions such as eating, breathing, voice and sight and furthermore of striking aesthetic deformity. Mutilation of this highly functional collection of organs is more keenly felt than that of any other region of the body. It is vital, therefore, that the surgeon keeps up with the recent achievements of functional surgery in order to offer the best service to his patients.

Cancer of the larynx is no exception. Despite newer techniques of radiotherapy and chemotherapy, surgery still gives the best oncological results. This requires a wide spectrum of operations varying from minimal ablation to total laryngectomy. With regard to conservation of laryngeal function two approaches seem to be most promising. The first is the use of magnifying and illuminating endoscopes, which permit early detection of cancer. This may permit cancer prevention by mass screening of high risk groups, by demonstrating premalignant stages and cancer in the preclinical stage. Thus, it may enable functional partial resections to replace radical operations in a higher percentage of cases. It also allows verification of recurrence.

The second basis of advanced conservation surgery of the larynx is clinical pathology. Sophisticated partial laryngectomies are only justifiable if a histopathologist is readily available to examine the excised specimen. He must be fully familiar with the surgical anatomy of the larynx and neighbouring organs, must know the patterns of cancer spread in this region and must feel a sense of responsibility for the individual patient.

Techniques of partial laryngectomy have developed rapidly during the last decade. There have been controversial discussions at recent meetings: ambitious concepts based on narrow approaches to the primary tumour or discrete handling of the regional lymphatic tissues have been recommended and compared with approved strategies of radical ablative surgery. Looking through our own collection of laryngeal specimens removed by total larnyngectomy some 10 years ago, we were both surprised and embarrassed to realise that today a partial resection could have been performed with the same prognosis but with retention of the patients voice.

More and more, the classical principle of resecting an affected area with a broad safety margin following well-defined anatomical structures, and then waiting for possible recurrence, is giving way to techniques based on knowledge of the spread of an individual tumour. Both larynx and neck are meticulously checked with numerous intraoperative biopsies taken for frozen section, and the resected specimen is checked by scrupulous histopathological examination. The patient must be warned of a possible second-stage procedure and of long-term endoscopic follow-up using cytological smears and precise biopsies.

The new surgical techniques of open or endoscopic partial resections of the larynx using microsurgery of the CO_2 laser are only possible and justified if the above requisites (endoscopic staging, intra- and postoperative histology and cooperation of the patient, who must be willing to risk an immediate second operation and to undergo strict endoscopic follow-up) are fulfilled.

This type of "explorative surgery" was and is condemned by many prudent and well experienced laryngologists who emphasise the contrast between "risky and conservative" versus "safe and radical". Cancer surgery does not tolerate compromise. However, the management of facial basal cell carcinomas has taught us to give priority to histological verification of tumour resection before completing the operation by reconstructive procedures. These lessons can be applied to oncological surgery of the upper aerodigestive tract with remarkable success in preserving important functional structures.

The Second Course on Head and Neck Surgery at the University of Erlangen-Nuremberg in 1979, dealt with the restoration of voice after laryngectomy and starred Professor Mario Staffieri from Brescia. The Third Course, in 1982, devoted to conservation surgery for carcinoma of the larynx, was initiated by Dr. Wolfgang Steiner, and organised by him and Dr. H. J. Pesch from the Department of Pathology at Erlangen. Their concept was a continuing dialogue illustrated by live operations and endoscopic demonstrations masterfully performed and presented by an international group of experts in conservation surgery of the larynx.

It transpired that this was not a symposion of conservative people, but of a very progressive faculty. The strict rules of resection of an advanced primary tumour with complete in-continuity eradication of the cervical lymphatics is giving way to a greater awareness of modern techniques of partial ablation of the larynx, regional functional neck dissection and numerous combinations of resection and reconstruction. This type of functional surgery is very refined but its microsurgical precision is radical, and both sophisticated and established from the oncological point of view. It is far from being conservative in the older sense.

The results reported by the various experts from 16 countries were presented frankly and discussed in a dynamic but always friendly atmosphere. It was fascinating to learn from so many outstanding personalities how they would handle the same problem. Witnessing both the philosophy and the convincing arguments of this faculty was the essence of the meeting and was even more stimulating than learning the details of craftsmanship of vertical and horizontal laryngectomies.

Agreement could not be reached on the indications for each procedure, and many questions remained unsettled, for example the value of combined radiotherapy and the avoidance of complications. It became apparent, however, that a lasting record of this course could be highly attractive to the international community of laryngologists. Thanks to the efforts of Springer-Verlag and to support by some below mentioned sponsors it has become possible to produce the proceedings in the form of this book.

It was not easy to collect all manuscripts in time and to ensure that they were of an appropriate length. Reviewing, slightly changing or rewriting paragraphs or tables was a necessary but pleasant task for the editors who learned many of the details only by rereading the passages. We have tried to facilitate comprehension by an attempt to coordinate medical and anatomical terms. Professor Stell of Liverpool has also taken over the burden of revising the texts of a number of the non-English-speaking authors. But it has been the aim of the editorial board not to standardise the contributions of different laryngologists from all parts of the globe, struggling with different problems and with varied experience.

A multi-author book has some disadvantages with regard to didactic principles and the avoidance of redundancy and controversial opinions. But this may be an advantage, in that it mirrors the present state of the art. This volume represents a great opportunity for the reader to compare various schools from different countries and keep up with all the achievements and pitfalls of contemporary surgery for carcinoma of the larynx.

It is hoped that it will provide young laryngologists with guidance to the numerous approaches and interest more advanced surgeons with its description of a wide variety of alternatives and experiences.

M. E. WIGAND

Acknowledgements

The following societies and authorities supported the IIIrd Course for Head and Neck Surgery: "Conservation Surgery for Carcinoma of the Larynx", held at Erlangen, June 29th–July 2nd 1982:

Deutsche Krebsgesellschaft
Deutsche Gesellschaft für Endoskopie
Deutsche Forschungsgemeinschaft
Bayerisches Staatsministerium für Unterricht und Kultus

The close collaboration of the Pathological Institute of the University of Erlangen-Nuremberg under its Head, Professor Dr. V. BECKER, was highly appreciated. The profound interest of Professor Dr. H. J. PESCH in the histopathology of laryngeal cancer and its spread has contributed greatly to the development of surgical treatment and to the success of the course.

Professor Dr. GIANPIETRO TEATINI of Ferrara, now Director of the Department of Oto-Rhino-Laryngology of the University of Sassari/Sardinia, is to be congratulated on his elegant moderation of the final panel discussion of the Course which summarized the pros and cons of advanced partial laryngectomy. Dr. ERWIN MÜNCH, Erlangen, undertook the difficult and onerous task of collecting and supervising the retyping of the manuscripts. He looked after the figures and photographs, and was invaluable as an Assistant Editor. Patients from several ENT Departments agreed to have their operations demonstrated live. We are grateful to them, and to the heads of the respective departments: Professor Dr. CH. BECK of Freiburg, Professor Dr. W. DRAF of Fulda, Professor Dr. W. KLEY of Würzburg.

The cooperation of Mrs. SIPPEL and Mrs. DUMMERT, who have taken care of the manuscript, is appreciated.

We are greatful to Mr. BERGSTEDT of Springer-Verlag for his encouragement and generous help in the production of this book.

We are indebted to the following companies who substantially supported the IIIrd International Course on Head and Neck Surgery and the publication of its proceedings:

Cooper-Laser Sonics, St. Clara, California
Ethicon GmbH, Hamburg-Norderstedt
Hoechst AG, Frankfurt am Main
Hoyer Med. Technik, Bremen
Immuno GmbH, Heidelberg
Pfrimmer & Co. GmbH, Erlangen
Richards Manufacturing GmbH, Tuttlingen
Karl Storz GmbH & Co., Tuttlingen
Richard Wolf GmbH, Knittlingen
Carl Zeiss, Oberkochen

THE EDITORS

Contents

A. Introduction into Conservation Surgery of the Larynx

Anatomy of the Larynx with Reference to Functional Cancer Surgery
Y. Guerrier. With 8 Figures 3

Histology of Laryngeal Carcinoma – Past and Present. A Historical Review
E. Grundmann. With 4 Figures 9

Historical Development of Reconstructive Surgery in Laryngeal Carcinoma
H. J. Denecke 15

B. Basics of Diagnosis and Planning of Therapy

I. Clinical Diagnosis of Laryngeal Carcinoma 21

Clinical Diagnosis of Laryngeal Carcinoma. W. Steiner. With 2 Figures 21

Microlaryngoscopy. J. Olofsson. With 6 Figures 27

II. Diagnostic Techniques of Clinical Pathology 31

Histopathology of Early Laryngeal Carcinoma. L. H. Weiland. With 7 Figures . . . 31

Histologic Grading – Early Lesions. J. Olofsson 37

III. Early Detection of Cancer in the Upper Aero-Digestive Tract: Mass Screening . . . 39

Experiences with Screening of Oto-Rhino-Laryngological Cancer in Hungary
L. Faragó 39

Laryngological Screening of Industrial Workers (Galvanizers, Spray Painters, Enamellers). J. Wilke. With 1 Figure 42

Prevention and Early Detection of Cancer of the Upper Aerodigestive Tract. Results of Endoscopic Mass Screening. W. Steiner 44

Screening for Upper Respiratory Tract Cancer. Sputum Cytologic Diagnosis
H. Bryan Neel III 48

Endoscopic Screening for Multiple Squamous Cell Carcinoma of the Upper Digestive and Respiratory Tracts (Oncologically Oriented Upper Aero-Digestive Pan-Endoscopy)
M. Savary, R. Pasche, and Ph. Monnier. With 4 Figures 51

IV. Radiological Diagnosis 59

Radiology of the Larynx. W. Strupler. With 6 Figures 59

The Value of Computerized Tomography in Conservative Surgery of Glottic Cancer
E. Meyer-Breiting. With 1 Figure 63

Computed Tomography in the Diagnosis of Laryngeal Carcinoma. J. Olofsson
With 3 Figures 66

V. Clinical and Histological Staging 69

The Systems of UICC and AJC for Staging of Laryngeal Carcinomas. J. A. KIRCHNER
With 5 Figures 69
What is the Glottis? P. M. STELL and R. P. MORTON. With 3 Figures 74
Staging of Laryngeal Carcinoma. J. OLOFSSON. With 3 Figures 79
The TNM-Classification with Regard to Surgical Planning of Partial Resections
of the Larynx. K. W. HOMMERICH. With 5 Figures 82
Correlation Between Clinical and Histological Staging in Laryngeal Cancer
D. F. N. HARRISON 86

C. Vertical Partial Resection of the Larynx

I. Surgical Techniques and Modifications of Vertical Partial Laryngectomy 89

History, Indications and Techniques of Vertical Partial Laryngectomy. J. LABAYLE
With 12 Figures 89
The Role of Laryngoplasty in Vertical Partial Laryngectomies. H. J. DENECKE
With 9 Figures 95
Selection of Treatment for In Situ and Early Invasive Carcinoma of the Glottis:
Surgical Techniques and Modifications. H. BRYAN NEEL III 104
Partial Glottic Laryngectomy (Moser's Modification). J. WILCKE. With 3 Figures .. 106
Experiences with Vertical Partial Laryngectomy with Special Reference to Laryngeal
Reconstruction by Sternohyoid Fascia. Z. KRAJINA and F. KOSOKOVIC
With 5 Figures 108
The Use of Cervical Fascia After Vertical Resection of the Larynx. D. COLLO
With 7 Figures 112
A Vascular Pedicled Flap of the Thyroid Gland and Its Application in Vertical Partial
Laryngectomy. E. MOZOLEWSKI, P. MAJ, P. WDOWIAK, K. JACH, and C. TARNOWSKA .. 116
Extended Frontolateral Partial Laryngectomy. C. NAUMANN. With 2 Figures 117
Vascular Pedicle Flap of the Thyroid Gland in the So-Called 3/4-Laryngectomy
E. MOZOLEWSKI, P. MAJ, P. WDOWIAK, K. JACH, and C. TARNOWSKA 119
Surgical Technique in Frontolateral Laryngectomy and Cordectomy. P. FEDERSPIL
With 2 Figures 119
Transoral Microsurgical CO_2-Laser Resection of Laryngeal Carcinoma. W. STEINER .. 121

II. Posttherapeutic Histology and Microstaging in Vertical Partial Laryngectomy .. 127

Vertical Partial Resections of the Larynx – Posttherapeutic Histology, Microstaging
J. A. KIRCHNER. With 8 Figures 127
Glottic Carcinoma – with Special Reference to Tumors Involving the Anterior
Commissure and Subglottis. Posttherapeutic Histology
J. OLOFSSON. With 4 Figures 131
Histomorphological Behaviour of the Tumour Growth in the Glottic Region
K. W. HOMMERICH. With 6 Figures 134
Posttherapeutic Histopathology of Laryngeal Carcinoma. L. H. WEILAND
With 3 Figures 138
Squamous Cell Carcinomas of the Anterior Wall of the Larynx. E. MEYER-BREITING
With 1 Figure 140

III. Oncological and Functional Results as the Basis of Surgical Indications 145

Vertical Partial Laryngectomy – Results. Y. GUERRIER and N. JAZOULI
With 1 Figure 145

Indications for Surgery or Radiotherapy for Glottic Cancer and Their Oncological
Results. J.-J. PIQUET. With 6 Figures 150

Phonatory Function Following Unilateral Laser Cordectomy. Z. KRAJINA 152

Oncological and Functional Results After Vertical Partial Laryngectomy
E. MOZOLEWSKI, P. MAJ, P. WDOWIAK, K. JACH, C. TARNOWSKA, and M. WASILEWSKA . 153

Laryngofissure and Partial Vertical Laryngectomy for Early Cordal Carcinoma:
Outcome in 182 Patients. H. BRYAN NEEL III 154

Vertical Partial Resection. Oncological and Functional Results. L. TRAISSAC
With 9 Figures 156

Endoscopic Therapy of Early Laryngeal Cancer. Indications and Results. W. STEINER
With 2 Figures 163

Oncological Results of Vertical Partial Laryngectomy. W. STEINER 170

Indications for Moser's Glottic Partial Resection. J. WILKE 173

Voice and Respiration Before and After Partial Laryngeal Resections
G. KITTEL 174

D. Horizontal Partial Resection of the Larynx

I. Surgical Techniques and Modifications 179

Horizontal Partial Laryngectomy. Historical Review and Personal Technique
J. E. ALONSO REGULES 179

Horizontal Supraglottic Laryngectomy: Surgical Technique
C. CALEARO, G. P. TEATINI, and A. STAFFIERI. With 5 Figures 183

My Personal Surgical Technique of Supraglottic Horizontal Laryngectomy. I. SERAFINI
With 7 Figures 186

Conservation Surgery for Supraglottic Carcinoma
M. F. VEGA, B. SCOLA, and M. CATALÁ. With 8 Figures 189

Horizontal Glottic Laryngectomy (Horizontal Glottectomy): Surgical Technique
C. CALEARO and G. P. TEATINI. With 4 Figures 195

Modifications of Supraglottic Resection of the Larynx. J. CZIGNER. With 6 Figures . . 197

Vascular Pedicle Flap of the Thyroid Gland in Horizontal Supraglottic Laryngectomy
E. MOZOLEWSKI, P. MAJ, P. WDOWIAK, K. JACH, C. TARNOWSKA, and M. WASILEWSKA 203

Three Quarters Laryngectomy. G. P. TEATINI. With 4 Figures 204

II. Posttherapeutic Histology and Microstaging in Horizontal Partial Laryngectomy . . 209

Horizontal Partial Resections of the Larynx. Posttherapeutic Histology and
Microstaging. J. A. KIRCHNER. With 3 Figures 209

Supraglottic Carcinoma – Posttherapeutic Histology. J. OLOFSSON. With 2 Figures . . 211

Histological Examination of the Excised Specimen After Supraglottic Laryngectomy
I. SERAFINI. With 6 Figures 214

III. Oncological and Functional Results of Horizontal Partial Resections as the Basis of Surgical Indications 219

Horizontal Supraglottic Laryngectomy: Results. A. STAFFIERI 219

Results of Supraglottic Horizontal Laryngectomy. I. SERAFINI 223

Oncological and Functional Results of Horizontal Partial Laryngectomy. M. F. VEGA . . 226

Horizontal Glottectomy: Results. A. STAFFIERI 228

Phonatory Function of the Larynx Following Partial Laryngectomy
S. VECERINA and Z. KRAJINA 230

Oncological Results of Supraglottic Horizontal Partial Laryngectomy
(Alonso Operation). W. STEINER 232

Oncological Results of Horizontal Partial Laryngectomy. J. WILKE 234

Horizontal Supraglottic Laryngectomy with Total Glossectomy – Oncological and
Functional Results. P. KOTHARY and R. DEV. With 3 Figures 235

Cineradiographic and Manometric Measurements of Deglutition Following Horizontal
Partial Laryngectomy. E. MOZOLEWSKI, K. JACH, M. SULIKOWSKI, and R. WYSOCKI . . 242

E. Surgical Management of the Lymphatic System

Why Perform a Functional Neck Dissection? C. CALAERO, G. P. TEATINI,
and A. STAFFIERI. With 8 Figures 247

Surgical Treatment of the Cervical Lymph Node System in Laryngeal Carcinoma
W. STEINER. With 1 Figure 253

Surgical Management of the Lymphatic System with Regard to Supraglottic Resections
of the Larynx. H. BRYAN NEEL III 264

F. Radiotherapy and Chemotherapy

Sequential Chemotherapy and Radiotherapy in Advanced Head and Neck Cancer
P. M. STELL, J. E. DALBY, P. STRICKLAND, J. G. FRASER, P. J. BRADLEY,
and L. M. FLOOD. With 3 Figures 269

Combined Radiation Therapy and Surgery for Limited Carcinoma of the Larynx
R. SAUER. With 2 Figures 274

Vertical and Horizontal Partial Resections of the Larynx After Radiotherapy
J. CZIGNER. With 1 Figure 280

Radiotherapy and Partial Laryngectomy. H. J. DENECKE 284

Radiotherapy and Partial Supraglottic Resection. C. CALEARO and A. STAFFIERI 285

Aspects of Adjuvant Chemotherapy in Combination with Horizontal Partial
Laryngectomy. J. THEISSING 286

G. Postoperative Course After Vertical and Horizontal Partial Laryngectomy

I. Complications After Partial Resections of the Larynx 291

Postoperative Care After Partial Resections of the Larynx. P. FEDERSPIL 291

Early and Late Complications After Laryngofissure or Vertical Partial Laryngectomy
H. BRYAN NEEL III 293

Early and Late Complications After Partial Resections of the Larynx. M. F. VEGA . . . 295

Early and Late Complications After Supraglottic Partial Resection of the Larynx
J. CZIGNER. With 2 Figures 298

Functional Complications After Supraglottic Laryngectomy
P. M. STELL, R. P. MORTON, and S. D. SINGH 301

Late Complications and Recurrences After Partial Resections of the Larynx. Z. KRAJINA   305

II. Early Detection and Management of Recurrences   309

Follow-up Examination After Partial Laryngectomy. Early Detection of Recurrences
W. STEINER 309

Early Detection of Recurrent Tumours After Previous Treatment of Laryngeal
Carcinomas. J. OLOFSSON 310

Early Detection and Management of Recurrences After Vertical Partial Laryngectomy
H. BRYAN NEEL III 315

Early Detection and Management of Recurrences After Vertical Partial Laryngectomy
Y. GUERRIER. With 6 Figures 316

Treatment of Recurrences After Supraglottic Horizontal Laryngectomy (S.H.L.)
M. F. VEGA 320

H. Final Synopsis of Conservating Surgery for Carcinoma of the Larynx

Resumé of the Course on Conservation Surgery for Carcinoma of the Larynx,
Erlangen 1982. G. P. TEATINI 325

A. Introduction into Conservation Surgery of the Larynx

Anatomy of the Larynx with Reference to Functional Cancer Surgery

Y. GUERRIER, Montpellier

Before starting a review of the surgical anatomy of the larynx a definition of what we understand by the term pharyngo-laryngeal cancer appears mandatory. The hypopharynx must be included in every oncological discussion of this area. Also, the standards of surgery for malignancies of the larynx must be recapitulated beforehand, because our aim will be to demonstrate the orientation of contemporary laryngeal surgery towards both the physiological functions and the anatomical compartments of this organ.

Pharyngo-laryngeal Cancer

Cancers of the larynx must be separated from those of the epilarynx and of the hypopharynx. According to the UICC the supraglottic region can be divided into the epilarynx or marginal compartment and into the vestibulo-epiglottic region. Unfortunately, the international anatomical term "laryngeal aditus" was not included. The occasional restriction of the term pharyngo-laryngeal cancer to cancer of the epilarynx including the free margin of the epiglottis, the region of the three folds, and of the ary-epiglottic folds appears unjustified.

Surgical Treatment of Pharyngo-laryngeal Cancer

There are total or partial laryngectomies. Partial vertical resections are used for the glottis, partial horizontal laryngectomy may remove the supraglottic compartments or may be restricted to the glottic region (Calearo's operation). In addition, we have adopted subtotal removal of the larynx with reconstruction to the treatment of certain T_2 tumours for which conventional partial laryngectomy was not safe enough, while total laryngectomy would overtreat the disease.

Resection of the hypopharynx can also be total or partial. The operations of Trotter or of Alonso such as supraglottic hemipharyngo-laryngectomy aim at the ablation of the piriform sinus. Partial pharyngectomy may be associated with partial or total removal of the larynx. A total pharyngectomy is technically feasible, but uncommon for practical reasons.

There are rare forms of laryngeal carcinomas, at least rare in France, originating in the crico-arytenoid region. They may be successfully removed, but I prefer irradiation. With their exception, the indications for total pharyngectomy for tumours of the piriform sinus with involvement of the postcricoid region are exceptional. Because of their bad prognosis in spite of surgery, their treatment by pharyngo-laryngectomy appears to be unreasonable.

The classical subdivision of the pharynx is:
1. nasopharynx
2. oropharynx and
3. hypopharynx.

In my experience the separation of the posterior pharyngeal wall as a fourth segment is justified, because in this wall no anatomical barrier exists, neither in the mucosa nor in its submucosal layers which would permit a subdivision into three levels. Malignant tumours of the posterior pharyngeal wall can, therefore, spread easily. An abdominal surgeon, accustomed to retrocolonic surgery, would be astonished to learn about our interpretation and results of pharyngolaryngeal surgery.

Important Anatomical Facts

A) The hypopharynx and the supraglottic larynx have a common branchiogenic origin. Their principal structures are explained in the sketches of Fig. 1 and 2. It could be proven by anatomical and radiological studies that the bottom of the piriform sinus never reaches below the level of the glottis. This plane functions as a lymphatic barrier hindering vertical tumour propagation, what was proved by the investigations of the anatomist Rouvière, the radiologist Baclesse and by the surgeon Alonso:

"At the free margin of the vocal cords only a very fine network of lymphatic vessels exists, arranged parallel to the direction of the vocal cords. They form a barrier between the supra- and subglottic regions. No injection into one of these regions entered the other by trespassing the intermediary network of the true vocal cord" (Rouvière 1932).

"Supraglottic carcinomas may grow considerably. But even if they occupy the whole vestibule, or infiltrate the pre-epiglottic space anteriorly, they don't invade the level of the vocal cord continuously. The invasion of the subglottis, rarely observed, takes place in the depth, between the ventricle and the thyreoidal lamina, at the roof of Morgagni's ventricle, stopping at the side of the glottis as if here existed an obstacle" (Baclesse 1938).

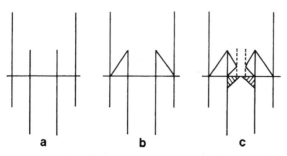

Fig. 1a–c. The pharyngo-laryngeal unit. **a** The axes of respiration and digestion. **b** The junction of both axes and the formation of the piriform sinus. **c** The principle of endolaryngeal and hypopharyngeal levels

Introduction into Conservation Surgery of the Larynx

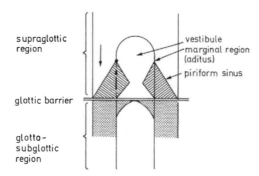

Fig. 2. The pharyngo-laryngeal unit with regard to regions and lymphatic barriers

"If nature almost always stops supraglottic cancer at a frontier above the bottom of the ventricle, why not exstirpate the tumour along this line, marked by a more prudent hand than ours" (J. M. Alonso 1961).

Since we can prove that a safe removal of vestibuloepiglottic cancer may be accomplished by following an inferior resection plane of few millimeters distant to the tumour, while maintaining a superior clearance of some centimeters, in our opinion a horizontal partial laryngectomy is a true segmental resection.

B) The thyroid cartilage loses its quality as a barrier at the sites of its ossification. These spots open the door to translaryngeal proliferation of cancer. The fibrous cartilage of the epiglottis, on the other hand, is perforated by a number of vessels.

C) The preepiglottic space is paired into two by a median partition. The anatomical features of this separation could be demonstrated by horizontal serial sec-

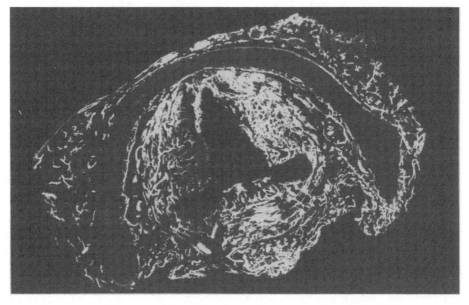

Fig. 3. Microangiography of the larynx (child). Horizontal section through the glottic plane. The cartilage forms a barrier between the endo- and extralaryngeal regions

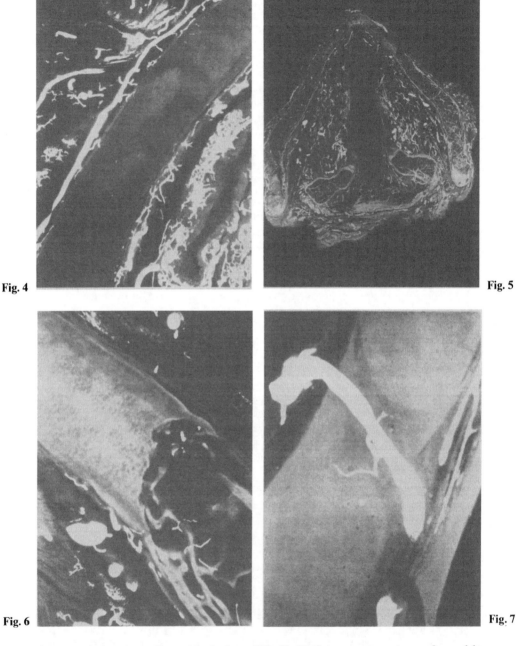

Fig. 4 Fig. 5

Fig. 6 Fig. 7

tions, carried out together with Andrea (Fig. 8). Both compartments are framed by the medial thyrohyoidal ligament anteriorly, and by the thyrohyoid membrane below the thyroid cartilage and its internal perichondrium.

In a vertical slide the preepiglottic space has a triangular form with a caudal tip. It is bounded by the broad hyo-epiglottic ligament above, anteriorly by the thyrohy-

Fig. 4. Microangiography of the larynx (same preparation as Fig. 3). With higher magnification the absence of vessels within the thyroid cartilage, and their predominance in the external perichondrium can be observed

Fig. 5. Microangiography of the larynx (adult). Horizontal section through the glottic plane. The vascularization of the ossified thyroid cartilage is demonstrated

Fig. 6. Microangiography of the larynx (same preparation as Fig. 5). With higher magnification details of the rich vascularization of the ossified thyroid cartilage are demonstrated

Fig. 7. Microangiography of the larynx. With high magnification the perforation of the epiglottis by blood vessels is visible. Communication between the endolarynx and the preepiglottic space is normal

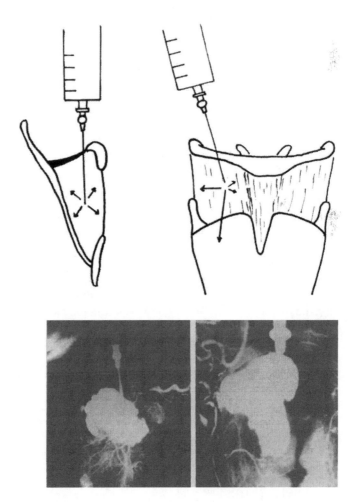

Fig. 8. The preepiglottic space visualized by injection technique. Even with large quantities of contrast medium no escape into the adjacent regions was observed. Note the existence of two separated preepiglottic spaces

oid membrane. A fixation to the posterior face of the hyoid bone, and to the superior horns of the thyroid cartilage was always noted. The practical importance of these facts is evident: Surgical removal of a carcinoma of the laryngeal aditus or of a piriform sinus includes resection of the preepiglottic space. While in these cases the ablation of one or both superior thirds of the thyroid wings is necessary, the resection of the hyoid bone depends on the case.

D) The elastic internal structures of the endolarynx can be observed in a frontal section. The conus elasticus forms a subglottic dome. Its cranial extension forms the vocal ligament which is connected to the vocal process of the arytenoid, dorsally, and to Broyles's ligament anteriorly. The fibrous tissue ends in the floor of the ventricle. Broyles's ligament originates in the thyroid angle and inserts in a shallow grove at the internal face which is often marked by an external hump in the thyroid crest. This ligament collects fibres of the internal perichondrium of the thyroid cartilage, and forms the fibrous anchor of the base of the epiglottis, of the vocal cords and of the ventricular folds.

Mucous glands may perforate the conus elasticus, which restricts its function as an oncological barrier against tumour spread. But the fibres of the connective tissue can also be split by tumour cells. Besides the ligament of Broyles the crico-thyroid membrane is an important oncological frontier. The crico-arytenoid articulation and the posterior edge of the thyroid cartilage form a secure barrier against the posterior spread of glottic cancer.

E) One important precondition of advanced pharyngolaryngeal resections is the maintenance of the undisturbed function of

respiration,
phonation, and
swallowing.

Three anatomical units are necessary for their display:

The cricoid ring for respiration,
an isthmus of mobile construction for phonation, and
a valve system, steered by sensitive and motor nerves for deglutition.

In my opinion the third aspect, the valuable mobility of a valve structure, is most important for a successful functional surgery of the larynx. It can be provided by the "arytenoid unit", which means the coordination of the movements of both the pharyngo-epiglottic and aryepiglottic folds together with their contents. The latter includes not only vessels and nerves, but also different muscle bundles with their proper innervation. All these various anatomical structures must be considered if oncological surgery is to preserve pharyngo-laryngeal functions in addition to ablating the tumor.

References

Guerrier Y, Andrea M (1973) Les loges épiglottiques. Nuovo Arch Otol 1:3–21
Guerrier Y, Andrea M (1977) La vascularisation des cartilages du larynx. Son importance clinique. Ann Otolaryngol (Paris) 94:273–290

Histology of Laryngeal Carcinoma – Past and Present. A Historical Review

E. Grundmann, Münster

Every scientist likes to discuss the novelties in his own field, and "New Aspects of Larynx Research" would be a popular title. My historical review rather has to look back, but when I prepared the text I duly realized how much is still to be learnt from older aspects, too. More, in fact, than a 15 minute lecture can hold, and so I shall focus on three problems for which the relevance of history is readily understood:
1. The value and biological significance of biopsy diagnosis,
2. Causal pathogenesis,
3. Prognostic aspects.

The 19th century left us a good number of weighty volumes on diseases of the larynx which we may reopen not only for the sake of curiosity, but also for useful information. 1883 Gottstein published a textbook "Diseases of the Larynx" of whose 428 pages only 18 were devoted to laryngeal tumors. To be exact, laryngeal carcinoma was dealt with in 2 pages, the rest was about other tumor types; 40 pages dealt with laryngeal tuberculosis, 12 with syphilitic lesions of the larynx. When Schech wrote his textbook "Diseases of the Larynx and Trachea" in 1903, a mere 8 pages of its 331 were about laryngeal cancer, 20 about tuberculosis, and 13 about syphilis. We are well aware how much the proportions have shifted in the meantime and why.

Yet, laryngeal carcinoma had been clearly described in the second century A.D. already by Galenus, and mentioned at least, as early as 91 B.C. by Asklepiades of Bithynia. Whether Boerhave's case of "cancerous angina" was actually a carcinoma of the larynx or rather of the hypopharynx invading the larynx, is hard to decide. But it is certain that the nestor of pathology, Morgagni, did write the first autopsy report of a laryngeal carcinoma, in Latin, of course:

"Plures autem in pharynge et ad summam laryngem tumores conspiciebantur qui carcinomatis habebant naturam".

He had performed the autopsy on a man of 50 who died with symptoms of aphonia and impaired swallowing.

The first exact differentiation of benign from malignant tumors of the larynx was established by v. Rokitansky, while the first reliable histologic diagnosis was pronounced by Rudolf Virchow.

1) Virchow's name leads us to the first problem, the *value and biological significance of biopsy diagnosis.*

Well known and paradigmatic is the case of Frederic III, the German Emperor. The story may be taken from the "Official Documentation" published 1888 by the Imperial Stationers (Reichsdruckerei) in Berlin, and from Sir Morell Mackenzie's replique published shortly after in the same year. According to the official German documentation, the German physicians consulted in this case, especially Professors Gerhardt and von Bergmann, had agreed quite early that the Crown Prince's disease was a carcinoma of the larynx. Dr. Mackenzie, consulted as an English expert, felt uncertain and insisted on the microscopical examination of an excised piece of tissue, to be performed by Virchow himself. The biopsy specimen was taken May 21st, 1887. Virchow's report reads: "There is only an irritative process; some isolated nests of epithelial cells in concentric layers are found amoung proliferating epithelia. This is most probably a case of pachydermia laryngis". Virchow did ask whether the excision had really been taken from the tumor itself. Two days later another excision by "sharp forceps" was attempted without success, leaving the patient almost completely voiceless. The failure aroused some controvery about whether Mackenzie had happened to damage the right vocal cord that had been unaffected so far. The tumor's localization on the left cord had been safely ascertained. Hereafter thermocauterization was repeated several times, also insufflation with a powder composed of morphium, bismut, Catechu and sugar. The patient had to endure daily thermocauterization for quite some time.

Again two pieces of tissue were excised on June 8th, 1887, and Virchow's diagnosis was again "pachydermia verrucosa", but he added: "Wheather this diagnosis is justified for the entire disease cannot be verified from the two excised specimens". Upon this verdict, Mackenzie refused to agree with the cancer diagnosis pronounced unanimously by all the other physicians, and so the extirpation recommended by v. Bergmann was not performed.

The patient's fate is history, he died June 15th, 1888, a few weeks after his succession to the throne. The autopsy, performed by Virchow and Waldeyer, resulted in the unequivocal diagnosis: "Extensive carcinoma of the larynx with metastases". The facts were so plain that Virchow closed his report with the words "No epicrisis is needed".

The factual evidence, however, did not prevent a prolonged and heated public controversy about the adequacy and appropriateness of the therapeutic measures taken. That the outcome of surgical intervention was far from secure at the time, may be inferred from Wassermann's 1889 publication about a Congress held in 1881 in London on larynx extirpation as a surgical method. Up to 1881 this operation had been performed in 41 cases of whom only 3 had been free from recurrencies for 3 years. 80 laryngectomies were recorded between 1881 and 1889, 5 of them being free from recurrency for 3 years. Details of Wassermann's compilation are shown on Table 1.

Table 1. Results of total laryngectomy (Wassermann 1889)

Follow-up	Before 1881	After 1881
Surviving less than 2 weeks	22	19
Surviving less than 2 months	3	9
Recurrencies	11	29
Death during later follow-up	2	9
Free from recurrencies for 3 yrs.	3	5
Follow-up too short	–	9
	41	80

The first total laryngectomy had been performed by Billroth in 1873. The general state of the art is aptly illustrated by Wassermann's dictum of 1889: "Radical surgery of malignant larynx tumors is at present as unsatisfactory as the mere treatment of symptoms is inefficient" (p. 225 of his book). We know the positive changes and improvements achieved in the past hundred years. It is not for me to recall the current rates of successful surgery, but some aspects of a comparison may be interesting.

When Mackenzie tried to excise pieces of larynx tissue by forceps the technique of specimen sampling was less well developed than that of histological diagnosis. In view of such drawbacks, the modern pathologist will understand why Rudolf Virchow was unable to pronounce a positive diagnosis of cancer: Pieces pinched from the mucosal surface give no clue to the in-depth invasion of a tumor, nor do they substantiate the diagnosis carcinoma or no carcinoma. Any pathologist familiar with the daily routine of larynx biopsies will know the particular difficulties hampering the correct diagnosis of cancer in these tissues (cf. Kleinsasser 1963; Grundmann 1973; Pesch and Steiner 1979, and others).

Even benign squamous epithelium may occasionally extend its cones into the underlying connective tissue; there is also the keratoakanthoma of the larynx whose basal parts are not readily differentiated from cancer, especially by the unexperienced diagnostician. In the larynx, like in other mucosal tissues and in the epidermis, precancerous lesions and in-situ carcinoma have to be distinguished from carcinoma (Steiner and Pesch 1977; Pesch and Steiner 1979, and others). Backed by the present wealth of detailed and substantial knowledge, we can but admire our predecessors and their fundamentally correct diagnoses that had to be based on the limited technical facilities of their time.

For illustration we may confront Sendziak's table of the age distribution in laryngeal carcinoma of 1897 with our own table of 1979 (Fig. 1). The recent curve shows a shift to the right, but the age peak is at 60 in both statistics. Maybe the shift is due to the higher general life expectancy of our generation; on the other hand, certain benign tumor types such as atypical papilloma, may have been counted

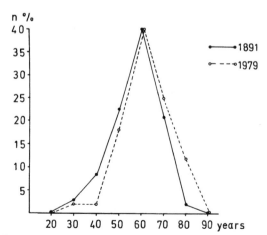

Fig. 1. Age distribution of laryngeal carcinoma. Comparison between Sendziak's table (1891) and current data of 1979

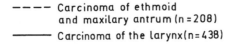
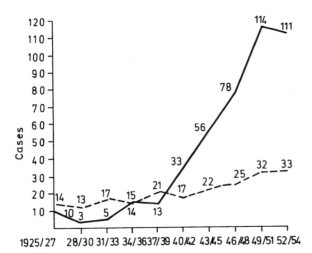

Fig. 2. Comparison of incidence rates of laryngeal carcinoma and ethmoid and maxillary cancer, 1925–1954 (Blümlein 1956)

among the carcinomas by Sendziak's contemporaries. This would also explain the comparably high incidence among the 30–40-year-olds recorded in the older table.

2) This leads to our second problem, *causal pathogenesis*. In an interesting study from Erlangen University, Blümlein (1956) published a curve (Fig. 2) illustrating the enormous increase of larynx carcinoma incidence in comparison to that of ethmoidal and maxillary cancer. The rise begins in 1937/39; we know for sure that laryngeal carcinoma affects predominantly smokers, and that its rapid increase is mainly associated, in analogy to bronchial carcinoma, with the inhalation of cigarette smoke. Some studies of the Münster group can be cited in this context (Müller and Krohn 1980): Squamous epithelial hyperplasias as well as metaplasias, dysplasias, in-situ carcinomas, and finally invasive carcinomas, are found significantly more often in heavy smokers than in non-smokers. Even ex-smokers, abstinent for at least 5 years, have a markedly higher proportion of dysplasias and carcinomas than non-smokers (Fig. 3). The correlation is universally accepted today, and it is also known that chromate industry workers, or those exposed to other carcinogenic agents, have an increased incidence of laryngeal carcinoma.

The larynx offers an almost perfect example for the historical debate on histogenesis in context with carcinogenesis. Mackenzie, for instance, held the thermocauterization performed prior to his first bioptic excisions responsible for causing the Emperor's ultimately verified carcinoma. Virchow's term "irritation carcinoma" played a considerable role at the time, referring mainly to unspecific irritants. A favorite subject for discussion was whether benign tumors were liable to turn malignant, especially in the larynx. A few singular publications such as the much-discussed papers of Semon (1889) and Barth (1898) were and are cited again and again. They related cases where carcinomas had been found in the vicinity of papillomas. Although today nobody would claim that cauterization could induce carcinoma in the larynx, nobody would deny either that scar carcinomas may occur also in the larynx, even if very rarely. Their biological significance is the same in the larynx as in the lungs or epidermis, and exogenous carcinogenic agents are sure to play an important role.

This is the place for a historical curiosity, namely some data trailed through the literature for quite some time as "proof" for the induction of malignant neoplasia,

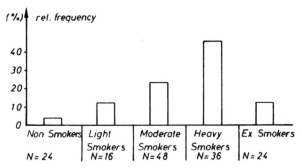

Fig. 3. Compared frequencies of dysplasia, in-situ carcinoma, and carcinoma of the larynx in groups with similar smoking habits (Müller and Krohn 1980)

especially in the laryngopharyngeal region, by the mere superficial transfer of cancer cells. The story must have started with Baratoux' report of 1888 about two brothers, one of whom had larynx carcinoma. For "painting" the throat of the healthy brother he happened to use the brush he had previously employed for the other brother's throat; the healthy brother later developed a retrolingual carcinoma. That this was a mere coincidence could be verified in later years, but the story survived and served for years as a pointer to cancer infection in general, and to infection by laryngeal carcinoma in particular.

3) The last of my topics is *prognosis* which depends, like in other tumor sites, on the grading and staging of the individual lesion. Although these two aspects need not be discussed in detail just now, it may be of interest that our colleagues from the past century were already aware of the better prognosis of glottis carcinoma in contrast to the worse outlook for supraglottic lesions.

Recent studies have emphasized the role of perifocal inflammation in particular for laryngeal cancer. In our Münster work group Blaeser (1975) verified the rate of ^{3}H-thymidine incorporation in a collective of 50 resected carcinomas. According to the respective tumor cell labeling rates the cases were divided in two groups, one of high growth rates (average: 38% labeled tumor cells), the other of low growth rates (average: 7% labeled tumor cells). The most interesting result of these studies was that the number of "inflammatory mesenchymal cells" in the immediate surroundings of the tumor, was inversely proportional to that of labeled tumor cells: Rapidly growing tumor cells are surrounded by fewer inflammatory mesenchymal cells than the slowgrowing tumors (Fig. 4). These mesenchymal cells were identified as lymphocytes, plasma cells, histiocytic monocytes, adventitial cells, and mast cells. If

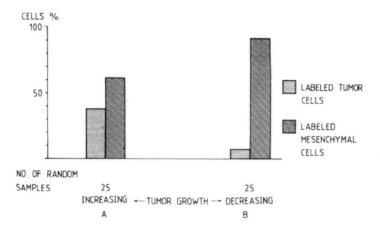

Fig. 4. Inverse correlation between tumor growth and inflammatory mesenchymal cells in 50 laryngeal carcinomas. Left: No. of labeled nuclei after incubation with ^{3}H-thymidine. Group A = fast-growing tumors, Group B = slow-growing tumors. Right: Percentage of cell types surrounding carcinomatous areas. LY = lymphocytes, PL = plasma cells, HIS = histiocytes. The second columns for PL and HIS marks the ^{3}H-thymidine index in these cells (Blaeser 1975)

thymidine labeling is analysed separately for each of these cell types, lymphocytes are found unable to incorporate ^{3}H-thymidine, while some 5% of plasma cells are able to do so – a finding that still needs to be confirmed (Fig. 4). The presence of proliferating plasma cells in tissue around the tumor had not been noticed, so far. Independent of this particular detail, Blaeser's results clearly support the concept of an inverse correlation between tumor growth and the amount of perifocal inflammation in laryngeal carcinoma.

Looking back at the past hundred years of larynx pathology we realize that truly reliable diagnosis of larynx carcinoma is an achievement only of the last two decades. Great admiration, therefore, is due to our colleagues from the 1880s for their courage and ability to pronounce a correct diagnosis in what was obviously the majority of cases. Larynx carcinoma is a good instance for both progress and backslides in research on the causal pathogenesis of cancer, ranging from the theory of "irritation cancer" to the "infectiousness" of tumor cells. How much the prognosis of laryngeal carcinoma has been improving since the days of Frederic III. is common knowledge and a challenge for further studies.

References

Baratoux J (1888) Du Cancer du Larynx. Paris
Barth E (1898) Zur Kasuistik des Übergangs gutartiger Kehlkopfgeschwülste in bösartige. Arch Laryngol Rhinol Vol. 7
Blaeser B (1975) Proliferationskinetik im peritumoralen Entzündungsfeld menschlicher Kehlkopf-Carcinome. Diss. Med. Fak. Münster
Blümlein H (1956) Zur Frage der Häufigkeit des Kehlkopfkrebses. Z Laryngol Rhinol 35:267–270
Gottstein J (1893) Die Krankheiten des Kehlkopfes. Deuticke, Leipzig-Wien

Grundmann E (1973) Die Bedeutung der präcancerösen Zell- und Gewebsveränderungen in Experiment und Klinik. Arch klin exp Ohren-Nasen-Kehlkopfheilk 205:55–67

Kleinsasser O (1963) Die Klassifikation und Differentialdiagnose der Epithelhyperplasien der Kehlkopfschleimhaut aufgrund histomorphologischer Merkmale. Laryngol Rhinol Otol (Stuttg) 42:339–362

Mackenzie M (1888) Friedrich der Edle und seine Ärzte. Antwort auf die Berliner Broschüre: Die Krankheit Kaiser Friedrich III. A. Spaarmann, Styrum-Leipzig

Müller KM, Krohn BR (1980) Smoking habits and their relationship to precancerous lesions of the larynx. J Cancer Res Clin Oncol 96:211–217

Offizielle Dokumentation (1888) Die Krankheit Kaiser Friedrich des Dritten, dargestellt nach amtlichen Quellen und den im Königlichen Hausministerium niedergelegten Berichten der Ärzte. Kaiserliche Reichsdruckerei, Berlin

Pesch HJ, Steiner W (1979) Die Bedeutung der Dysplasien an der Kehlkopfschleimhaut. Verh Dtsch Ges Pathol 63:105–111

Schech P (1903) Die Krankheiten des Kehlkopfes und der Luftröhre. Deuticke, Leipzig-Wien

Semon F (1889) Die Frage des Übergangs gutartiger Kehlkopfgeschwülste in bösartige, speziell nach intralaryngealen Operationen. Int Centralbl Laryngol Rhinol 6:209–227

Sendziak J (1897) Die bösartigen Geschwülste des Kehlkopfes. J.F. Bergmann, Wiesbaden.

Steiner W, Pesch HJ (1977) Vor- und Frühstadien des Kehlkopfkarzinoms. Prospektive endoskopisch-histologische Untersuchungen. Verh Dtsch Ges Pathol 61:364

Wassermann M (1889) Über die Extirpation des Larnyx. Dtsch Z Chir 29:H 5 und 6

Historical Development of Reconstructive Surgery in Laryngeal Carcinoma

H. J. Denecke, Heidelberg

Partial resection of the larynx was developed about 100 years ago, particularly in France and Italy. Since the mutilating operation of total laryngectomy was regarded as intolerable for the patient, partial laryngectomy was preferred. At that time, partial resection could only be justified in tumors of limited extent, especially since the radicality of the excision would have suffered. In addition, appreciable disturbances of air passage and deglutition with potentially fatal aspiration pneumonia would have occurred without reconstruction in resection of larger tumors.

According to the literature, the first surgeon to have carried out reconstruction in partial resection of the larynx was Gluck. At the beginning of this century, he used a pedicle skin flap "to avoid infections of the raw area, to prevent stenoses and to improve deglutition" after hemilaryngectomy. This reconstructive procedure reduced the danger of aspiration pneumonia which was a frequent, severe and potentially fatal complication up to that time. In special situations in the region of the laryngostoma, he resorted to double-flap reconstruction as described by Balassa (1844) for closure of fistulae after laryngeal injuries. Gluck considered that the flap reconstruction of Velpeau (1832), which had likewise been developed for surgical treatment of laryngeal injuries was not appropriate for reconstruction after tumor surgery.

In the 1920's, J. Soerensen recommended that mucosal defects in the region of the aryepiglottic fold and the arytenoid cartilage should be covered with mucosa in resection of carcinomas by means of "laryngotomy". He emphasized that the laryngeal mucosa is especially suitable for "suturing the defects" in this region due to its good mobility. In large mucosal defects, he detached the mucosa from the piriform sinus in order to use it for resurfacing, a technique which derives from Wilms.

Besides the mucosal flaps, J. Soerensen has also used pedicle skin flaps and bridge flaps to cover the raw areas after resection of carcinomas by means of laryngotomy. He was thus able to prevent the development of stenoses and to improve glottal closure. J. Soerensen called this "wallpapering of the laryngeal defects". In his opinion also tubed flaps, introduced by Ganzer (1917) and Gillies (1920) could be used for laryngeal reconstruction. – Free skin grafts or free mucosa grafts have been hardly used in surgery of laryngeal carcinomas because of the poor chances of healing in and the tendency to shrinkage of the raw areas.

In order to ensure a safe excision of the tumor far into healthy tissue and to avoid discrediting partial laryngectomy due to recurrences, J. Soerensen already recommended working with a head light for better illumination of the surgical field.

Most surgeons who have worked with partial laryngectomy and reconstruction of the resection defects in the course of the last 60 years have used an intralaryngeal or intratracheal dressing with cannula for the postoperative phase. Only in this way was it possible to fix the sutured flaps in position and to prevent aspiration pneumonia. J. Soerensen referred to "Mikulicz tamponade" of the larynx and the trachea.

Since the 1930's, the indication for total extirpation could be appreciably restricted in favor of partial resection of the larynx. This was made possible on the one hand by the introduction of magnification surgery with head light and binocular loupe or with surgical microscope, and on the other hand by refinement of reconstructive techniques. Magnification surgery ensures more safety for excision of tumors into healthy tissue. Accordingly, larger defects result and necessitate more extensive reconstructive measures. This applies both to glottic-subglottic and to supraglottic tumors.

After resection of relatively small and superfical glottic-subglottic carcinomas, it is sufficient to mobilize the surrounding mucosa and to suture it as sliding flap over the resulting defect as recommended and carried out by J. Soerensen in the 1920's and readopted by De Amicis in 1962. However, this mucosal displacement is not sufficient to cover larger superficial defects. For these cases, the Author has good experience for more than 25 years with pedicled mucosa flaps from the subglottic region, the false vocal cord or the posterior wall of larynx and trachea. These flaps can be turned over the defect and sutured to its edges without tension.

The pedicle skin flaps from the neck introduced by Gluck and J. Soerensen are suitable for filling deeper resection defects. However, these flaps have to be modified according to modern criteria depending on the position and size of the defects. Thus A. Réthi (1965) described pedicle skin flaps which he has used ingeniously to widen the lumen and to improve function in laryngeal stenoses after hemilaryngectomy. In 1961, Conley reported on the attempt to form a kind of vocal cord on the skin flap turned into the larynx and in this way to improve glottal closure. In the course of the last 30 years, the author has also developed a series of laryngoplasties using pedicled skin flaps for covering large resection defects and to improve laryngeal function after partial laryngectomies. Details on the current state of development of this surgery are described in Volume V, 3 of the Kirschner Operationslehre.

Alonso introduced supraglottic partial laryngectomy for treatment of supraglottic carcinomas in the 1940's. Whereas an open granulating pharyngostome was originally left behind in this technique, in the 1950's Alonso recommended that the resection defect at the larynx inlet should be covered with mucosa and that the larynx should be fixed by sutures cranially against the hyoid bone or the base of the tongue in order to improve deglutition. The pharynx was primarily closed. Since the mucosa from the vicinity of the resection defect is either not sufficient in extensive resections or must be sutured under tension and then tears open later, there is danger that the perivascular sheath is exposed to the pharynx lumen postoperatively. As the branches of the external carotid artery or the external carotid artery itself are often ligated or severed in the simultaneous neck dissection, there is danger of severe arrosion hemorrhage into the pharynx with possible aspiration of blood or bleeding into death. This danger is present especially in preirradiated patients. For this reason, the author has since 1955 always formed a temporary epithelialized pharyngostome by turning in a thick pedicle skin flap over the perivascular sheath into the pharyngeal defect. In this way reliable protection of the vessels is achieved. In addition, the formation of pharyngeal stenosis with the concomitant swallowing difficulties can be avoided even in extensive resection defects. However, a second operation is necessary two or three weeks later to close the pharyngostome. The combination of this surgical technique with the cricopharyngeal myotomy introduced into partial laryngectomy by the author in 1953 has proved to be especially advantageous in extensive supraglottic tumors. The significance of myotomy in this field could be confirmed by Ogura in 1959. These surgical techniques are also described in Volume V, 3 of the Kirschner Operationslehre.

The advantage of reconstructive measures in connection with partial laryngectomies is obvious. They were introduced by Gluck at the beginning of this century and have been continuously refined until the present day. They allow restoration of the functions of the larynx despite extensive resections. Laryngeal stenoses as well as synechias in the region of the anterior commissure are avoided and the mobility of the arytenoid cartilages remains largely undisturbed. Under the pedicle skin flap, cartilage from the ear or the rib can be transplanted in deeper defects and brings about an improvement of glottal closure with the familiar favorable consequences. The disadvantage of the use of pedicle skin flaps for reconstruction is that several – in most cases two – operations are necessary up to closure of the larynx or the pharynx. In extensive tumors which would have made total laryngectomy necessary on the basis of traditional indications, the patient is willingly prepared to accept this disadvantage.

Some authors object to reconstruction of resection defects with skin flaps in that possible recurrencies are only recognized late. But it must be borne in mind that recurrences are very rare with appropriate care and experience of the surgeon. In addition, if there is a recurrence it can penetrate more rapidly to the surface through a skin flap than through scar tissue which offers more resistance to the spreading of carcinomas.

The reconstructive measures require of the surgeon great knowledge and experience in the field of plastic surgery, since perfect function after closure of the larynx or pharynx must be guaranteed.

References

Alonso JM (1947) Conservative surgery of cancer of the larynx. Trans Am Acad Ophthalmol Otolaryngol 53:633

Alonso JM (1950) La chirurgie conservatrice pour le cancer du larynx et de l'hypopharynx. Ann Otolaryngol Chir Cervicofac 67:567

Alonso JM (1957) A propos de la chirurgie fonctionelle du cancer du larynx (Laryngectomie partielle horizontale). Ann Otolaryngol Chir Cervicofac 74, 75

Balassa: zit. nach Th. Gluck u. J. Soerensen, Handb. der spez. Chir. des Ohres ect. (s. unten) S 69

Conley JJ (1961) Glottic reconstruction and wound rehabilitation. Procedures in partial laryngectomy. Arch Otolaryngol 74:239

De Amicis et al.(1962) La laringofissura con chiusura postoperatoria immediata nella chirurgia endolaringea. Ann Laringol 61:545

Denecke HJ (1953) Die oto-rhino-laryngol. Operationen. In Allgemeine und spezielle chirurgische Operationslehre, begr. von M. Kirschner, Bd. V. Springer, Berlin, Göttingen, Heidelberg

Denecke HJ (1960) Versorgung von Mesopharynxdefekten nach Exstirpation maligner Tumoren dieses Gebietes. Arch klin exp Ohr-Nas-Kehlk-Heilk 176:645

Denecke HJ (1961) Der Einfluß der laryngoplastischen Eingriffe und der Antibiotica auf die Indikation zur Larynxexstirpation. Arch klin exp Ohr-Nas-Kehlk-Heilk 178:288

Denecke HJ (1965) Teilresektion des Larynx. Monatsschr Ohrenheilk 99:415

Denecke HJ (1967) Plastische Eingriffe am Hals unter Berücksichtigung des Larynx. Z Laryngol Rhinol Otol 46:415

Denecke HJ (1970) Laryngoplastiken mit gestielten Hautlappen bei der partiellen Laryngektomie. Arch klin exp Ohr-Nas-Kehlk-Heilk 196:212

Denecke HJ (1980) Die oto-rhino-laryngologischen Operationen im Mund- und Halsbereich. In: Allgemeine und spezielle Operationslehre, Bd. V, 3. Springer, Berlin Heidelberg New York

Gluck TH, Soerensen J (1922) Die Exstirpation und Resektion des Kehlkopfes. Handb. der spez. Chir. des Ohres ect. In: Katz L, Blumenfeld F (Hrsg) Bd. IV. Leipzig: Kabitzsch, S 68 ff

Réthi A (1956) Hemilaryngektomie und plastische Beseitigung der konsekutiven Kehlkopfstenose. Z Laryngol Rhinol Otol 35:101

Soerensen J (1930) Die Mund- und Halsoperationen. Urban & Schwarzenberg, Berlin Wien

Wilms (1930) zit. nach J. Soerensen, Die Mund- und Halsoperationen. Urban & Schwarzenberg, Berlin Wien, S 257

B. Basics of Diagnosis and Planning of Therapy

I. Clinical Diagnosis of Laryngeal Carcinoma

Clinical Diagnosis of Laryngeal Carcinoma

W. STEINER, Erlangen

Laryngoscopic Examination Methods

Indirect Laryngoscopy

The disadvantages of the indirect mirror examination of the larynx are: the small field of view, inadequate illumination, and an unfavourable viewing angle, particularly in the presence of anatomical variations, for example an overhanging, U-shaped epiglottis.

Indirect Microlaryngoscopy

Microscopic magnification of the mirror offers only minor advantages. The field of view is still limited, and the image inverted and in some regions incomplete.

Direct Laryngoscopy

The development of *direct laryngoscopy* (suspension and supported laryngoscopy) (Kirstein 1895; Killian 1911; Seifert 1922) has considerably improved the view of the endolarynx.

The next logical step was the introduction of the microscope into direct laryngoscopy ("Microlaryngoscopy" by Kleinsasser, 1968/76) under general intubation anaesthesia. Endolaryngeal microsurgery was accepted throughout the world, and has been applied to excisional biopsy and removal of very early cancer lesions.

The most important modification is non-intubation microlaryngoscopy employing jet ventilation (Stange et al. 1974).

Special laryngoscopes with distending blades have been developed by Storz (Weerda et al. 1979) and by Wolf (1982). The larger proximal and distal openings permit better operating conditions; and these laryngoscopes are also suitable for jet ventilation and laser surgery.

Transconioscopy

Transconioscopy has been recommended for the direct inspection of the subglottic region and trachea. It is, however, a surgical intervention that is not without a certain risk, and is therefore not suitable as a routine method.

Flexible Laryngoscopy

The advantages of the new short and small-calibre Olympus and Wolf endoscopes are that they permit both transnasal and transoral inspection of the larynx and trachea, even in the presence of anatomical or pathological obstacles, and undisturbed assessment of function. They can frequently be used transnasally, in young children to assess the larynx.

Their disadvantages are the relatively small field of view, which makes their use rather difficult, the absence of magnification, and the difficulty or impossibility of carrying out simultaneous local diagnostic measures such as swabs or biopsies; also the quality of the photographic or film documentation is not optimal in comparison with the rigid 90° angled telescopes.

Further disadvantages are the relatively high price and repair costs, and complicated cleaning and disinfection.

In consequence, this technique is not suitable for routine use as a replacement for the mirror examination; nevertheless, for certain indications the flexible endoscope represents an excellent addition to endoscopy with rigid 90° angled telescopes.

90°-Telescopes Introduced Orally Without Anaesthesia

Indirect Hopkins Laryngo-Pharyngoscope[1] (Berci and Ward 1974). This instrument consists of two parts: a metal sheath having a diameter of 8.5 mm, with built-in fibres, and a telescope which is introduced through the sheath. In order to increase magnification an Endo-Magnifier can be attached.

Hopkins Tele-Laryngo-Pharyngoscope[1]. This advanced model of the above-mentioned instrument provides up to fourfold magnification, depending on the object distance. The built-in focusing device is operated by a lever – and is only for focus adjustment. Increased magnification reduces depth of focus.

Ward and Berci (1974), who introduced the Hopkins 90° telescopes in the USA for examination of the pharynx and larynx, considered that despite its advantages, the endoscope had no chance of being used in routine work.

Stomato-Pharyngo-Laryngoscope[2]. The construction permits simple inspection of the pharynx and larynx. It is a fixed-focus system, of 8 mm diameter.

Magnifying Laryngo-Pharyngoscope[2] (v. Stuckrad and Lakatos 1975). The special Lumina lens system of this endoscope provides a zoom-lens effect without being a real zoom. The outer diameter of this one piece laryngoscope is 9 mm. Lens system, light carrier and antimisting tube are integrated in the sheath, thus achieving simple handling and maintenance. A noteworthy feature is the built-in magnifying device which enables the user to change over easily from panoramic vision to close-up vision simply by moving the lever. The object seen through the endoscope is auto-

---

1 Manufactured by K. Storz, Tuttlingen, FRG
2 Manufactured by R. Wolf, Knittlingen, FRG

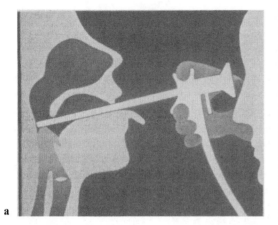

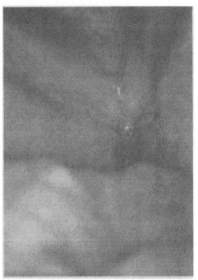

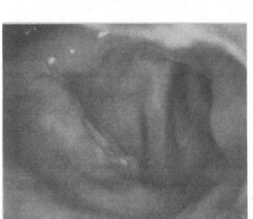

Fig. 1. a Endoscopy of the larynx with the magnifying laryngoscope in the conscious patient (schematic representation). b Supraglottic carcinoma ($pT_{1b}N_0M_0$), 50-year-old male. Ulcerating tumour of the laryngeal epiglottis, localized mainly on the right (magnifying laryngoscopy, survey). c The tumour, restricted to the supraglottis is an indication for horizontal partial resection. Determination of the (macroscopic) extent of the tumour in the conscious patient with the 90° telescope (magnifying laryngoscope; detail)

matically focussed when the magnification lever is used. Magnification depends on the object distance ($\times 2.5 - \times 8$) (Fig. 1).

Since 1975 we have gained experience in the use of the magnifying endoscope in more than 40,000 test subjects and patients (Steiner, 1976/83). Its advantage in comparison with indirect mirror laryngoscopy and direct laryngoscopy under anaesthesia, may be summarized as follows: the examination is technically simple, it can be carried out rapidly and without anaesthesia in the conscious patient allowing assessment of function and is easily tolerated, stressing neither the patient nor the examiner.

The examiner can see more and see better thanks to the features of direct vision (the image is not inverted) (Fig. 1)
- better illumination
- magnification
- the 90° viewing angle
- "wide-angle viewing", which permits a better overview.

Photo, cine or video documentation with the aid of direct adaption of the camera to the endoscope, is relatively simple, technically uncomplicated, quick, requires no anaesthesia, and is of high quality (Steiner 1978).

In our opinion, magnifying endoscopy is a routine examination technique which can replace conventional mirror examination in general, and microlaryngoscopy for purely diagnostic purposes in numerous cases. Microlaryngoscopy under anaesthesia is increasingly being reserved for microsurgical interventions with therapeutic intent. This means less effort and reduced stress for patient and physician and less burden on the hospital.

The tasks of laryngeal endoscopy – detection, clarification, treatment and monitoring of benign, premalignant and malignant lesions – are best carried out with a combination of magnifying endoscopy in the conscious patient and microlaryngoscopy under anaesthesia. In individual cases, in particular for tumour aftercare, the use of thin flexible laryngoscopes has proved successful. Neither indirect microlaryngoscopy nor transconioscopy has any practical importance in modern diagnostic laryngoscopy.

Importance of Magnifying Endoscopy in the Diagnosis of Laryngeal Carcinoma

Establishing Biological Status

Thanks to direct vision and low-power magnification, *diagnostic measures* are simpler and more reliable.

Swab cytology and forceps or needle *biopsy* after superficial anaesthesia with a spray can be carried out selectively and make possible a reliable clarification of suspicious lesions in the larynx (Fig. 2). Swab cytology performed in the conscious patient with the aid of magnifying laryngoscopy, is an elegant, non-stressful procedure which, provided its capabilities and limitations are properly understood, has proved its value as a primary preoperative diagnostic technique.

A biopsy specimen is obtained via magnifying laryngoscopy or microlaryngoscopy with the patient under general anaesthesia. It must always be done prior to primary radiotherapy, and whenever cytology is negative.

Establishing the Extent of the Tumour

In most patients with carcinoma of the larynx, pre-therapeutic inspection with the magnifying endoscope permits the extent of the tumour to be established so that a decision can be made as to the type of surgery required (partial resection or laryngectomy, the most expedient approach, etc.) (Fig. 1).

In our opinion, neither multiple biopsies removed from the neighbourhood of the tumour during microlaryngoscopy, nor computerized tomography or other methods, are suitable to establish the true extent of tumour spread, in particular, into the submucosa before treatment. The definitive decision as to whether partial resection is still possible, or whether laryngectomy is needed, is taken during surgery, on the basis of the macroscopic and histologic findings.

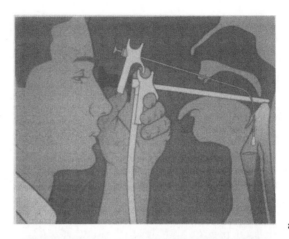

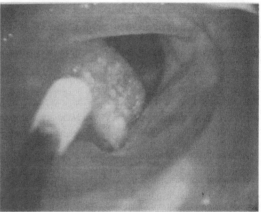

Fig. 2a, b. Cytological laryngeal swab under magnifying laryngoscopic control. Carcinoma diagnosis without anaesthesia. **a** Schematic representation of the examination method. **b** Cotton wool carrier in place in a T_3 laryngeal carcinoma on the right. Cytological results: Pap. V

Diagnostic Concept for Carcinoma of the Larynx

Suspected Advanced Cancer (T_2, $T_{3/4}$) UICC-Classification

Surgery planned. (Vertical partial resection, e.g. hemilaryngectomy, horizontal partial resection or laryngectomy)

Diagnostic procedure
Endoscopy with the magnifying laryngoscope in the conscious patient
– photodocumentation
– determination of the tumour extent
– swab cytology

Positive cytology (Papanicolaou IV/V)
is an adequate basis for surgery and is justified because so far no false positive cytology has been recorded, the sole differential diagnosis is tuberculosis (Fig. 2).
Histological grading, typing and staging is carried out post-operatively on the resected material.

Negative or unclear cytology (Papanicolaou I to III)
Biopsy under magnifying endoscopic control
false negative rate ca. 30% (Steiner, 1979).

Prior to surgery endoscopy of the upper aerodigestive tract is carried out under anaesthesia looking for a second primary tumour.

Radiotherapy Planned as Primary Treatment (Exception). The same measures as already mentioned, but generally *biopsy* for pre-therapeutic histological grading and typing;

additionally, if possible X-ray tomography/computed tomography to demonstrate cartilage infiltration and extralaryngeal spread.

For improved pre-treatment determination of the extent of the tumour (staging), CT can, depending on size and location of the lesion, prove useful in some cases (see Olofsson, page 66 and Meyer-Breiting, page 63).

$T_{3/4}$: Endoscopy of the upper aerodigestive tract under anesthesia
- better determination of tumour spread
- exclusion of simultaneous second primary (see Savary, page 51).

Suspected Carcinoma In Situ or Early Cancer (T_1, T_2 UICC-Classification)

Circumscribed – vocal cord mobile
   Magnifying laryngoscopy in the conscious patient
- photodocumentation
- swab cytology

Cytology findings:
Pap. I–III Microlaryngoscopy – excisional biopsy
Pap. IV–V Microlaryngoscopy – therapeutic resection (laser)

The smaller the lesion and the less clear its biological status, the less justified is the use of the laser for diagnostic excision (Steiner 1980). The diagnostic procedure for early cancer in the larynx is described in detail (Steiner, page 163).

Microlaryngoscopic excisional biopsy of circumscribed lesions (irrespective of their clinical status) which as the diagnostic method of choice is always performed if at all possible, in our opinion obviates additional diagnostic measures such as intravital staining with toluidine blue or stroboscopic examinations, in particular since the rate of false positive findings (16% and 10% respectively) and false negative findings (23% and 30% respectively) has, in our own investigations, proved to be relatively high (Steiner 1979).

Microlaryngoscopy under intubation anaesthesia represents the method of choice for the excision of lesions, and, in the case of precursor and stages of cancer, can at one and the same time be both diagnostic and therapeutic.

References

Kleinsasser O (1968/1976) Mikrolaryngoskopie und endolaryngeale Mikrochirurgie. Schattauer, Stuttgart
Pesch H-J, Ernst M, Steiner W, Ortkras M (1983) Zytodiagnostik im Bereich der oberen Luftwege. 13. Deutscher Zytologie-Kongreß, Freiburg (Abstractband) 38

Stange G, Gebert E, Loo C van de (1974) Intubationslose Narkose bei direkter Laryngoskopie. Z Laryngol Rhinol 5:339
Steiner W (1976) Krebsfrüherkennung in Mund, Rachen und Kehlkopf. Dtsch Ärzteblatt 73:3159
Steiner W (1979) Techniques of diagnostic and operative endoscopy of the head and neck (Part 1). Endoscopy of ear, cerebellopontine angle, nose, paranasal sinuses, larynx, nasopharynx, oro- and hypopharynx. Endoscopy 1:51
Steiner W (1979) Vergleichende Beurteilung endoskopischer Diagnostik- und Therapieverfahren beim Kehlkopfkrebs und seinen Vorstadien. Habilitationsschrift, Erlangen
Steiner W (1980) Fortschritte in der endoskopischen Larynxdiagnostik. Ther Umsch 12:1021
Steiner W, Jaumann MP, Pesch H-J (1980): Früherfassung des Kehlkopfkrebses. Ther Umsch 12:1087
Steiner W (1983) Untersuchungen zur Erkennung von Risikogruppen für Tumorerkrankungen im Kopf- und Halsbereich. Forschungsbericht, Bundesministerium für Jugend, Familie und Gesundheit 9/10: 573/629
Steiner W (1983) Endoskopie von Pharynx und Larynx. Arzt im Krankenhaus
Stuckrad H v, Lakatos I (1975) Über ein neues Lupenlaryngoskop (Epipharyngoskop). Z Laryngol Rhinol 54:336
Ward PH, Berci G, Calcaterra TC (1974) Advances in endoscopic examination of the respiratory system. Ann Otol Rhinol Laryngol 83:754
Weerda H, Pedersen P, Wehmer H, Braune H (1979) Ein neues Laryngoskop für die endolaryngeale Mikrochirurgie. Arch Otorhinolaryngol (NY) 225:103

Microlaryngoscopy

J. OLOFSSON, Linköping

The clinical examination of the larynx includes mirror laryngoscopy, which may be complemented by the use of the operating microscope to achieve a magnified view, which has proved to be especially valuable for indirect evaluation of superficial lesions of the vocal cords and can be furnished with stroboscopic equipment. Telescopic examination has in some departments entirely replaced the mirror examination. Palpation of the larynx and neck should not be forgotten. Especially for major lesions the radiographic examination adds important information about both vertical and deep tumour extension. The surface extension is best assessed by laryngography and the deep extension by computed tomography.

A direct laryngoscopy should be performed using the operating microscope – microlaryngoscopy – a technique introduced in the 1960's by Kleinsasser (1968). Intubation anesthesia, jet-technique or the use of HFPPV (High Frequency Positive Pressure Ventilation) may be used. The microlaryngoscopy is complemented by inspection using 90° optical instruments for examining the sub-surface of the vocal cords and the area below the anterior commissure and other parts of the subglottis as well as the ventricles, a part of these may be examined by lifting the false vocal cords by small hooks. The microlaryngoscopic technique is a great asset in the laryngological diagnosis of e.g. premalignant lesions of the vocal cords. Microlaryngoscopy has improved the possibilities of obtaining representative biopsy specimens and considerably facilitated endolaryngeal surgery. The photographic documen-

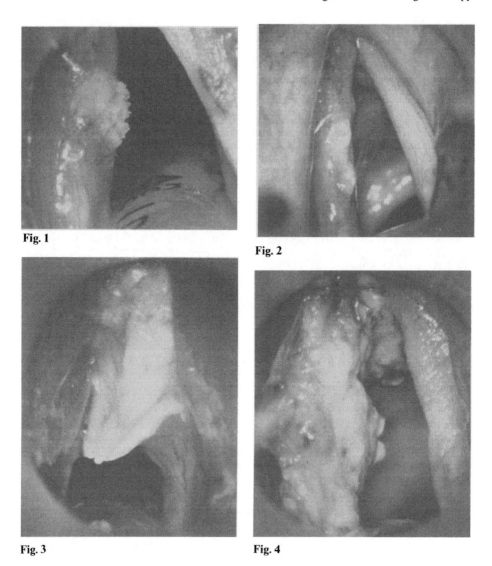

Fig. 1. Localized, keratotic lesion with warty appearance (carcinoma in situ) at the mid-portion of the left vocal cord and amenable to endoscopic excision

Fig. 2. Leukoplakia at the mid-portion (moderate dysplasia) and erythroplakia anteriorly (microinvasive carcinoma) of the left vocal cord. Multiple biopsy specimens or a major excision of the mucosa with step serial histologic sections are necessary to obtain a correct diagnosis

Fig. 3. Verrucous carcinoma occupying the anterior part of the right vocal cord. Note the characteristic papillary, keratinized appearance. Endoscopic excision and laser surgery proved to be adequate treatment in this case

Fig. 4. Carcinoma involving the full length of the left vocal cord and the anterior commissure and extending down subglottically

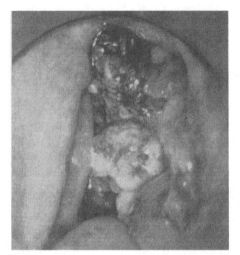
Fig. 5

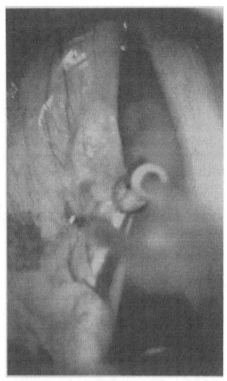
Fig. 6

Fig. 5. Extensive, exophytic tumour of the right hemilarynx nearly completely obliterating the airway. Radiography proved useful to assess the vertical and especially the caudal extent of this tumour

Fig. 6. Minor surgical measures, such as stripping of the vocal cord, is adequate treatment for localized premalignant lesions

tation, especially of superficial vocal cord lesions has been improved and movie and video recording have become easier.

The microlaryngoscopic technique has increased the number of premalignant lesions diagnosed in relation to invasive carcinomas (Kleinsasser 1976) and thus being a valuable aid in the diagnosis but also in the treatment of early laryngeal lesions. The appearance of premalignant lesions varies from a grayish-white keratotic lesion with sometimes a warty appearance (Fig. 1) to an erythroplakia or a mixture of both (Fig. 2). The erythroplakia more often represents severe dysplasia-CIS with or without microinvasion than do a keratotic lesion. Verrucous carcinomas exhibit specific microlaryngoscopic (Fig. 3) and microscopic features (van Nostrand & Olofsson 1972). An exact mapping of squamous cell carcinomas is essential for a correct classification and appropriate treatment (Fig. 4). Extensive tumours may be difficult to assess microlaryngoscopically (Fig. 5) and radiological examination is a necessity.

The final diagnosis should never be based on the microlaryngoscopic picture alone but on the histologic examination of representative material. Localized lesions may be removed entirely by excision or stripping of the vocal cord using cup forceps and a pair of scissors (Fig. 6) or a knife. The use of laser has further widened the possibilities of endolaryngeal surgery.

Supravital stains have for many years been used as a complement in the early diagnosis of malignant lesions. Toluidine blue is usually regarded as a nuclear stain but is also diffused between the cells (Strong et al. 1968). In a prospective study we evaluated the strength and weakness of toluidine blue as an aid in the diagnosis of glottic lesions. The staining results and the histologic findings in 272 biopsy specimens from the vocal cords were compared (Lundgren et al. 1979). 75 of the specimens were taken from patients who had received radiotherapy. Biopsies were taken from all positively stained areas and from all microlaryngoscopically suspect areas, irrespective of the staining result. The sensitivity of the staining in detection of moderate and severe dysplasia and carcinoma was 91% (135/148). Of the 13 false negative staining results, there was keratosis in 11. The overall specificity, represented by the proportion of negative staining reactions in the benign group of lesions, was 52% (64/124) for the whole group and 62% (50/81) for the non-irradiated group. False positive staining reactions occurred in inflammatory reactions, ulcerations, granulation tissue, bleeding surfaces and in post-irradiation changes without atypia. Toluidine blue vital staining should be considered a complement in the microlaryngoscopic diagnosis and provides an increased chance to obtain a representative biopsy specimen from minor lesions which may be overlooked or in diffuse lesions.

Smear cytology is another aid in the microlaryngoscopic diagnosis of laryngeal lesions. Smear cytology has not gained the same position in laryngology as in gynecology. In a prospective study the reliability of laryngeal smear cytology was evaluated in comparison with the histologic diagnoses in 520 lesions (Lundgren et al. 1982). The sensitivity of smear cytology in the detection of invasive carcinoma was 93% (137/147) and for severe dysplasia-CIS 83% (59/71) but only 45% (17/38) for moderate dysplasia. False negative cytology reports were more frequent following radiotherapy. The specificity of smear cytology in the detection of histologically "benign" lesions was 80% (210/264). The cytologic test is easy to perform and may be of diagnostic value especially in screening examinations. It has to be stressed that smear cytology never can replace the histologic examination as a base for therapeutic decisions.

References

Kleinsasser O (1968) Mikrolaryngoskopie und endolaryngeale Mikrochirurgie. Technik und typische Befunde. Schattauer, Stuttgart

Kleinsasser O (1976) Mikrolaryngoskopie und endolaryngeale Mikrochirurgie. Technik und typische Befunde. Schattauer, Stuttgart, p 43

Lundgren J, Olofsson J, Hellquist H (1979) Toluidine blue. An aid in the microlaryngoscopic diagnosis of glottic lesions? Arch Otolaryngol 105:169–174

Lundgren J, Olofsson J, Hellquist H, Strandh J (1982) The role of smear cytology in laryngeal diagnosis. J Otolaryngol Otol 11:371–378

Strong MS, Vaughan CW, Incze JS (1968) Toluidine blue in the management of carcinoma of the oral cavity. Arch Otolaryngol 87:527–531

van Nostrand AWP, Olofsson J (1972) Verrucous carcinoma of the larynx. A clinical and pathologic study of 10 cases. Cancer 30:691–702

II. Diagnostic Techniques of Clinical Pathology

Histopathology of Early Laryngeal Carcinoma

L. H. WEILAND, Rochester (Minnesota)

To be amenable for conservative laryngeal surgery the malignancies contained within this anatomic structure must be limited in size and in extent of growth. In a relative sense this is equivalent to an early stage of the cancer. In absolute terms the duration of the tumor may represent months or even years. Most "small" and "early" laryngeal carcinomas are discovered at an early stage of their evolution because they produce symptoms. Hoarseness is the hallmark symptom of laryngeal cancer and in particular those of the vocal cords. Therefore, the remainder of this discussion is directed at early cancer of the true vocal cords. This group of tumors is representative of those that are most acceptable for conservation surgery.

For practical purposes nearly all laryngeal malignancies are carcinomas that have their origin from the squamous or ciliated pseudostratified epithelium of the mucous membranes (Fig. 1). Carcinomas from minor salivary gland tissue and sar-

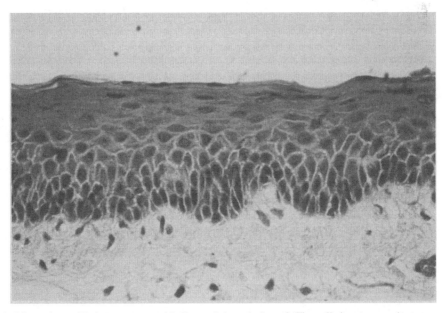

Fig. 1. Normal stratified squamous epithelium of the vocal cord. The cells have normal maturation from the basal layer to the prekeratinized superficial layers. HE, ×250

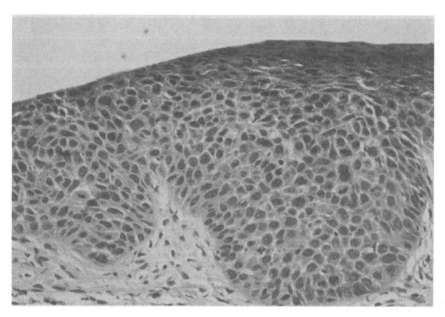

Fig. 2. Carcinoma in situ of the vocal cord. The most striking feature is the lack of normal maturation. Nearly the entire thickness is replaced by cells that are large, have an increased nuclear cytoplasmic ratio, nuclear pleomorphism and hyperchromatism. These changes are of sufficient degree to place it in the malignant rather than dysplastic category even though some maturation is present on the very surface. A line of condensed collagen, the so called basement membrane is intact. HE, ×250

comas from the various connective tissues of the larynx are relatively rare and will receive no further discussion.

It is very likely that carcinoma of the larynx is preceded in most instances by a condition of "cancer susceptibility" of the epithelium that may express itself morphologically as keratosis or dysplasia. These are epithelial changes that are relatively well known to pathologists because of their common occurrence in the epidermis and in the uterine cervix. It is also likely that carcinogenic factors exert influence on laryngeal epithelium. However, documentation of such factors has been elusive. To date only the smoking of tobacco and the ingestion of alcohol have withstood the scrutiny of epidemiological studies.

Carcinoma in situ is the earliest morphologically recognizable form of laryngeal cancer (Fig. 2). It is defined as a neoplastic condition in which malignant cells as determined by microscopic examination replace the normal cells in the laryngeal epithelium. The malignant cells may be variable in appearance. This variation usually reflects changes and alterations in the cytoplasm. For practical purposes, however, carcinoma in situ is defined as a lack of maturation and a disorderly proliferation of cells that usually have a similarity in size and structure to the basal cells of this epithelial layer. There is nuclear hyperchromatism, increased nuclear cytoplasmic ratio, increased mitotic activity and other nuclear abnormalities. The cytoplasm of malignant cells is capable of differentiation, a change that is manifest in laryngeal epithelial cells by keratin production. Thus, carcinoma in situ of the larynx may appear to have malignant basal cells near the "basement membrane", yet have abundant keratin production at its surface. This feature often leads inexperienced pathologists to underdiagnosis in laryngeal carcinoma since most are accustomed to the criteria that a full epithelial thickness must be occupied by undifferentiated cells before a diagnosis of carcinoma in situ can be made.

The distinction between severe epithelial dysplasia and carcinoma in situ is frequently difficult or impossible on a morphologic basis alone. There is a significant degree of interpathologist variation in interpretation. Even the same pathologist may interpret the evidence somewhat differently and on the same specimen make a diagnosis of severe dysplasia on one day and carcinoma in situ on another date. These seemingly great discrepancies become quite minor if the laryngologist believes in conservative therapeutics. It makes little difference whether a vocal cord lesion is severely dysplastic, carcinoma in situ, or even early invasive carcinoma. Such lesions, if small, can all be treated by the same techniques and in a most conservative and effective way. This approach has been used for a decade or more on lesions of the uterine cervix where the relationships between dysplasia, carcinoma in situ, and minimally invasive carcinoma are similar to those of the larynx.

Most laryngeal carcinomas have a moderate degree of differentiation and therefore a moderate degree of keratin production even when they become invasive and when they metastasize (Fig. 3). This statement applies to carcinoma of the vocal cord but is less appropriate for carcinomas of the noncordal larynx. This feature has some therapeutic implication; in general, keratinizing and well differentiated tumors are less responsive to radiation therapy than some of the anaplastic car-

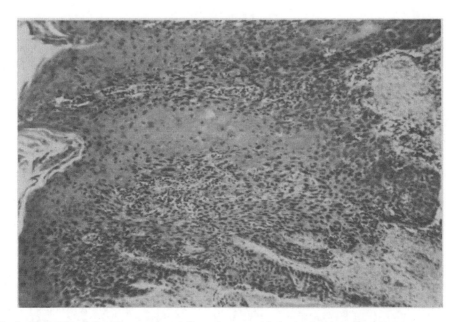

Fig. 3. Well differentiated squamous cell carcinoma with beginning invasion. Carcinoma of the vocal cord usually produces an abundance of keratin. This attempt at differentiation and maturation may result in "underdiagnosis" by pathologists. Here, the depth and the irregularity of the lower tumor border are evidence of infiltration. HE, ×250

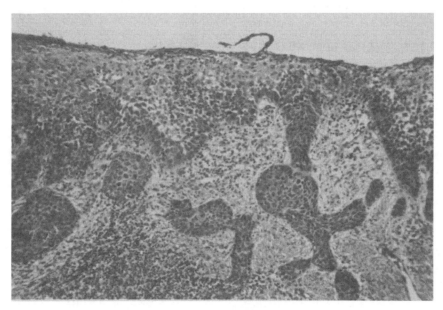

Fig. 4. Invasive carcinoma of the vocal cord. Numerous finger like projections of well differentiated squamous cell carcinoma extend beyond the "basement membrane" and into the subepithelial stroma. Here the tumor has access to lymphatic vessels; note the response of chronic inflammation. HE, ×250

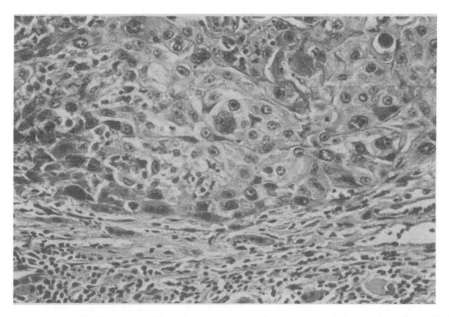

Fig. 5. A "pushing" margin of invasive squamous cell carcinoma of the vocal cord usually indicates that the tumor has a relatively slow growth rate and is less likely to have metastasized. HE, ×250

cinomas. When epidermoid carcinoma becomes invasive it must do so in a very focal manner and not as a broad expanse of invasiveness. This statement is based on personal experience in examining numerous sections of individual cases. Invariably the earliest evidence of invasion is focal and consists of single cells or small clusters of cohesive cells penetrating the region of the basement membrane (Fig. 4). Once the cancer has crossed this territorial boundary it gains access to a region of immediate lymphatic supply and the possibility for metastatic spread to lymph nodes exists.

Although most vocal cord carcinomas are quite similar in morphological characteristics some variability may occur. The variability includes, in addition to the degree of differentiation, differences in growth patterns and differences in the tissue response to the invasive tumor. Differences in growth pattern can be observed at the margin were the tumor edge butts on the normal tissues. The majority of the well differentiated tumors have a sharp and discrete border that suggests a slow expansion of the tumor mass (Fig. 5). Frequently the more poorly differentiated tumors exhibit an infiltrative margin that suggests more rapid tumor growth as well as inherent qualities of the cytoplasmic membrane that allows this infiltration to occur (Fig. 6). As with malignant tumors in other anatomic sites the presence of a "pushing" margin imparts a slightly more favorable outlook than an "infiltrative" margin. Tissue response to invasive carcinoma varies from an absence of reaction to one of intense desmoplasia (Fig. 7). A third response is the presence of variable amounts and various types of inflammatory cells. These reactions should, in teleological theory, be favorable to the host in controlling the spread of the cancer. If this is their purpose it seems relatively ineffective since little prognostic significance can be placed on the presence, type or absence of this reaction. Occasionally the inflamma-

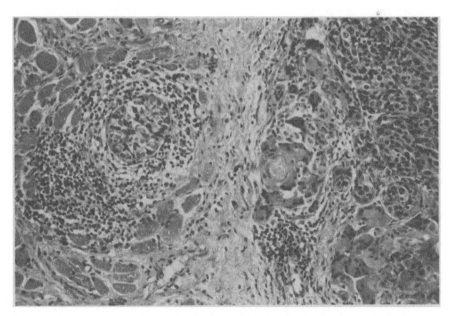

Fig. 6. This squamous cell carcinoma has a poorly defined and "infiltrative" border of invasiveness. Note the projection of tumor, surrounded by inflammatory cells, within the vocalis muscle. HE, ×250

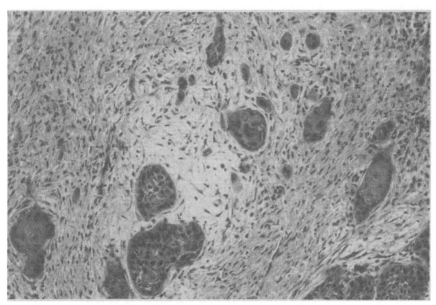

Fig. 7. Invasive laryngeal carcinoma with an intense desmoplastic tissue reaction. This reaction is of unknown cause but may be related to biochemical substances produced by the tumor. As a "defense mechanism" this reaction is ineffective. Similar tissue response can result from radiation therapy. HE, ×250

tory response is granulomatous and histiocytic, probably a reaction to keratin. Undoubtedly, ulceration of some of the larger tumors accounts for many of the acute inflammatory reactions seen in laryngeal cancer.

Lymphatic permeation, as seen on microscopic examination, is rare with small laryngeal carcinomas. With bulky tumors its presence is directly related to the intensity with which it is sought. When found, the regional lymph nodes will invariably harbor metastatic tumor.

In summary, histopathological examination of laryngeal carcinoma should include the type of carcinoma, its size, whether it is associated with an acceptable "premalignant" condition of the mucous membranes, the extent of the tumor to involve adjacent anatomic and microanatomic structures (this includes a statement as to whether it is in situ or invasive), whether or not lymphatic permeation is seen in the specimen and the reaction of the tissues to the malignancy. This information can be derived from routine examination of the specimen. It provides the necessary and desirable information so that the treatment can be appropriately planned.

Histologic Grading – Early Lesions

J. OLOFSSON, Linköping

The non-invasive epithelial lesions of the larynx include keratosis, hyperplasia, dysplasia and carcinoma in situ (CIS). Most of these lesions are diagnosed on the vocal cords. Comparison of the reports on non-invasive epithelial lesions of the larynx is complicated by the inconsistency of the nomenclature and definitions used by different workers.

The classification used should be based on the degree of atypia as this has a bearing on the prognosis. The classification proposed by a panel of pathologists at the Centennial Conference on Laryngeal Cancer in Toronto (1974) was keratosis, keratosis with atypia, CIS and CIS with microinvasion, which is very much in line with the classification presented by Kleinsasser in 1963a. Kleinsasser's Group I (Simple hyperplasia – Einfache Plattenepithelhyperplasie) would correspond to keratosis; Group II (Restless hyperplasia – Plattenepithelhyperplasie mit vereinzelten örtlichen Zellatypien) to keratosis with atypia, and Group III (CIS – Präkanzeröses Epithel) to CIS with or without microinvasion.

An impression of the probability that invasive carcinoma will develop from the different non-invasive epithelial lesions can be obtained from the figures reported in literature. Kleinsasser (1963b), Delemarre (1970), and Lubsen (1980) using the same nomenclature and taking biopsy excisions only reported development of invasive carcinoma in (mean values) 9.2% for Group I, 23.6% for Group II and in 57.8% for Group III (Hellquist 1981). Lumping together various materials where excision, stripping, cordectomy or radiotherapy had been used the corresponding figures were 3.9%, 8.8% and 13.6% for the different groups (Hellquist 1981).

A follow-up study was performed of 161 patients treated in Linköping. The material was divided into three groups following the guidelines above. Group I: Hyperplasia and/or keratosis with or without mild dysplasia; Group II: Moderate dysplasia and Group III: Severe dysplasia – CIS. Invasive carcinoma developed in 2/98, 3/24 and 9/39 in the different groups and up to 13 years after the initial diagnosis (Hellquist et al. 1982).

A differentiation of severe dysplasia in well and moderately to poorly differentiated forms proved to have prognostic importance. It was the well differentiated form that presented the greatest difficulty with a higher incidence of recurrence and development of carcinoma than the moderately to poorly differentiated ones. Diffuse forms of severe dysplasia-CIS had a worse prognosis than localized lesions.

References

Centennial Conference on Laryngeal Cancer, Toronto (1974) Workshop No. 2. Premalignant laryngeal lesions, carcinoma in situ, superficial carcinoma – definition and management. (Chairmen Miller AH, Batsakis JG). Can J Otolaryngol 3:513–575
Delemarre JFM (1970) De betekenis van de plaveiselcellige hyperplasi van het larynxepitheel. Academisch proefschrift, Amsterdam

Hellquist H (1981) Dysplasia of the vocal cords. Linköping University Medical Dissertations, No. 105, Linköping

Hellquist H, Lundgren J, Olofsson J (1982) Hyperplasia, keratosis, dysplasia and carcinoma in situ of the vocal cords – a follow-up study. Clin Otolaryngol 7:11–27

Kleinsasser O (1963a) Die Klassifikation und Differentialdiagnose der Epithelhyperplasien der Kehlkopfschleimhaut auf Grund histomorphologischer Merkmale. Z Laryngol Rhinol Otol 42:339–362

Kleinsasser O (1963b) Über den Krankheitsverlauf bei Epithelhyperplasien der Kehlkopfschleimhaut und die Entstehung von Karzinomen. Z Laryngol Rhinol Otol 42:541–558

Lubsen H (1980) De plaveiselcellige hyperplasie van de larynx en het papilloma inversum van de neus en de neusbijholten. Academisch proefschrift, Amsterdam

III. Early Detection of Cancer in the Upper Aero-Digestive Tract: Mass Screening

Experiences with Screening of Oto-Rhino-Laryngological Cancer in Hungary

L. Faragó, Szombathély

Screening for oto-rhino-laryngological cancer, performed in an outpatient department of the Hungarian capital in 1966, revealed a higher prevalence of precancerous and cancerous conditions in the upper airways among workers in certain branches of industry than in the general population (Faragó 1966; Faragó 1967; Faragó 1970). This prompted us to investigate the possible relationship between air pollution, a known carcinogenic factor, and prevalence of precancerous and cancerous lesions of the upper airways (Faragó et al. 1970).

The screening procedure was carried out by an oto-rhinolaryngologist in the workplace of the persons to be screened; traditional instruments were used and endoscopy was done. The tests for air pollution were performed by Dr. Mórik, National Institute of Hygiene. Dust samples collected in the workplace were analysed for carcinogens, especially for tar and 3.4-benzyprene content. Screening and dust sampling were conducted simultaneously. 90.78% of the employees attended the screening, 6.81% were absent because of illness and 2.41% refused to participate.

In accordance with authors in Hungary and abroad, adult type papilloma, pachydermia, leucoplakia and chronic hyperplastic laryngitis were regarded as precancerous conditions (Alföldi and Duchon 1965; Epstein 1952; Faragó and Nagy 1966; Jackson 1931; Morgenroth 1962).

29,900 persons were examined including urban and rural subjects and workers in factories with low and high degree of air pollution. In this paper the results obtained in persons working in factories with high air pollution are described.

3586 persons (70.1% men, 29.9% women) working in bus garages were examined, 220 of them had positive findings (6.13%). In aluminium foundries 835 persons (85.98% men and 14.02% women) were examined. 110 of them (13.17%) showed some pathological abnormality. The oral cavity was the most affected site (168 persons in the bus garages, 79 persons in the aluminium foundries), the second most affected site was the larynx: 69 in garages, 48 in foundries. Some persons had more than one precancerous lesion: 237 garageworkers and 131 foundryworkers. Cancer was detected in 8 garageworkers and 4 foundryworkers (Table 1).

Because of the role of smoking and alcohol in the pathogenesis of malignancy of the upper aerodigestive tract the history of these factors was taken from the persons having positive findings. Among the 220 persons screened in the bus garages 195

Table 1. Results of screening in persons working in places with high degree of air pollution

	Bus garages	Aluminium foundries
Number of persons examined	3586	835
men	70.71%	85.98%
women	29.29%	14.02%
Number of persons with positive		
findings	220	110
percentage	6.13%	13.17%
Localisation, number of patients		
oral cavity	168	79
larynx	69	48
Cancer	8	4
Praecancerous lesions	237	131

Table 2. Age, duration of employment, smoking and drinking habits of persons with positive findings

	Bus garages	Aluminium foundries
Persons with positive finding	220	110
Age 41–60 years	128	56
Mean duration of employment	12 yrs	10 yrs
Smokers	195 (88.64%)	95 (86.37%)
21–60 cigarettes per day	93 (47.69%)	69 (72.63%)
Heavy alcohol drinkers	82 (37.37%)	41 (37.37%)

Table 3. Results of dust analysis

	Bus garages	Aluminium foundries
Heating loss, %	29.90	19.60
Benzene soluble compartm., %	7.87	0.67
3.4-benzpyrene, ng/g dust	8.13	17.70

(88.64%) were smokers; 93 of these (47.69%) consumed 21–60 cigarettes per day. The corresponding figures in the aluminium foundries were as follows: of 110 patients with suspect lesions 95 were smokers (86.37%), 69 consuming 21–60 cigarettes per day (72.63%). 82 persons out of 220 with positive findings were heavy drinkers (37.37%) in the bus garages while 41 persons (37.27%) out of the 110 patients working in an aluminium foundry with positive findings, could be regarded as heavy drinkers (Table 2).

About 80% of the persons did not know about their pathological condition and were free of symptoms; the remainder had minor complaints but did not attribute any importance to them.

Table 3 shows the results of dust analysis: in the dust samples collected in the bus garages the heating loss was 29.9%, the benzene soluble compartment was 7.87% and the 3.4-benzpyrene content was 8.13 ng/g dust. In the aluminium foundries the values were: 19.60%, 0.67% resp. 17,7 ng/g.

Statements

1. An increasing 3.4-benzpyrene concentration was found in village streets, town streets, bus garages and aluminium foundries.
2. In nearly 30,000 persons examined a precancerous lesions was found in 4.6%.
3. The lowest prevalence was found in villages, it was somewhat higher in urban dwellers in certain occupations, and the highest values were found in industrial workers employed by factories with pronounced air pollution.
4. The prevalence among men was four times higher than among women.
5. Clustering of positive cases occurred in persons between 31 and 60 years of age, especially in the fifth and sixth decades.
6. In this paper only the results obtained in work places with high air pollution are described.
7. The overall prevalence of laryngeal cancer in the Hungarian capital was 0.11%, in bus garages 0.22%, and in aluminium foundries 0.47%.
8. This is the first investigation in Hungary of the question of possible relationship between upper respiratory cancer and fuel consumption. In other countries a higher rate was found with high population density and increased fuel consumption.
9. From our figures no causal relationship between the prevelance of precancerous and cancerous conditions on the one hand, and 3.4-benzpyrene pollution of the air, cigarette and alcohol consumption on the other hand can be established. But, we would like to draw attention to these possible aetiological factors (Hueper 1950).
10. Detection of early cancer is now a world problem.
11. Regular screening of populations at risk for oto-rhino-laryngological cancer has been justified by this study; also elimination of chemical carcinogens is desirable. Lack of specialists, time and money cannot be reasons for neglecting these tasks.

References

Alföldi J, Duchon J (1965) Frühdiagnose des Larynxkrebs mit dem Jodtest nach Schiller. Zeitschrift für Laryngol Rhinol Otol (Stuttg) 44:71–75

Epstein AA (1952) Organisieren der Frühdiagnose des Krebses. Sovjet ref onk 8:28–40

Faragó L (1966) Über einen seltenen Fall von maligner Entartung eines kindlichen Larynxpapilloms. Monatsschr Ohrenheilk 100:131–134

Faragó L (1967) Bericht über 22 697 Hals-Nasen-Ohren-Reihenuntersuchungen Carcinome betreffend. Frül-Orr-Gégegyóg 13:101–110
Faragó L (1968) Bericht über oto-rhino-laryngologische Krebsreihenuntersuchungen. Monatsschr Ohrenheilk 102:588–601
Faragó L (1970) Workmen's serial examination for cancer of the larynx. Magy Onkol 14:97–104
Faragó L, Kertészné SM, Mórik J (1970) The results of oto-rhino-laryngo-logical carcinoma screening tests in the light of the 3.4-benzpyrene pollution of the air. Az Egészségtudomány 14:284–298
Hueper WC (1950) Arch Ind Hyg 2:325
Jackson CH (1931) Fragen der praecancerosen Zustände im Kehlkopf. Proc Reg Soc Med 24:301
Morgenroth K (1962) Praeceröse Veränderungen in der Mundhöhle. Vortrag am VIII. Internationalen Krebskongress in Moskau

Laryngological Screening of Industrial Workers (Galvanizers, Spray Painters, Enamellers)

J. Wilke, Erfurt

The incidence of laryngeal cancer in the German Democratic Republic was determined as 5.5 per 100,000 inhabitants. In industrial cities, however, the figures increased to 6.2 to 8.9 per 100,000 people. From these observations a screening project for high risk groups appeared reasonable. In a first attempt 424 industrial workers (366 males and 58 females) were submitted to laryngoscopy. They were employees of industrial workshops occupied with galvanization, spray painting or enameling. Depending on their job they were exposed to:
  hydrocyanic acid and cyanides,
  chromate compounds,
  nitro dilutions,
  hydrochloric acid,
  phosphoric acid,
  sulphuric acid,
  nickel salts,
  tin compounds,
  trichloroethylene and other organic solvents,
  aldehyde resin varnish,
  benzene, toluene, xylene.

The investigations were carried out near the workplace. Persons with suspected laryngeal findings were asked for thorough examination in the clinic. Our main interest was the detection of chronic inflammation and of laryngeal tumors.
The laryngoscopical findings were divided into four groups:
Group 1 consisted of 91 people with normal endolaryngeal mucosa. Group 2 had 92 persons with hyperemic mucosa, and incidental teleangiectasia of the vocal cords. Group 3 included increased hyperemia and the features of chronic catarrhal

Table 1. Endoscopic results of laryngological screening in relation to the time of occupation

Time of occupation (Years)	Normal endolarynx or slight hyperemia (%)	Chronic laryngitis (%)
0– 5	48	52
6–10	41	59
11–15	38	62
16–20	40	60
21–25	48	52
26–30	30	70
31–40	29	71

laryngitis (123 persons). Group 4 was divided in two sub-groups: 98 persons with circumscribed hyperemia and swelling, diagnosed as hyperplastic laryngitis, belonged to category 4a, while hyperplastic laryngitis of the entire endolarynx was defined as sub-group 4b (20 persons). Additional attention was given to smoking. The correlation of mucosal findings with the time duration of employment is given in Table 1. Figure 1 shows the distribution of presenting symptoms in the screened population.

The results can briefly be summarized:
- In 57% of all examined persons there was macroscopical evidence of chronic laryngitis.
- Pathological findings were significantly more frequent in smokers than in non-smokers.
- There was no difference in the prevalence of mucosal lesions between galvanizers and enamellers.
- The time of employment had no measurable influence on the degree of pathological changes.
- Cancer or precancer was not observed in the population examined.

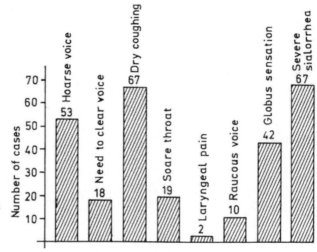

Fig. 1. Presenting symptoms in the screened population of 424 industrial workers

Prevention and Early Detection of Cancer of the Upper Aerodigestive Tract. Results of Endoscopic Mass Screening

W. STEINER, Erlangen

Although the conditions for the early detection of cancer in the upper aerodigestive tract are extremely favourable, in particular in the oral cavity and larynx, an analysis of the international literature reveals a predominance of the advanced stages of cancer. While the early detection of cancer would provide an excellent chance of effecting a cure with function-preserving forms of treatment, extensive carcinomas require aggressive combined therapy, which often results in mutilation and early disablement or death.

There are various reasons why these tumours are able to grow to an advanced stage before detection, and these may be organ-, tumour-, patient- or physician-related (Steiner 1982a). A diagnostic work-up oriented only to the presenting symptoms, is far from adequate to achieve any appreciable improvement in the early recognition of cancer.

Moreover, there is a marked increase in the incidence of, and the mortality from, cancers in the oral cavity, pharynx, and larynx. This can be clearly recognized in the statistics of the regional cancer registries in the Federal Republic of Germany, of the Federal Statistical Office in Wiesbaden, and of the Health Authorities in the USA and France (Steiner 1982b, 1983). In all probability, this increase in cancers of the mucosa in the upper aerodigestive tract can be referred to the increasing consumption of tobacco and of alcohol.

Despite vigorous campaigns designed to show the dangers of smoking and excessive alcohol consumption, it appears virtually impossible to influence people's smoking and drinking habits – more and more women and young people are taking up cigarette smoking in the USA[1] and in the Federal Republic of Germany. In view of this fact preventive and screening examinations might lead to a more frequent detection of precancerous lesions and early cancers in the upper aerodigestive tract, too.

A start was made on the first examination programme in 1975, at the Erlangen ENT Department, with the aim of investigating the practicability and effectivity of endoscopic mass screening examinations (Steiner 1976; Steiner et al. 1976).

Examination Group 1975–1976

The mouth, pharynx and larynx were examined in a total of 6432 people during a 6-month trial screening programme (1975/76). About 50% were men, and 80% of the group were relatively uniformly distributed between the ages of 30 and 70.

---

1 US Department of Health (1979/80)

Results. Roughly every fifth person examined had a finding that required further diagnostic and therapeutic measures. Within the total group the percentage of oral and laryngeal lesions suspected of being precancerous was 2.3%; the histological work-up verified carcinomas in 0.2%. In the high-risk group of smokers, which comprised 1574 persons, a precancerous lesion was found clinically in 7%, and a carcinoma diagnosed histologically in 0.7%.

Our results with respect to the histologically verified precancerous and early cancer stages, are given in table 1. While in the overall group the percentage of precancerous stages (dysplasias) in the oral cavity and larynx was 0.4%, and the percentage of early cancers 0.2% (together 6/1000), in the group of smokers, comprising 1574 subjects, the percentage of dysplasias increased to 1.4%, and early cancers to 0.6%. This means that in the *high-risk group of smokers, 20 out of 1000 presented with a histologically verifiable precancerous lesion or early cancer in the oral cavity or larynx.*

A further pilot study was carried out with the support of the Federal Ministry of Health (Steiner and Jaumann 1980; Steiner 1983).

Examination Group 1978–1980

Between 1978 and 1980, the upper respiratory tract of 6899 employees of the fur trade, textile, porcelain, timber, cigarette and metal-working industries, were examined endoscopically, and in some cases radiologically. The age peak in about one-third of the subjects was in the fifth decade, while about 80% of the employees were aged between 30 and 60. Women examined accounted for only 15%. About 46% of the subjects investigated were exposed to heat, dust, chemical vapours and irritating gases. Smokers predominated at 54% compared to non-smokers, while only 4% were ex-smokers. About 63% admitted to drinking alcohol regularly. Among the 4011 subjects (58%) with ENT symptoms, the majority reported hardness of hearing, impaired nasal breathing or headaches as the main symptom.

Results. The ENT examination turned up a pathological finding in about every fifth exployee. At 18%, the benign lesions formed the main group of diseases.

Chronic laryngitis was diagnosed in 1.5% of the test subjects. A precancerous lesion (leukoplakia, hyperplasia, etc.) in the oral cavity (n = 14), or in the larynx (n = 93) was suspected in 1.6% of all those examined. To data, only 28 lesions (approximately 0.4%) have been verified histologically as dysplasias, while squamous cell carcinomas in the larynx (n = 5) and in the oral cavity (n = 1) have been confirmed in about 0.1% of the cases.

With respect to the histologically confirmed dysplasias and carcinomas in the oral cavity and larynx, a greater prevalence (0.8% and 0.2%, respectively) can be seen in the high-risk group of smokers (N = 3712) (approximately 1%) (Table 1).

An analysis of the relationship between the chronic laryngitis, precancerous conditions and carcinoma in the larynx and oral cavity, and the smoking and drinking habits in the various occupational groups, reveals an unequivocal correlation with the consumption of tobacco and alcohol, but not with occupational exposure to noxious agents.

Table 1. Increase in prevalence rates for oro-laryngeal carcinomas and their precursor stages in the high-risk group of smokers in comparison with the overall group of subjects examined during the Erlangen field studies. a) screening at the Department[a] b) screening in the plants[b]

Findings in larynx/oral cavity	Clinical diagnosis suspected precancers (%)	Histological diagnosis Dysplasia (%)	Carcinoma (%)	Dysplasias and Carcinomas (%)
1975/76 (GRA) (n=6432)	2.3	0.4	0.2	0.6
Smokers (n=1574)	7.4	1.4	0.7	2.1
1978/80 (FMH) (n=6899)	1.6	0.4	0.1	0.5
Smokers (n=3712)	2.8	0.8	0.2	1.0

[a] Supported by GRA = German Research Association
[b] Supported by FMH = Federal Ministry of Health

The number of parameters – age and sex distribution of the groups, smoking and drinking habits, occupational exposure to toxins, the reasons for carrying out the examinations, the methods employed, etc. – make it difficult to directly compare the examination results presented here with those established by various workers in Germany, India, Austria, Hungary, and in the USA in stomatological and/or laryngological mass screening examinations (Bick 1980; Farago 1968 (1984 see page 39); Klein 1975; Mehta et al. 1969/82; Neel et al. 1981 (1984 see page 48); Schnieder 1979; Toth 1966, Wilke (1984 see page 42); Wodak 1965).

With respect to the incidence of findings and the correlation with smoking and drinking, the greatest agreement is found with the results of screening examinations carried out by Farago (1968) in Budapest in factories and plants (the results are very similar).

Table 2. Increase prevelance for carcinoma in the oral cavity and larynx in various high-risk groups

High-risk groups				Carcinomas in the oral cavity and larynx per 1000
Erlangen field studies (n=5300)	male/female		smokers	4/1000
"Mayo Lung Project" (n=9500)	male	more than 45 years	smokers	6/1000
American Department of Health (estimated figures)	male	more than 40 years	smokers/alcohol abuse	8/1000

A detailed discussion of the reports in the literature and the consequences for the introduction of cancer screening examinations of the oral cavity, pharynx and larynx is presented by Steiner (1983).

To summarize our findings it may be said that: among the general population, there is considerable interest in such a mass screening programme. The examination methods currently available, including endoscopy using a 90° angled telescope (magnifying laryngopharyngoscope described by von Stuckrad and Lakatos 1975), are suitable for carrying out such a screening programme. The examination can be performed rapidly and with no stress either to the patient or the examining physician; the test is inexpensive and reliable, and the diagnostic yield relatively high, and, if such examinations are concentrated on high-risk groups, also economically practicable and justifiable.

References

Bick W (1980) Erfahrungen über Krebsvorsorgeuntersuchungen in Kiefer- und Gesichtsbereich. In: Pape K (Hrsg) Acta Chirurgiae Maxillo-Facialis, Bd 5. Johann Ambrosius Barth, Leipzig

Faragó L (1968) Bericht über oto-rhino-laryngologische Krebsreihenuntersuchungen. Monatsschr Ohrenheilk 102:588

Klein HD (1975) Routine telescopic laryngoscopy. Am Fam Physician 11:86

Mehta FS, Pindborg JJ, Odont D, Gupta PC, Daftary DK (1969) Epidemiologic and histologic study of oral cancer and leukoplakia among 50915 villagers in India. Cancer 24:832

Mehta FS, Gupta MB, Pindborg JJ, Bhonsle RB, Jalnawalla PN, Sinor PN (1982) An intervention study of oral cancer and precancer in rural Indian populations: a preliminary report. Bull WHO 60:441

Neel HB, Sanderson D, Fontana RS, Taylor WF, Woolner LB (1981) Sputum cytologic diagnosis of upper respiratory tract cancer. Ann Otol Rhinol Laryngol 90:312

Schnieder EA (1979) Erfahrungen und Ergebnisse mit Reihenuntersuchungen zur Früherkennung von Malignomen in Larynx und Hypopharynx. Vortrag auf dem Deutschen Endoskopiekongreß, Erlangen

Steiner W, Bierl F, Köstler R, Jaumann MP, Panis R (1976) Krebsfrüherkennung im Mund-, Rachen- und Kehlkopfbereich. Arch Otorhinolaryngol 213:430

Steiner W (1976) Krebsfrüherkennung in Mund, Rachen und Kehlkopf. Dtsch Ärzteblatt 73:3159

Steiner W, Jaumann MP (1980) Untersuchungen zur Erkennung von Gefährdungsgruppen für Tumorerkrankungen im Kopf- und Halsbereich. Forschung im Geschäftsbereich des BMJFG, Jahresbericht 1978/79, Kohlhammer, Stuttgart, Bd 88, S 171

Steiner W (1982a) Krebsfrüherkennung und Vorsorge im oberen Aero-Digestivtrakt. Munch Med Wochenschr 123:194

Steiner W (1982b) Krebsfrüherkennung und Vorsorge im oberen Aero-Digestivtrakt. Verh Dtsch Krebs Ges, Bd 3, Fischer, Stuttgart New York, S 73

Steiner W (1983) Untersuchungen zur Erkennung von Risikogruppen für Tumorerkrankungen im Kopf- und Halsbereich. Forschungsbericht. Bundesministerium für Jugend, Familie und Gesundheit

Stuckrad H von, Lakatos I (1975) Über ein neues Lupenlaryngoskop (Epipharyngoskop). Laryngol Rhinol Otol (Stuttg) 54:336

Toth E (1966) Laryngologische Erfahrungen in der Krebsdurchlese der Männer. Fül-Orr-Gegegyog 12:61

U.S. Department of Health, Education and Welfare (1979) Smoking and health: a report of the Surgeon General

U.S. Department of Health and Human Services (1980) The Health Consequences of Smoking for Women: a report of the Surgeon General

Wilke J (1984) Laryngological Screening of Industrial Workers. In: Wigand ME, Steiner W, Stell PM (Hrsg) Functional Partial Laryngectomy. Springer, Berlin Heidelberg New York Tokyo, p 42.

Wodak E (1965) Über die Bedeutung der Vorsichtsuntersuchungen im Hals-, Nasen-, Ohren- und Kehlkopfbereich. Krebsarzt 20:424

Screening for Upper Respiratory Tract Cancer. Sputum Cytologic Diagnosis

H. BRYAN NEEL III, Rochester (Minnesota)

Screening for cancer is a common issue for debate because few, if any, evaluations of the screening process have been conducted on a long-term, prospective basis with use of concomitant, unscreened controls. Periodic sputum cytology has been incorporated in screening programs designed to detect presymptomatic lung cancer in chronic smokers of excessive numbers of cigarettes (National Cancer Institute 1975; Neel et al. 1981; Sanderson and Fontana 1975; Taylor and Fontana 1972; Taylor et al. 1981). Cytologic examination has led to identification of cancers in the upper respiratory and alimentary tracts of the head and neck region. This observation comes as no surprise, because cigarette smoking is an etiologic factor common to both upper and lower respiratory tract cancers.

Materials and Methods

During recruitment of subjects for the Mayo Lung Project, 9211 patients were randomized into a participant (screened) group and a control (comparison) group. The participant (screened) subjects had roentgenographic and cytologic rescreening at 4-month intervals. The patients in the control (comparison) group were advised to have annual rescreening. Intensive efforts were made to secure compliance in the participant (screened) group. Those in the control (comparison) group were merely sent letter-questionnaires once a year that did not mention roentgenography or sputum cytology.

All patients were men older than 45 years who were smoking one package of cigarettes or more daily or had done so within the previous year. Almost all had smoked heavily for more than 20 years. All patients had a complete medical examination, including a standard 36- by 43-cm chest roentgenogram and cytologic examination of a 3-day pooled specimen of sputum.

The specimens for sputum cytology in each patient were pooled, 3-morning collections of spontaneous deep-cough sputum fixed in 50% alcohol and 2% Carbowax (Doak Pharmacal Company, Inc., Westbury, NY) (Neel et al. 1978; Saccomanno et al. 1963).

The cytologic diagnosis of squamous cell cancer was based on conventional cellular criteria for malignancy. Generally, a squamous cell carcinoma arising in the upper portion of the respiratory tract could not be distinguished cytologically from one developing in the lower portion.

Results

From Nov. 1, 1971, through July 1, 1980, tumors in the upper respiratory and alimentary pathways were detected in 30 patients in the participant (screened) group and 24 patients in the control (comparison) group (Neel et al. 1981). Lung cancer was found in 120 participants and 83 control subjects. All but one of the tumors in the upper respiratory and alimentary passages (upper airway) were squamous cell carcinomas.

Among the 30 participant (screened) subjects, the search for cancer in the upper airway was undertaken because of abnormal sputum cytologic findings in 12 and symptoms (for example, hoarseness, sore throat, and sore in the mouth) in 17. In the remaining patient, the tumor was found during a routine head and neck examination for an inflammatory ear problem. Among the 24 control (comparison) subjects, the search was begun because of symptoms in 21. Two control subjects had abnormal sputum cytologic findings and concurrent development of symptoms, and one tumor was found on a routine head and neck examination.

In the same period when the search for upper airway tumors was prompted by abnormal sputum cytologic findings in the 12 participant (screened) patients, 12 other screened patients with abnormal results of sputum cytology were found to have roentgenographically "occult" lung cancer (Taylor et al. 1981). Therefore, half the patients with abnormal findings on sputum cytology had "occult" cancer in the upper airway and half had "occult" cancer in the lower airway (lung). This finding emphasizes the importance of the otorhinolaryngologic examination in screening programs for airway cancer.

Survival. Of the 30 participants, 18 are alive and free of tumor and 12 have died; 9 of the 12 died from their upper airway tumors. Among the 24 controls, 20 are alive and free of tumor and 4 have died; all 4 died from their upper airway tumors. Of the nine participants who died, four had had positive results and five had had negative results on sputum cytology.

For analysis of survival from the time of first detection, the 24 controls were compared with the 30 participants. For controls, the four deaths due to upper airway cancer occurred during an exposure time of 814 person-months, a rate of five deaths per 1000 months. For participants, the findings were somewhat different; there were nine deaths in 934 person-months, a rate of 10 deaths per 1000 months. Contrary to our expectations, there is no evidence that survival of screened subjects is better than that of control patients (Neel et al. 1981).

Discussion

It is well known that patients who are at risk for lung cancer are also at risk for squamous cell carcinoma of the head and neck region. This is illustrated by the observation that 54 of the 257 patients (21%) in the project who were found to have cancer through July 1, 1980, had tumors in the head and neck region (excluding the lip). The 17 screened patients in whom symptoms developed and the one asymptomatic patient who had an otorhinolaryngologic examination for an unrelated problem had *negative* results of sputum cytology on one or more occasions before the otorhinolaryngologic examination at which their tumors were detected (Neel et al. 1981). Thus, sputum cytology may yield negative results at the same time that cancer can be readily detected by a thorough examination of the upper respiratory and alimentary passages; the patient may or may not have symptoms. Furthermore, the stages of tumors (by the American Joint Committee for Staging and End-Results Reporting) seemed to be comparable in the participants in whom tumors were detected cytologically and in those in whom they were detected because of symptoms. Similarly, when all participant (screened) and control patients were compared, the various stages of the cancer were about equally represented in the two groups.

Contrary to our expectations, survival in the participant (screened) patients, including those whose examinations were prompted by abnormal results of sputum cytology, was not better than that in the control (comparison) patients. Perhaps the similarity of the survival data is related to the fact that the distribution of patients among the various disease stages in the two groups was similar. Also, the onset of symptoms closely approximated the time that results of sputum cytology became abnormal in many of the patients. Questioning high-risk patients about symptoms and performing a thorough examination of the upper respiratory and alimentary passages are the usual approaches for early diagnosis. Sputum cytology helps reveal some of these tumors in high-risk patients, but it does not seem to improve survival over that achieved by localization of the tumor after symptoms develop.

References

National Cancer Institute (1975) Cooperative Early Lung Cancer Group: Manual of Procedures, Jan 1
Neel HB III, Sanderson DR, Fontana RS, Taylor WF, Woolner LB (1981) Sputum cytologic diagnosis of upper respiratory tract cancer: Second report. Ann Otol Rhinol Laryngol 90:312–315
Neel HB III, Woolner LB, Sanderson DR (1978) Sputum cytologic diagnosis of upper respiratory tract cancer. Ann Otol Rhinol Laryngol 87:468–473
Saccomanno G, Saunders RP, Ellis H, Archer VE, Wood BG, Beckler PA (1963) Concentration of carcinoma or atypical cells in sputum. Acta Cytol (Baltimore) 7:305–310
Sanderson DR, Fontana RS (1975) Early lung cancer detection and localization. Ann Otol Rhinol Laryngol 84:583–588
Taylor WF, Fontana RS (1972) Biometric design of the Mayo Lung Project for early detection and localization of bronchogenic carcinoma. Cancer 30:1344–1347
Taylor WF, Fontana RS, Uhlenhopp MA, Davis CS (1981) Some results of screening for early lung cancer. Cancer 47:1114–1120

Endoscopic Screening for Multiple Squamous Cell Carcinoma of the Upper Digestive and Respiratory Tracts (Oncologically Oriented Upper Aero-Digestive Pan-Endoscopy)

M. SAVARY, R. PASCHE, and PH. MONNIER, Lausanne

When it appears in the same organ system, the tendency towards tumor multifocality suggests the probability of common etiological factors (Wynder et al. 1977). For cancer of the mouth, pharynx and oesophagus, the epidemiology is similar. It resembles that of the larynx, trachea and bronchi (Cahan 1977). There exists, therefore, considerable overlap between high risk groups for upper and lower respiratory tract (larynx, trachea, bronchi) and upper digestive tract (mouth, pharynx, oesophagus) cancers (Fontana and Sanderson 1975; Savary et al. 1979).

In a retrospective study, we have shown that out of 951 patients housing an ENT cancer, 138, that is 14.5%, developed at one point or another in their evolution simultaneous or successive multifocal cancers (Table 1), located on the upper digestive or lower respiratory tract (Pasche et al. 1981). Sixty percent of these second site cancers were in the ENT region. The oesophagus and the tracheo-bronchial tree were concerned to an equal degree, each representing 20% (Fig. 1). When the primary cancer was bucco-pharyngeal, second sites were especially frequent (17%), and were located 8 out of 10 times in the digestive tract and 2 out of 10 times in the respiratory tract. However, when the primary cancer was laryngeal, multifocality was

Table 1. Multiple foci squamous cell carcinoma of the upper digestive and lower respiratory tracts (mouth – pharynx – oesophagus – larynx – bronchi): 951 ENT primary cancers. Overall rate of multiple primary cancers of the upper digestive and respiratory tracts in 951 patients with buccal, pharyngeal or laryngeal carcinoma

ENT primary cancers: 951	
Simultaneous second primary cancers:	61 (6.4%)
Successive second primary cancers:	77 (8.1%)
Total:	138 (14.5%)
– Double	117 = 117 Tumors
– Triple	15 = 30 Tumors
– Quadruple	4 = 12 Tumors
– Quintuple	1 = 4 Tumors
– Sextuple	1 = 5 Tumors
	168 Tumors

ENT Clinic, CHUV, Lausanne (Switzerland) – (1. 01. 1967–31. 12. 1980)

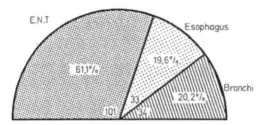

Fig. 1. Sites of 168 second primary tumors appearing synchronously or metachronously in 138 patients with cancer of the mouth, pharynx or larynx (1967–1980)

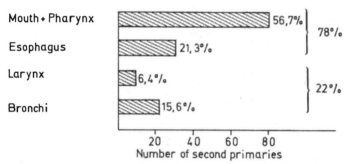

Fig. 2. Site of 141 second primaries in 114 patients with primary bucco-pharyngeal cancer

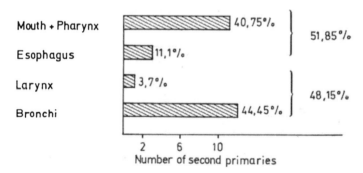

Fig. 3. Site of 27 second primaries in 24 patients with primary laryngeal cancer

Table 2. Second primary cancers: relationship with the location of the primary tumor. When the primary cancer was bucco-pharyngeal, multifocality was especially frequent (17%). When the primary tumor was laryngeal, multifocality was distinctly less frequent (8.6%)

Primary cancers of *mouth and pharynx:*	672
Second primary cancers:	141 tumors for 114 patients (17%)
Primary cancers of *the larynx:*	279
Second primary cancers:	27 tumors for 24 patients (8.6%)

ENT Clinic, CHUV, Lausanne (Switzerland) – (1967–1980)

distinctly less frequent (8.6%), the second site tumor appearing 48% of the time in the respiratory tract. *The digestive tract remained, in 52% of the cases, the site of the second tumor when the primary cancer was laryngeal (Table 2, Figs. 2 and 3).*

The search for a second primary cancer should be considered an essential step in the work-up of all patients presenting with an upper aero-digestive tract carcinoma. *Screening endoscopy constitutes therefore one of the fundamental techniques that the head and neck surgical team must master* (Savary et al. 1979).

This *endoscopic screening technique* is based on our present knowledge of squamous cell carcinogenesis in this region. The basic requirements are the following:

1. The entire epithelial surface which is submitted to the carcinogenic risk must be explored, that is the buccal cavity, the pharynx and the oesophagus on one hand; the larynx and the tracheo-bronchial tree on the other.
2. Particular attention must be paid to high risk zones, which correspond to regions where the carcinogens remain in contact with the mucosa for the longest time (floor of the mouth, gingivoglossal grooves, retromolar spaces; vallecular and piriform sinuses; supra-stenotic zones for the oesophagus – at or below the secondary bronchi for the bronchial tree – (Ledermann 1964; Vaughan 1972).
3. The manipulation of the instruments must allow visualisation of the complete epithelial surface. For the upper digestive tract, this implies the use of the rigid endoscope equipped with a distal bevel which permits the smoothing out of the mucosa.
4. The optical quality of the instruments must be excellent, so as to detect lesions in the first macroscopic stages (Hopkins Optics).
5. Histo-cytological sampling methods must be adequate. For the oesophagus, an abrasive balloon equipped with silicate cristals in its distal portion provides endoscopically the harvesting of exfoliated cells from each distinct lesion (Monnier 1981).
6. The use of detection techniques such as vital staining with Lugol 3% or Toluidine Blue 1% is indispensable, because of the possible occurrence of an "occult" type of early squamous cell carcinoma in the mouth, pharynx or oesophagus (Tumor Prevention 1977; Monnier et al. 1981).

Practically speaking, this oncologically oriented endoscopy is performed on an out-patient basis, for all patients who have, or are suspected of having an ENT cancer.

Examination of the oral cavity is carried out using a surgical microscope, before and after Toluidine Blue gargle.

For the pharyngo-larynx, the surgical microscope and laryngeal mirror or the von Stuckrad indirect laryngoscope provide a detailed dynamic examination of the high risk zones, with the use of vital staining (Steiner 1979). The patient then undergoes general anesthesia. The bronchoscopy is performed using first a rigid bronchoscope, then a fibroscope.

Finally, hypopharyngo-oesophagoscopy is accomplished using a rigid oesophagoscope equipped with Hopkins Optics. Toluidine Blue is systematically applied with cotton swabs and washing (Savary 1980).

Vital Staining (Lugol 3%; Toluidine Blue 1%)

Early cancer can escape visualization in spite of the best optical conditions, especially in the mouth, pharynx and oesophagus (Tumor Prevention 1977; Monnier et al. 1981).

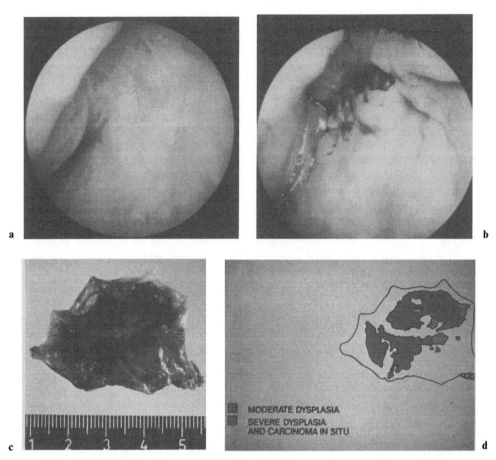

Fig. 4a–d. Intraepithelial carcinoma of the right piriform sinus discovered during a pre-therapeutic upper aero-digestive pan-endoscopy in a 47 year-old patient with invasive carcinoma of the mouth. **a** the discretion of the macroscopically visible mucosal alteration: colour change with no surface irregularity. **b** the clear appearance obtained with Toluidine Blue staining. **c** the multicentric mapping of the lesions with satellite foci on the stained surgical specimen. **d** the good correlation between the surgical specimen stained with Toluidine-Blue and the histological examination by step sections (5/cm^2)

A 3% Lugol solution marks negatively the suspicious lesion (Voegeli, 1966). Toluidine Blue has an affinity for the cell nuclei. Its penetration power in the dysplasic or carcinomatous squamous epithelium is between five and six cell layers (Monnier et al. 1981).

The technique is composed of three distinct stages:
A) Mucolysis: washing or multiple swabbing with 1% acetic acid
B) Staining: one minute's washing or swabbing with 1% Toluidine Blue
C) Decoloration: thorough rinsing with 1% acetic acid.

The method is very efficient on the smooth areas of the upper digestive squamous mucosa. False positives are numerous especially in zones where the mucosa presents crypts, papilla or folds. The decoloration is of utmost importance in avoiding most of these false positive results. Two false negatives are known:
- severe dysplasia with parakeratosis which prevents the stain penetrating the dysplastic epithelium
- submucosal extension of an invasive cancer.

The method cannot be applied on respiratory mucosa. The smooth mucosa of the pharynx and oesophagus is ideal for Toluidine Blue staining, which facilitates the screening of "early" second primary cancers devoid of macroscopic signs (Fig. 4 a–d).

Morphological Aspects of "Early" Cancer

Aside from the special techniques involved, screening endoscopy requires a perfect knowledge of the morphological aspect of early cancer. For the mouth, the pharynx and the oesophagus, the endoscopic morphology of "early" cancer is based on
a) the aspect of the fundamental lesion
b) The mapping of the lesion (Monnier et al. 1981)

The fundamental lesion can be characterized by both a colour change and a surface alteration. The mapping takes into account the topografical distribution of the lesions and their relationships to each other (Table 3).

Table 3. Endoscopic morphology of "early" squamous cell carcinoma (mouth, pharynx, esophagus). An elevated lesion is generally associated with a whitish colour change, whereas a depressed lesion usually presents as an erythroplasia. In the mouth, the pharynx and esophagus, a carcinoma "in situ" can be flat (surface alteration=0) and show no colour change. For the pharynx and esophagus, the topography of dysplasia, carcinoma "in situ" and microinvasive cancer is multicentric in 90% of the cases (presence of satellite lesions).

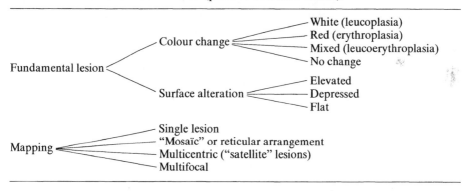

Fundamental Lesion

In the pharynx and the oesophagus, the most common form of "early" cancer is a flat or slightly depressed zone of *erythroplasia*. Such a lesion is difficult to detect with the naked eye, as well as through an endoscope, although it is usually multicentric, often forming a mosaic pattern. When occurring in the lower part of the oesophagus, these erythroplastic changes often escape the fibroscope or may be confused with the reddish erosions of stage I reflux oesophagitis (Savary et al. 1980).

The whitish, elevated, plaque-like lesion is a rare form of "early" cancer of the pharynx and oesophagus. It presents most often as a solitary lesion, but can occasionally associate with the flat, multicentric erythroplastic type of "early" cancer.

The invisible form of dysplasia or carcinoma in situ also occurs in the mouth, in the pharynx and in the oesophagus. This "occult" type of "early" cancer can only be detected by vital staining techniques and probably corresponds to a forerunner form of depressed erythroplastic type (Monnier et al. 1982).

Mapping of the Lesions

In most cases (90%) the topographic distribution of the "early" cancerous lesions is multicentric in type, for the pharynx as well as the oesophagus (Monnier et al. 1982). From the start, the squamous cell carcinogenesis presents as a pathological process concerning a *segment* or *zone,* and has a multilesional character within the given segment even in the very early stages. When a dominant lesion exists (in situ carcinoma or microinvasive carcinoma), the surrounding sites of dysplasia appear distinctly as sattelite lesions. They are sometimes connected to one another by delicate grooves and thus present a reticular or mosaic pattern.

The histological examination of these early lesions performed by serial sections shows that the invasive nature (that is, the tendency to cross the basement membrane) can also be multicentric (Monnier et al. 1982).

Conclusion

Since we have begun to perform, as a pre-therapeutic work-up for all ENT cancer patients, this type of oncologically oriented upper aerodigestive pan-endoscopy, the average incidence of simultaneous multiple site tumors has increased from 6.4% to 25% (Tables 1 and 4).

Sixty-two percent of these tumors are located in the ENT region, 12% in the tracheo-bronchial tree and 26% in the oesophagus (Table 5). Eighty-nine percent of these simultaneous second primaries were T_{IS} or T_1 cancers (Table 6).

Table 4. Synchronous second primary cancers (primary ENT malignancies). Upper aerodigestive cancers: simultaneous second primary cancers discovered by oncologically oriented upper aerodigestive pan-endoscopy. Toluidine-Blue staining has been systematically used since the beginning of 1980

Year	Primary cancers	Simultaneous second primary cancers	%
1977	69	8	11.5
1978	97	11	11
1979	88	11	12.5
1980	108	27	25
1981	113	33	29
→ 30. 6. 82	58	17	29
Total	533	107	19.6

ENT Clinic, CHUV, Lausanne (Switzerland)

Table 5. Sites of second primary tumors (107 cases) (1. 1. 1977 – 30. 6. 1982). Upper aero-digestive cancers: sites of the simultaneous second primaries. 26% of them were located in the esophagus

62%	ENT
26%	Esophagus
12%	Bronchi

ENT Clinic, CHUV, Lausanne (Switzerland)

Table 6. Staging of simultaneous second primaries (107 cases) (1. 1. 1977 – 30. 6. 1982). Upper aero-digestive cancers: staging of the simultaneous second primary tumors discovered by pre-therapeutic screening endoscopy. 89% of these second primaries were T_{1s} or T_1 cancers

T_{1s}	24%	⎫ 89%
T_1	65%	⎭
T_2	6%	
T_{3-4}	5%	

ENT Clinic, CHUV, Lausanne (Switzerland)

We do not know yet whether or not this systematic pre-therapeutic screening proposed to all patients with an ENT cancer will modify the long term prognosis. This program has enabled us, however, to describe in detail the endoscopic morphology of early cancer of the upper digestive tract bearing squamous cell epithelium.

References

Cahan WG (1977) Multiple primary cancers of the lung, esophagus, and other sites. Cancer 40:1954–1960

Fontana RS, Sanderson DR (1975) The Mayo lung project for early detection and localization of bronchogenic carcinoma: a status report. Chest 67:511–521

Ledermann M (1964) The anatomy of cancer with special reference to tumors of the upper air and food passages. J Laryngol Otol 78:181–208

Monnier PH (1981) Le diagnostic au stade "précoce" du carcinome épidermoïde de l'oesophage. Med Hyg 39:2937–2945

Monnier PH, Savary M, Pasche R (1981) Contribution of toluidine blue to bucco-pharyngo-oesophageal cancerology. Acta Endoscopica 11:299–315

Monnier PH, Savary M, Pasche R (1981) Intraepithelial carcinoma of the oesophagus: endoscopic morphology. Endoscopy 13:185–191

Monnier PH, Savary M, Pasche R, Anani P (1982) Endoscopic morphology of microinvasive squamous cell carcinoma of the oesophagus. Clin Oncol 1:559–570

Pasche R, Savary M, Monnier PH (1981) Multifocalité du carcinome épidermoïde sur les voies digestives supérieure et respiratoire distales: technicité du diagnostic endoscopique. Acta Endoscopica 11:277–291

Savary M (1980) L'oesophagoscopie: indication et apport en oncologie. In: Veronesi U, Emanuelli H, De Lena M, Guzzoni A, Rilke T, Spinelli P. Progressi diagnostici in oncologia, Casa Editrice Ambrosiana, Milano. p 9–23

Savary M, Crausaz PH, Monnier PH (1979) La place de l'endoscopie totale aéro-digestive supérieure en cancérologie. Schweiz Med Wochenschr 109:838–840

Savary M, Monnier PH (1980) Le reflux gastro-oesophagien: l'apport de l'endoscopie dans l'indication opératoire et les contrôles post-opératoires. Helv Chir Acta 47:693–706

Steiner W (1979) Tracheoscopy, bronchoscopy, oesophagoscopy, mediastinoscopy, interdisciplinary panendoscopy. Endoscopy 2:151–157

Tumor Prevention, Treatment and Research Group, Chengchow, Honan, China (1977) Pathology of early oesophageal squamous cell carcinoma. Chin Med J [Engl] 3:180–192

Vaughan CW (1972) Carcinogenesis in the oral cavity. Otolaryngol Clin North Am 5:291–300

Voegeli R (1966) Schillersche Iodprobe im Rahmen der Oesophagusdiagnostik. Pract Otorhinolaryngol 28:230–334

Wynder EL, Dodo H, Bloch DA, Gantt RC, Moore OS (1969) Epidemiologic investigation of multiple primary cancer of the upper alimentary and respiratory tracts. I. A retrospective study. Cancer 24:730–739

IV. Radiological Diagnosis

Radiology of the Larynx

W. STRUPLER, St. Gallen

Radiological examination of the larynx does not compete with endoscopy but is a complementary procedure in the investigation of laryngeal tumours. Both of these methods have their advantages and limitations. As a rule, the radiodiagnosis must follow clinical examination and noninvasive laryngoscopy, and must precede biopsy. This sequence is of particular importance when contrast laryngography is carried out. Endoscopy and some X-ray examinations, e.g. laryngography, provide knowledge of the extent of tumours, of superficial mucosal alterations and functional impairment. Other radiological procedures give more information about the volume and the depth of tumour invasion.

In addition, computerized tomography of the larynx and the soft tissues of the neck serves as the most valuable diagnostic tool available. When considering voice preserving laryngeal tumour surgery the three dimensional preoperative evaluation of the extent of the tumour is of particular importance. In centres where computertomographic facilities are not available, conventional X-ray-diagnostic procedures of the larynx are still useful. They will, therefore, be described briefly.

The *conventional lateral view of the larynx* delineates the airway cavities of the pharynx, larynx and trachea from the surrounding structures of higher density, e.g. epiglottis, aryepiglottical folds, ventricle, tracheal wall etc. (Fig. 1). The laryngeal cartilaginous skeleton becomes more visible with increasing calcification (Fig. 2) and ossification.

A pathological process can be recognized by a deformation of the mucosal surface or of the laryngeal skeleton (Fig. 3). Lateralisation of the lesion, however, is not possible.

The *lateral xeroradiogram* of the larynx provides an essential improvement in diagnosis because of the simultaneous display of soft tissue, cartilaginous and osseous structures. There is a wide range of contrast by the recording of small density variations, excellent contours by the so-called edge-effect, and an astonishing transparency, allowing good judgement of structures of different radiodensity.

The X-ray-picture of the larynx in the postero-anterior *projection* has a very limited diagnostic value for laryngeal tumour detection because of the superimposed cervical spine.

A *contrast laryngography* is performed under surface anesthesia by coating the mucosal surface with a suspension of a contrast medium. In both p-a and lateral projections a surface image is obtained. This allows functional diagnosis. Typical se-

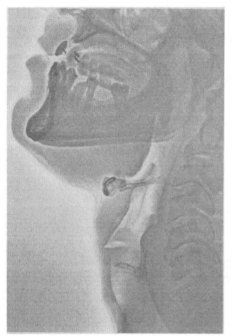 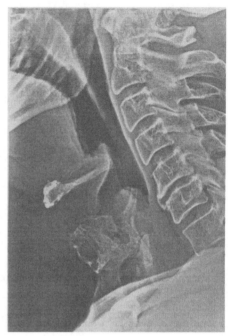

Fig. 1 **Fig. 2**

Fig. 1. Lateral view of pharynx, larynx and cervical trachea with normal findings (black and white copy of a positive xeroradiogram)

Fig. 2. Lateral view of pharynx and larynx in a case of an endolaryngeal carcinoma recurrence after X-ray treatment. Edema of laryngeal structures, especially of the epiglottis, arytenoid and postcricoid area, and stenosis by an intralaryngeal exophytic tumour are shown (black and white copy of a negative xeroradiogram)

quences may be recorded in single frames or with radiocinematography on conventional film or taped on TV. This manoeuvre allows depiction of endoscopically difficult or nonaccessible areas of the larynx (Fig. 4).

The *conventional multidirectional tomography* (Fig. 5) of the larynx is usually done in a frontal plane at 2–3 mm intervals, but can also be performed on a lateral view. There is no doubt that before the development of CT conventional tomography was the most precise radiodiagnostic method for laryngeal evaluation.

Fig. 3. Lateral view of the pharyngo-larynx and the cervical trachea. Narrowing of the laryngeal entrance by a preepiglottic cyst, involving both the free epiglottic portion and the preepiglottic space (black and white copy of a negative xeroradiogram)

Fig. 4. Lateral and postero-anterior views of a pharyngo-esophagogram in a patient with an infiltrating carcinoma of the right glottic-supraglottic area. The right piriform sinus is narrowed.

Fig. 5. p-a Tomogram of the same larynx as in Fig. 4, showing the remarkable size and extension of the tumour, involving not only the supraglottic but also the paraglottic and subglottic region

Radiological Diagnosis

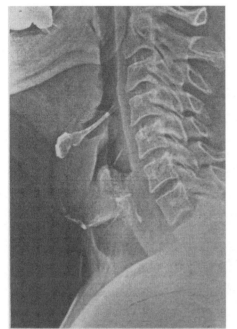

Fig. 3

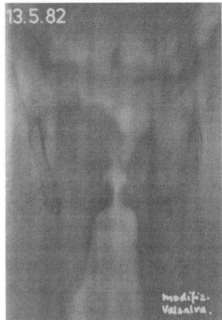

Fig. 5

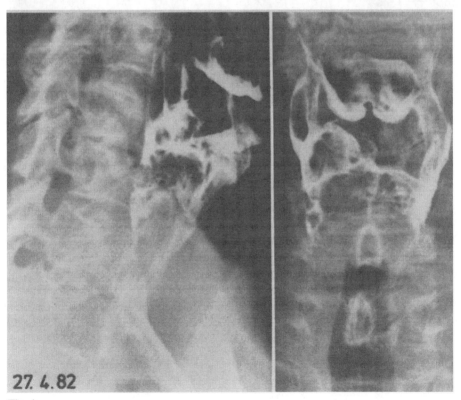

Fig. 4

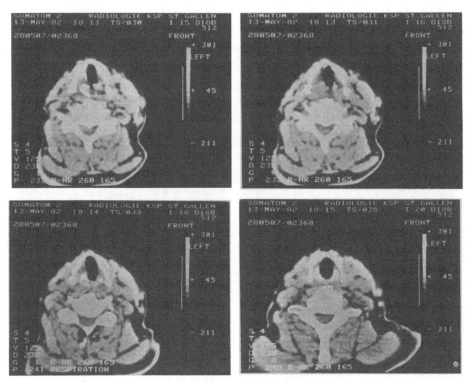

Fig. 6. Axial computer tomograms of the neck from the patient of Fig. 4 and 5, showing the deep infiltration of the lateral laryngeal compartments, the right arytenoid region and the right ary-epiglottic fold

Xeroradiographic tomography is superior to conventional tomography. The airway borders are distinctly delineated; in p-a-projection asymmetrical structures will become evident.

During the last few years *computerized tomography* (CT) has been developed. Transverse CT-scanning of the neck has acquired great importance and attention, particularly in the area of the larynx and the adjacent soft tissues. CT-scanning definitely gives more information. The high sensitivity of small variations in density provides better imaging of the morphologic structures and their pathologic alterations. The invasion of a tumour into the tissues beneath the mucosa or into the cartilage, or neoplastic infiltration into the surrounding soft tissues, e.g. the preepiglottic space, the postcricoid region or the paralaryngeal structures may be recognized much better by the more pronounced contrast differences (Fig. 6). If necessary, demonstration is enhanced by special methods, such as the "high resolution technique". When searching for lymph node metastases along the large cervical vessels, and enhancement in density by intravenous administration of contrast medium may be helpful.

# The Value of Computerized Tomography in Conservative Surgery of Glottic Cancer

E. MEYER-BREITING, Frankfurt

The histological T-classification (pT) of laryngeal carcinomas correlates well with the prognosis (Norris et al. 1970; Meyer-Breiting 1981). But the clinical T-classification often fails because the examination was limited to superficial findings and indirect signs. 1977 Mancuso and coworkers produced a first report about the use of computerized tomography (CT) for the investigation of laryngeal cancer. Since 1980 we have tested the availability of the computerized tomography for the investigation of laryngeal cancer in cooperation with various radiological institutes of the Frankfurt region. The radiological findings have been compared with our histological observations in serial whole organ sections of the completely or partially resected larynx. During this procedure we were interested in clarifying the following points:

1. of what value is the CT scan deciding on conservative surgery?
2. Which anatomical structures can help to reveal the extent of the tumor?
3. Where are the limits of CT for laryngeal tumors, and what are its consequences for conservative surgery of the larynx.

These questions are best answered by some examples. The computerized tomography shows different grades of *density for various tissues* in the larynx as demonstrated in Fig. 1. The density of fat is very low whereas that of squamous cell carcinoma is relatively high. Therefore tumours are very easily recognized in the preepiglottic space or supraglottic part of the paraglottic space.

Figure 1a shows a section through a *normal supraglottic larynx* and figure 1b a central epiglottic cancer with penetration into the *preepiglottic space*. The tumour appears endoscopically to be within the limits of supraglottic partial laryngectomy, and this is confirmed by CT. Figure 1c demonstrates the CT of a central epiglottic carcinoma involving the lower preepiglottic space – an essential borderline for supraglottic partial laryngectomy – and displacing the *petiolus* backwards. The mucosal surface of this petiolus was not suspicious as seen endoscopically. This would indicate treatment by supraglottic partial laryngectomy but CT findings revealed that total laryngectomy was necessary.

In a *normal* CT of the *glottic region* there is a higher density in the paraglottic than in the preepiglottic space caused by the thyreoarytenoid muscles. The fine hyperdense strips in the vocal margin correspond to the vocal ligaments. A typical triangular hypodense field can only be seen in front of and lateral to the arytenoid (Fig. 1d). Glottic cancer infiltrating less than 4 mm is not imaged by CT, and usually shows a tomogram of a normal larynx.

Only deeper infiltrations become recognizable by computerized tomography, e.g. the *frontolateral* glottic carcinoma in Fig. 1e involving both anterior thirds of the left paraglottic space. The posterior third including the above-mentioned hypodense triangle was free of pathological hyperdense structures. A reduction of vocal cord mobility was observed before operation. As a sign of no involvement of the

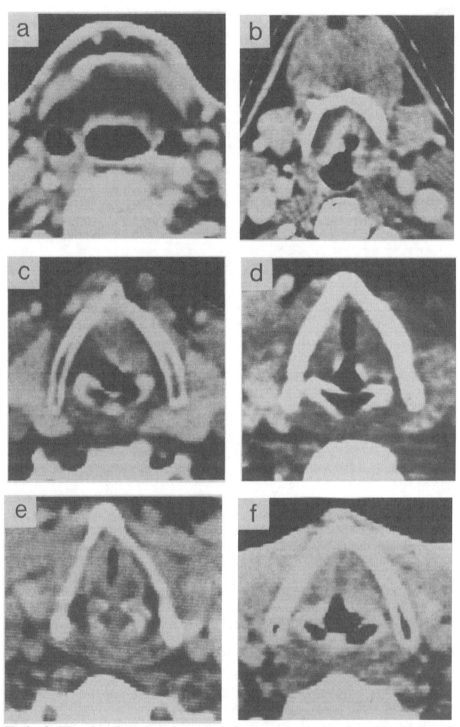

Fig. 1a–f. CT sections through the supraglottic (**a–c**) and the glottic region with normal (**a, d**) and pathological (**b, c, e, f**) findings. Note the hypodense triangular field in front of the arytenoid cartilage in **e** and its involvement by tumor in **f** *(right)*. For further details see text

thyroid cartilage a thin hypodense strip regularly lies between it and neighbouring hyperdense structures of the thyroarytenoid muscles or of a tumour.

Tumours growing around and near to the arytenoid cartilage diminish the feasibility of conservative surgery of the larynx. In Fig. 1f a glottic cancer is seen originating from both *posterior thirds* of the right vocal cord. The arytenoid cartilage is surrounded by hyperdense masses histologically showing a deeply infiltrating tumour. A partial laryngectomy seemed to be possible in this case but, in fact, was insufficient and had to be extended to a total laryngectomy. According to the CT the tumour was not completely resectable by removal of the arytenoid cartilage.

Computerized tomography is an expensive diagnostic procedure and should be kept in reserve for borderline cases with an unclear extent of infiltration, which could limit the practicability of conservative surgery as demonstrated before. But we must regard possible technical *sources of failure,* e.g. limited resolution, the possibility of tumourlike density and asymmetry of normal structures and the partial volume effect. The last is one of the causes of our failure in recognizing the tumour-penetration through the lower anterior laryngeal framework by CT. Most failures of CT examination occurred by interpreting framework findings (Meyer-Breiting et al. 1982).

Our preliminary experiences with computerized tomography of the larynx were:
1. Computerized tomography can give important information about borderline condition for conservative surgery.
2. The hypodense areas of the preepiglottic space, and of certain parts of the laryngeal skeleton are critical areas revealing early tumor infiltration.
3. To avoid failures of CT interpretation we have to emphasize the following points: a) No CT evaluation without exact anatomical and pathoanatomical knowledge of larynx and laryngeal cancer behaviour. b) CT evaluation only in connection with the laryngoscopic observations. c) No evaluation of only one section plane, d) and no evaluation of structures in the presence of artificial alterations.

References

Mancuso AA, Hanafee WN, Juillard GJF et al. (1977) The role of computed tomography in the management of cancer of the larynx. Radiology 124:243–244

Meyer-Breiting E (1981) Histologisches Verhalten und Prognose fortgeschrittener Plattenepithelkarzinome des Kehlkopfes. Arch Otorhinolaryngol (NY) 231:746–750

Meyer-Breiting E, Halbsguth A, Opritoiou G (1982) Die Bedeutung der Computertomographie für Diagnostik und Therapieplanung fortgeschrittener Kehlkopfcarcinome. Arch Otorhinolaryngol (NY) 235:689–691

Norris CM, Tucker GF, Burns KF, Pitser WF (1970) A correlation of clinical staging, pathological findings and five year end results in surgically treated cancer of the larynx. Ann Otol Rhinol Laryngol 79:1033–1048

Computed Tomography in the Diagnosis of Laryngeal Carcinoma

J. OLOFSSON, Linköping

The mucosal extent of laryngeal tumours can be fairly accurately assessed by laryngoscopy and conventional radiography i.e. plain films, tomography, contrast laryngography. These methods allow a functional study to be performed (Olofsson and Sökjer 1977, 1979). Deep infiltration is indicated by vocal cord fixation and more than 50% of glottic carcinomas with this feature invaded the laryngeal framework and/or spread outside the larynx (Olofsson et al. 1973; Olofsson and van Nostrand 1973). The detection of cartilage invasion by radiography is unreliable, the destruction of the anterior portion of the thyroid cartilage may be diagnosed by low-voltage lateral plain film examination. A better mapping of the deep extension of the tumours is a prerequisite to safer select the patients especially for conservation surgery but is certainly of importance too, when radiotherapy or surgery is discussed.

Computed tomography (CT) is a useful tool to be able to delineate the depth of the tumour invasion (Mancuso et al. 1978; Archer et al. 1978; Archer and Yeager 1979; Gregor et al. 1981; Sökjer and Olofsson 1981). CT has been suggested to replace all other radiologic methods for examining laryngeal carcinoma. However, we do not quite agree with this opinion.

Material and Methods

34 patients with mainly major laryngeal carcinoma have been examined by CT. The examination was performed with a Philips Tomoscan 300, slice thickness 3–6 mm and scanning time 2.4–9.6 s. In 24 patients undergoing laryngectomy the specimens were examined by the technique of whole organ sections and the CT-findings were compared with those at the histological examination.

Results and Conclusions (Figs. 1–3)

CT gives information on deep infiltration e.g. to the preepiglottic space and extension deep to the arytenoid cartilage (Fig. 1), which cannot be detected by ordinary radiological methods and often not by laryngoscopy. Such information has implications for a decision on conservation surgery but also when performing a total laryngectomy the entire mucosa of the piriform sinus should be included in the specimen to avoid a local recurrence.

The assessment of cartilage invasion and tumour spread outside the laryngeal framework is facilitated by CT (Fig. 1). Invasion of the anterior portion of the thyroid cartilage is a frequent finding for tumours involving the anterior commissure. Most often it is the ossified parts of the cartilage that are invaded. In men of more

Radiological Diagnosis

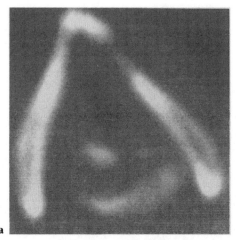 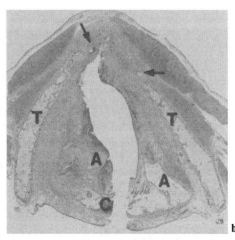

Fig. 1a, b. CT scan (a) and corresponding transverse histologic section (b) through the vocal cords. The tumour involves the full length of the right vocal cord and the anterior part of the left vocal cord. Invasion of the thyroid cartilage (*T*) is present anteriorly. Posteriorly the tumour invades the arytenoid cartilage (*A*) and the cricoid plate (*C*)

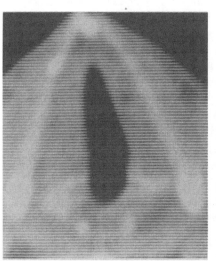 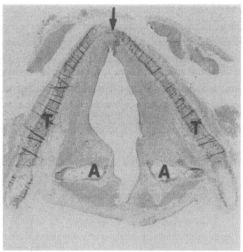

Fig. 2a, b. CT scan (a) and corresponding transverse histologic section (b) through the vocal cords. Microscopically invasion of the thyroid cartilage can be seen anteriorly which cannot be diagnosed on the CT scan

than 50 years of age the anterior part of the thyroid cartilage is usually ossified. Major invasion can be assessed by lateral low-voltage plain films in most cases. CT adds important additional information in many cases but the correct interpretation is not always easy. Minor invasion may be undiagnosed (Fig. 2).

Tumours crossing the anterior commissure often extend subglottically and then they may extend outside the larynx through the crico-thyroid membrane, what may be assessed by CT (Fig. 3).

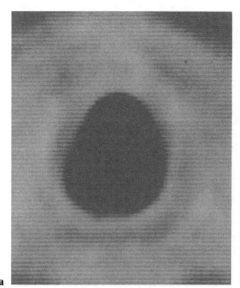 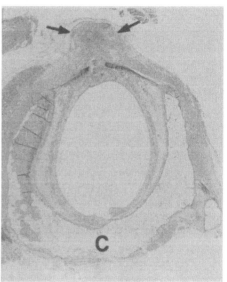

Fig. 3. CT scan (**a**) and corresponding transverse histologic section (**b**) through the crico-thyroid membrane. Tumour extension through the membrane (*arrows*) is seen on the CT scan. *C*, Cricoid cartilage

In conclusion CT should be considered a valuable complement in the radiologic diagnosis of laryngeal carcinoma (Gregor et al. 1981; Sökjer and Olofsson 1981). CT adds important information about the deep tumour invasion, cartilage destruction and extension of tumour outside the larynx. CT should be used especially for large T_2 tumours, T_3 and T_4 tumours and for tumours involving the anterior commissure, where there is a great risk for early cartilage invasion.

References

Archer CR, Friedman WH, Yeager VL, Katsantonis GP (1978) Evaluation of laryngeal cancer by computed tomography. J Comp Assist Tomog 2:618–624
Archer CR, Yeager VL (1979) Evaluation of laryngeal cartilages by computed tomography. J Comp Assist Tomog 3:604–611
Gregor RT, Lloyd GAS, Michaels L (1981) Computed tomography of the larynx: a clinical and pathologic study. Head Neck Surg 3:284–296
Mancuso AA, Calcaterra TC, Hanafee WN (1978) Computed tomography of the larynx. Radiol Clin North Am 16:195–208
Olofsson J, Lord IJ, van Nostrand AWP (1973) Vocal cord fixation in laryngeal carcinoma. Acta Otolaryngol (Stockh) 75:496–510
Olofsson J, van Nostrand AWP (1973) Growth and spread of laryngeal and hypopharyngeal carcinoma with reflections on the effect of preoperative irradiation. 139 cases studied by whole organ serial sectioning. Acta Otolaryngol [Suppl] (Stockh) 308:1–84
Olofsson J, Sökjer H (1977) Radiology and laryngoscopy for the diagnosis of laryngeal carcinoma. Acta Radiol [Diagn] (Stockh) 18:449–468
Olofsson J, Sökjer H (1979) Radiologic assessment of laryngeal carcinoma. A clinico-pathologic comparison based on whole-organ serial sections. Acta Radiol [Diagn] (Stockh) 20:789–814
Sökjer H, Olofsson J (1981) Computed tomography in carcinoma of the larynx and piriform sinus. Clin Otolaryngol 6:335–343

V. Clinical and Histological Staging

The Systems of UICC and AJC for Staging of Laryngeal Carcinoma

J. A. KIRCHNER, New Haven (Connecticut)

Staging

To evaluate various forms of therapy and to indicate prognosis in laryngeal cancer, a staging system is essential. Only by comparing similar lesions can surgeons, radiotherapists and medical oncologists compare their results.

The TNM system provides a common language for clinicians by assessing the extent of the primary tumor (T), the condition of the regional lymph nodes (N) and the presence or absence of distant metastases (M). The addition of numbers to these three components (T_1, T_2, etc.) indicates the local, regional and distant extent of the disease.

Although several systems of staging have been used, they are similar to one or both of the systems most commonly used, viz. that of the International Union Against Cancer (UICC) or the American Joint Committee. With the 1980 revisions by the AJC, the two systems are virtually identical. Anatomical regions and sites are the same for both systems. The "T" groups are equivalent and present no significant points of disagreement.

Cervical lymph node classifications differ somewhat, with the AJC specifying size as an important characteristic. But here again, the two systems are in basic agreement, since a metastatic node larger than 3 cm usually indicates rupture of the capsule and invasion of adjacent tissue.

On the basis of observations made on surgical specimens examined by serial section, the following comments on the TNM systems can be made:

Primary Tumor (T)

Supraglottic

T_1. This lesion is relatively superficial, and is usually curable by local excision or radiotherapy.

Supported by U.S.P.H.S. Grant No CA 22101-06 National Cancer Institute, DHHS

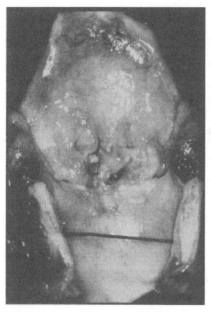

Fig. 1. Supraglottic cancer extending downward to the vocal cords, without vocal cord fixation. Under the UICC classification, this lesion is T_2. Histological examination of all such tumors, i.e. those that cross the anterior commissure in a vertical direction, show extensive invasion of the thyroid cartilage. This and similar lesions should be grouped in T_4

T_2. The AJC's "adjacent supraglottic sites" seems preferable to the UICC's "extending to the vocal cords without fixation." In our practice, this latter type of tumor is extraordinarily rare. The lesion that descends from the ventricular band to the vocal cord above and below the ventricle is usually associated with a fixed cord. And if the lesion descends below the anterior commissure, even if the vocal cord mobility is not entirely lost, the thyroid cartilage is usually destroyed by cancer invading forward into the soft tissues (Fig. 1) (Kirchner, Cornog, Holmes 1974).

T_3. The UICC classification includes "tumor limited to the larynx with fixation." This is too vague, since it does not specify which part of the larynx is fixed. If it refers to fixation of the epiglottis or ventricular bands, the description is acceptable, but if "fixation" refers to the vocal cords, the lesion is transglottic and the thyroid cartilage is invaded in about 75% of such growths over 3 cm's.

The AJC group includes tumors with "extension to involve post cricoid area, medial wall of pyriform sinus, or pre-epiglottic space." This description is useful because medial wall involvement does not preclude partial laryngectomy for surgical control, nor does pre-epiglottic space invasion contra-indicate horizontal supraglottic laryngectomy.

T_4. The AJC's "...destruction of thyroid cartilage" is desirable, since this indicates spread outside the larynx and it can be identified on preoperative CAT scan. It should, however, be kept in mind that in a serial section study of 63 supraglottic lesions, we have not observed invasion of the thyroid cartilage in a single case unless the tumor extends downward over the ventricle or anterior commissure or unless it is part of a pyriform sinus lesion (Kirchner and Som 1971).

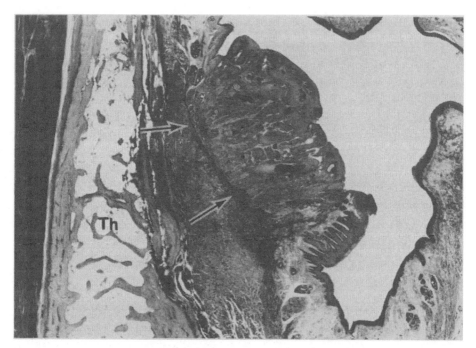

Fig. 2. T_1 glottic cancer showing the characteristic limitation by the conus elasticus, indicated by arrows. Th = Thyroid cartilage (ossified)

Glottis

T_1. Lesions associated with normal vocal cord mobility do not penetrate the conus elasticus, nor do they invade the underlying thyro-arytenoid muscle (Fig. 2).

T_2. Serial section evidence casts doubt on "supraglottic extension of tumor with normal or impaired mobility." Impaired mobility in such a lesion suggests that the growth has crossed the ventricle and that it is likely to have invaded the thyroid ala.

T_3. In both the AJC and UICC systems, fixation of the true cord is the main feature of the T_3 lesion. It usually indicates invasion of the thyro-arytenoid muscle, thus making it difficult to determine the extent of the tumor and its suitability for partial resection (Kirchner and Som 1971).

T_4. Extension beyond the confines of the larynx frequently occurs with those growths extending more than 1 cm below the level of the glottis. "T_3" glottic lesions that measure 3 cms or more invade the laryngeal framework in over 75% of cases. They should, therefore, be classified T_4.

Subglottis

The significance of subglottic extension depends largely on whether this occurs in the anterior or posterior portion of the glottis. Since the superior surface of the cricoid cartilage approaches the level of the glottis in its posterior portion, a glottic cancer extending 1 cm below free edge of the vocal cord in the anterior larynx may still be within the confines of the thyroid ala and well above the cricoid cartilage. By contrast, a posterior glottic cancer at the vocal process of the arytenoid needs only a

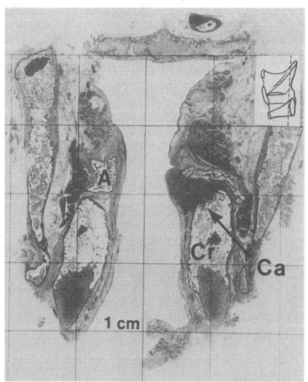

Fig. 3. Coronal section through posterior larynx (see insert). The 1 cm grid shows that only a few mm of subglottic extension in the posterior larynx is sufficient to allow cancer to invade the cricoid rostrum

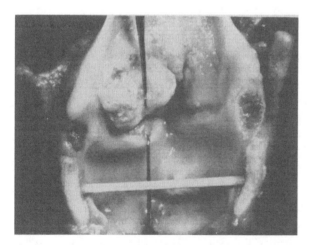

Fig. 4. This tumor illustrates the difficulty of accurate staging by inspection alone. The true cord could not be seen by indirect laryngoscopy because of overhanging tumor, and was considered to be fixed, with a T_3 classification. The true cord is not involved, and the lesion should have been staged T_2

few millimeters downward extension to reach the cricoid cartilage (Fig. 3). The degree of subglottic extension, then, is more important in the posterior glottis than in the anterior, since: 1. the proximity to the cricoid plate reduces the possibility of adequate resection by partial laryngectomy, and, 2. cancer invading the thin mucosal covering of the cricoid plate exposes the cartilage and bone to infection and damage during radiotherapy.

Computerized scanning has now facilitated identification of framework destruction, even though ossification patterns vary among individuals, and even between the corresponding areas in the two sides of the same individual larynx.

Accurate staging of the tumor may not be easy, so that similar lesions are not always being compared when results are reported from different treatment centers. This fact results in large discrepancies in published cure rates. A case in point is shown in Figs. 4 and 5. The lesion is a large T_2 supraglottic growth that had been staged T_3 by direct and indirect laryngoscopy. The true vocal cord could not be well

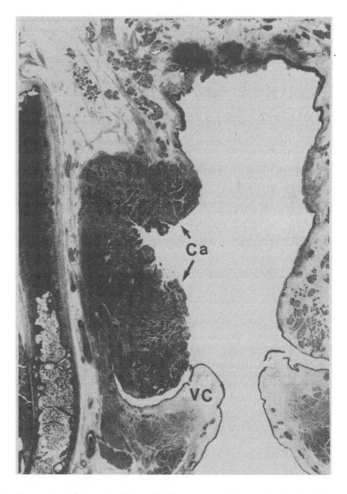

Fig. 5. Section of lesion similar to that shown in Figure 4. The true cord is not involved with tumor, but is being crowded from above. It should have been staged T_2, not T_3 as it was

seen by inspection, and was considered to be fixed. If this lesion had been successfully treated by radiotherapy, it would have been reported with other T_3 results, whereas it actually belongs in the T_2 category.

The clinician should use every necessary means of evaluating a lesion before treatment. This may require nothing more than indirect laryngoscopy, but it may, in some cases, require laryngography or computerized scanning. In this way, reported results of treatment are more likely to be accurate and useful.

References

American Joint Committee on Cancer (1980) Staging of cancer of head and neck sites and of melanoma. Chicago
International Union Against Cancer (1974) TNM classification of malignant tumors. Geneva
Kirchner JA, Cornog JL, Holmes RE (1974) Transglottic cancer. Arch Otolaryngol 99:247–251
Kirchner JA, Som ML (1971) Clinical and histological observations on supraglottic cancer. Ann Otol Rhinol Laryngol 80:638–645
Kirchner JA, Som ML (1971) Clinical significance of fixed vocal cord. Laryngoscope 81:1029–1044

What is the Glottis?

P. M. Stell and R. P. Morton, Liverpool

Introduction

The glottis is defined by the UICC and the AJC as consisting of the vocal cords, and the anterior and posterior commissures (1 and 2).

None of these structures is defined by the UICC or the AJC. The vocal cord has been defined for many years by anatomists, but the anterior and posterior commissures have never been defined. Both the UICC and the AJC define a glottic tumor as passing from T_1 to T_2 when it extends to the supra or subglottic regions, but neither body defines where this boundary lies.

Under the UICC scheme the vocal cord is mobile in stage T_1, but may be of impaired mobility in T_2. The case where the lesion is confined to the glottis with impaired mobility is not considered.

The vocal cord is defined as being attached anteriorly to the angle between the laminae of the thyroid cartilage, and posteriorly to the anterior end of the vocal process of the arytenoid cartilage. The vocal fold is confined to that part covered by tightly adherent squamous epithelium (Cunningham) and which comes together on phonation. The vertical height of this, the free border of the vocal cord, is 5 mm (Stell et al.).

The vocal folds form slightly more than half of the rima glottidis, the remaining part being formed by the body and vocal processes of the arytenoid cartilage. The anterior commissure has attracted great interest for 50 years at least. This term is a clinical term and not an anatomical one, and a definition of the term has never been

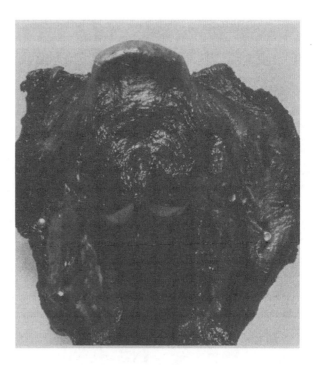

Fig. 1

universally accepted. Olofsson (1976) stated that the anterior commissure is an area anteriorly between the vocal cords with the same vertical extent as the anterior part of the vocal cords, bounded superiorly by the anterior angle of the ventricles and extending inferiorly for 2–3 mm. Laterally it extends for 2–3 mm to include the macula flava, the elastic condensation of the vocal ligaments. The anterior commissure tendon, described by Broyles, extending from the margin of the thyroid notch down to the insertion of the vocal ligaments, lies beneath the mucosa and does not enter into this definition.

If the mucosa of the larynx is stained selectively the vocal cords are seen to narrow anteriorly: the superior surface remains constant but the inferior surface slopes upwards, so that the anterior end of the vocal cord comes to a point (Fig. 1). The anterior ends of the two vocal cords may abut, or there may be a thin vertical strip of non squamous epithelium at this point (Stell et al.). This area forms the apex of the triangular anterior fixed part of the subglottis (Tucker). Tumors of the glottis extending to or across this point thus readily gain access to the subglottic space with its richer lymphatic drainage system, and vascular and glandular laminae (Bridger and Nassar) allowing the tumor to escape from the larynx by the cricothyroid membrane.

The posterior commissure has not been defined. Differential staining shows that the posterior commissure consists of a "Turkish saddle" of squamous epithelium, first defined by Virchow and more recently redefined by Stell et al. The saddle consists of a band of squamous epithelium 11 mm in height in men, and 9 mm in height in women, continuous laterally with the squamous epithelium overlying the vocal process of the arytenoid cartilage and the posterior end of the vestibular folds (Fig. 2).

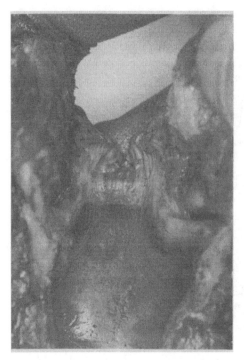

Fig. 2

From the above definitions it follows that:
a) Tumors arising from or involving the mucosa of the posterior half of the glottis cannot be classified fully.
b) The supra and subglottis begin at the superior and inferior margins of the free edge of the vocal cord. Tumors involving the upper or lower surface of the cord are not strictly confined to the glottis, and must therefore be classified as at least T_2 by both the UICC and AJC methods.

Some disagree with this definition. Ogura states that the glottis extends to a line 1 cm inferior to the free edge of the vocal cord, and Kirchner and Som state that it extends inferiorly to the superior border of the cricoid cartilage.
c) The anterior commissure is a point rather than an area and while tumors may cross this point they cannot arise from it.
d) Tumors confined to one vocal cord with impaired mobility (i.e. not complete fixation) cannot be classified.

The purpose of this paper is to examine the classification of a series of patients with glottic carcinoma and to assess the effect of unclear definitions in the accuracy of classification.

Patients

404 patients with a glottic carcinoma were seen between 1965 and 1982. Of these 185 had a tumor which had not fixed the cord completely and which was confined exclusively to the glottic structures.

These 185 patients are divided up into those arising from the vocal cord(s), those arising from the parts of the glottis not included by the UICC definition, and those affecting the "adjacent" areas of the upper and lower surfaces of the vocal cord, where classification may be in doubt.

Results

It can be seen from Table 1 that 134 of 185 glottic tumors (72%) could be classified accurately. The remainder were in some doubt because the tumor was confined to the vocal cord whose mobility was reduced, because the tumor arose from a part of the glottis which is not included in the UICC definition, or because the tumor extended to adjacent areas whose classification is in doubt.

Table 1. Glottic tumors

Confined to one vocal cord (T_{1a})	115
Confined to both vocal cords (T_{1b})	18
Arising from post commissure	1
Arising from vocal process	7
Arising from the vocal cord with involvement of the superior surface of the cord	27
Arising from the vocal cord with involvement of the inferior surface of the cord	13
Reduced mobility of the vocal cord	4

Recurrence

The overall recurrence rate was low – in a period ranging up to 16 years, 25 patients (13.5%) have suffered a recurrence of their disease, 21 at the primary site, 1 at the

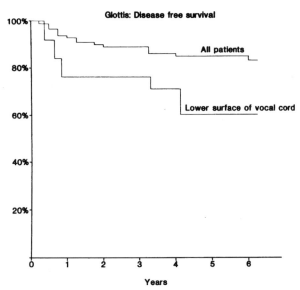

Fig. 3

primary site + the nodes, 2 in the cervical nodes and 1 at distant metastases. However, these figures conceal a very high recurrence rate for patients with subglottic extension of whom 5/13 suffered a recurrence, 4 at the primary site, and one in the lymph nodes.

Figure 3 shows the overall disease free survival, and disease free survival for the group with subglottic extension.

Survival

The overall 5 year survival rate calculated by the actuarial method was 89%. For the lesions confined to one completely mobile cord it was 87%, and for the unclassifiable lesions 91%. For those extending to the undersurface of the vocal cord it was 84%.

Discussion

The above results show that almost 30% of tumors arising from the rima glottidis cannot be classified accurately by the UICC or AJC scheme, because they arose from the muscoa over the vocal process of the arytenoid cartilage, because the vocal cord was not fully mobile, or because the tumor extended to the upper or lower surfaces of the vocal fold.

All patients had a good survival rate: indeed the patients with unclassifiable tumors did slightly but not significantly better than those with a tumor confined to a mobile cord. The patients with a tumor extending to the inferior surface of the vocal cord had a low disease free survival, of 60% at 5 years, but most of the patients with recurrence were salvaged by surgery.

The difference in interpretation of the classification may explain some of the differences in reporting of results. In 1974 the Centennial Conference on laryngeal cancer was held in Toronto. Results were collected from 17 centres around the world (Till). The proportion of patients with glottic tumors assigned to category T_1 varied from 18% for Milan to 62% for Liverpool. Such a vast difference may of course be due to differences of patterns of disease or referral, but this would probably not explain differences in 10% found on two occasions from different centres in the same city. Clearly those centres which classify equivocal cases as T_2 rather than T_1 will record better results, albeit legitimately.

References

American Joint Committe (1977) Manual for Staging of Cancer, Chicago p 39
Bridger GP, Nassar VH (1972) Cancer spread in the larynx. Arch Otolaryngol 95:497–505
Broyles FN (1943) The anterior commissure tendon. Ann Otol Rhinol Laryngol 52:342–345
Cunningham's Textbook of Anatomy (1943) Oxford University Press, London, 8th edition, p 666
Kirchner JA, Som ML (1971) Clinical significance of a fixed vocal cord. Laryngoscope 81:1029
Ogura JH, Mallen BW (1963) Carcinoma of the larynx. Postgrad Med 34:493

Olofsson J (1976) Specific features of laryngeal carcinoma involving the anterior commissure and the subglottic region. Centennial Conference on Laryngeal Cancer. Appleton-Century-Crofts, New York pp 626–640
Stell PM et al. (1978) Morphometry of the epithelial lining of the human larynx: I. The glottis. Clin Otolaryngol 3:13–20
Till JE et al. (1975) A preliminary analysis of end results for cancer of the larynx. Laryngoscope 85:1162–1172
Tucker GF et al. (1973) The anterior commissure revisited. Ann Otol Rhinol Laryngol 82:625–636
UICC (1978) TNM Classification of Malignant Tumors, Geneva, 3rd ed p 34
Virchow R (1887) Über Pachydermia laryngis. Berl Klin Wochenschr, pp 585–589

Staging of Laryngeal Carcinoma

J. Olofsson, Linköping

There are many problems involved in the classification and staging of laryngeal carcinoma. Some of these problems concern the exact delineation of the different laryngeal regions, that was highlighted at the Centennial Conference on Laryngeal Cancer in Toronto, 1974. Long discussions led to a definition of the glottic region to include the free margins and the horizontal surfaces of the vocal cords and the commissures. The lower lateral angle of the ventricles was considered the border between the glottic and supraglottic regions. The sub-surface of the vocal cords is a part of the subglottis (Fig. 1). Correct classification requires a detailed mapping of these parts of the cords. In the classification of small glottic lesions laryngography furnishes the most reliable mapping of the tumour and enables even a slight involvement of the sub-surface of the vocal cord to be assessed (Olofsson and Sökjer 1977).

The anterior commissure is another important area which is well assessed by laryngoscopy especially using 90° optical instruments and laryngography. Tumours involving the anterior commissure often extend subglottically changing a T_1 tumour to a T_2. When dealing with primary supraglottic carcinomas the lower margin of the tumour is important to assess to decide if a horizontal supraglottic laryngectomy can be performed (Olofsson 1975, 1982).

The anterior commissure area is also a common site for early cartilage invasion, which is difficult to assess with conventional radiographic methods. A low-voltage lateral plain film may show major invasion (Olofsson and Sökjer 1979). Computed tomography is the new diagnostic tool, which may provide additional information and thus changing a T_1 or T_2 tumour to a T_4 (UICC 1978; Sökjer and Olofsson 1981).

The surface extension of tumours is well assessed by clinical and conventional radiographic means. The deep extension, however, is difficult to assess (Figs. 2 and 3). Fixation is an important sign indicating deep invasion and in a high percentage invasion of the laryngeal framework and spread of tumour outside the larynx (Olofsson et al. 1973; Olofsson and van Nostrand 1973). The irregular ossification of

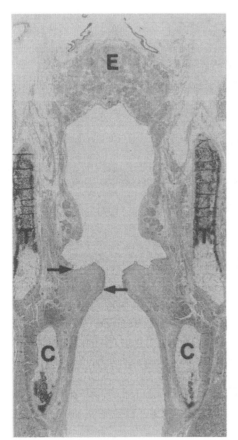

Fig. 1

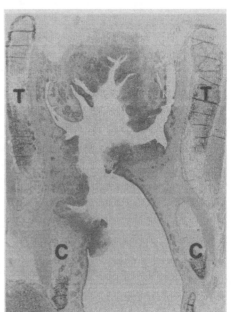

Fig. 2

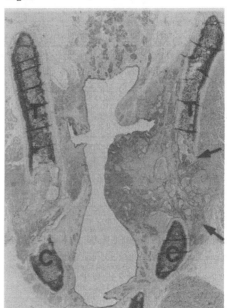

Fig. 3

Fig. 1. Coronal section of a normal adult larynx through the midportion of the vocal cords. The glottic region is marked by arrows. *C*, Cricoid cartilage; *E*, Epiglottis; *T*, Thyroid cartilage

Fig. 2. Coronal section through the anterior third of the vocal cords. Multiregional tumour (probably primary glottic) with involvement of both vocal cords, false vocal cords, base of epiglottis and with subglottic extension on the left side. No cartilage invasion or spread outside the larynx can be seen

Fig. 3. Coronal section through the midportion of the vocal cords. Glottic, sub- and supraglottic carcinoma invading the laryngeal framework and extending outside the larynx (*arrows*). This tumour is mainly growing beneath an intact mucosa. The vocal cord was fixed indicating deep invasion. Radiographic examination including computed tomography is necessary to be able to correctly assess this tumour

the thyroid alae makes the assessment of invasion difficult, at least with conventional radiographic methods (Olofsson and Sökjer 1979).

Computed tomography depicts the larynx in the transverse plane, and thus adds a new projection to the ordinary a.p. and lateral projections. Computed tomography is indicated for examination of tumours, where there is a risk of cartilage invasion or extralaryngeal extension (Sökjer and Olofsson 1981). The technique of whole-organ serial sectioning of laryngectomy specimens in the transverse plane affords unique possibilities for comparing computed tomography and the findings in the histologic sections. The diagnostic potential of computed tomography will be better evaluated by systematic studies using whole-organ serial sectioning in the same way as has been performed for laryngoscopy and conventional radiographic methods.

It is of great importance, that, when laryngeal cancer material is reported the classification used is strictly adhered to and that the anatomical regions are clearly delineated enabling a comparison to be made between different reports. We have to make full use of all our clinical and radiological examinations including computed tomography to achieve better accuracy in our pre-therapeutic staging, which is of utmost importance when selecting patients for voice and airway conservation surgery.

References

Centennial Conference on Laryngeal Cancer, Toronto (1974). Workshop No. 1. Classification, anatomy, growth, and spread of laryngeal cancer. (Chairmen Harrison DFN, van Nostrand AWP). Can J Otolaryngol 3:407–511

Olofsson J, Lord IJ, van Nostrand AWP (1973) Vocal cord fixation in laryngeal carcinoma. Acta Otolaryngol (Stockh) 75:496–510

Olofsson J, van Nostrand AWP (1973) Growth and spread of laryngeal and hypopharyngeal carcinoma with reflections on the effect of preoperative irradiation. 139 cases studied by whole organ serial sectioning. Acta Otolaryngol [Suppl] (Stockh) 308:1–84

Olofsson J (1975) Specific features of laryngeal carcinoma involving the anterior commissure and the subglottic region. Can J Otolaryngol 4:618–632

Olofsson J, Sökjer H (1977) Radiology and laryngoscopy for the diagnosis of laryngeal carcinoma. Acta Radiol [Diagn] (Stockh) 18:449–468

Olofsson J, Sökjer H (1979) Radiologic assessment of laryngeal carcinoma. A clinico-pathologic comparison based on whole-organ serial sections. Acta Radiol [Diagn] (Stockh) 20:789–814

Olofsson J (1982) Laryngeal carcinoma: problems in diagnosis and classification. J Otolaryngol 11:167–177

Sökjer H, Olofsson J (1981) Computed tomography in carcinoma of the larynx and piriform sinus. Clin Otolaryngol 6:335–343

Union Internationale Contre le Cancer (1978) TNM classification of malignant tumours (Larynx, classified 1972, confirmed 1978). Geneva

The TNM-Classification with Regard to Surgical Planning of Partial Resections of the Larynx

K. W. Hommerich, Berlin

Failures of partial resections of the larynx with subsequent early recurrence of cancer are due to an incomplete removal of the primary tumour with all of its processes. In my experience the laryngeal surgeon who based his surgical decisions merely on the present UICC tumour classification would run the risk of planning an oncologically unsafe operation. The reason is that the pre-operative inspection of the endolarynx cannot clarify the real extension of the lesion in the depth of the laryngeal muscles and superstructure. Our scepticism was nourished by the histological examination of serial sections of 130 larynx specimens, removed by total laryngectomy for advanced cancer. The results were given in the doctoral theses of Menke (1974), Weede (1974), Strüwind (1977) and Sparmann (1980).

These investigations, using a new histological technique (Hommerich et al. 1971) have realized or confirmed the concept and findings of Leroux-Robert (1936) and other authors (Kleinsasser et al. 1969; Harrison 1970; Kirchner 1969, 1977; Olofsson 1973). They revealed, among other conclusions, that the mode of ossification of the thyroid cartilage (see also Pesch 1981) would definitely enhance the masked proliferation of the carcinoma. Three factors contribute to the misinterpretation of a visible lesion:

1. Infiltration of the larynx superstructure by the tumour without clinical symptoms,
2. occult invasion of the soft tissues of the larynx, and
3. tumour growth into the adjacent paralaryngeal space.

Figures 1–4 illustrate these three phenomena which were observed by us and by other investigators. In supraglottic tumours e.g., the inferior extension lateral to the sinus of Morgagni into the glottic plane without involvement of the vocal cord itself was striking (Fig. 1).

Even in large transglottic tumours with destructive growth of all three levels of the larynx, microscopical examination could sometimes detect additional spread of the malignancy into the piriform sinus (Fig. 2). The inferior margin of the specimen might be free of carcinoma while processes of the lesion have already reached the paratracheal space.

Influenced by the repeated observations of such patterns of clinically hidden tumour growth, the method of postoperative staging was introduced, using a symbol "p" (pathology) in order to determine the histopathological features of the tumour extension of the individual case. This objective classification should facilitate the comparison of cancer treatment statistics.

In our own material the direction of tumour invasion to a certain extent followed the rules of probability. Of course there existed rare forms of spread. On the other hand, however, the invasion of certain laryngeal compartments by the lesion was commoner than that of other regions, obviously guided by structural peculiarities.

Clinical and Histological Staging 83

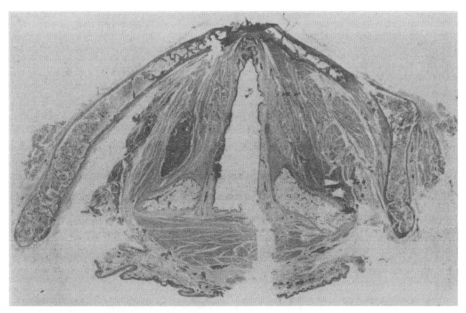

Fig. 1. Supraglottic tumor with inferior extension into the mass of the left vocal cord; note the tumor island near the arytenoid cartilage

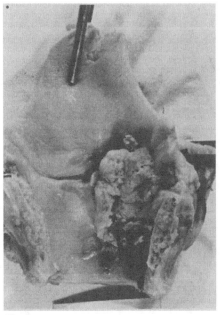

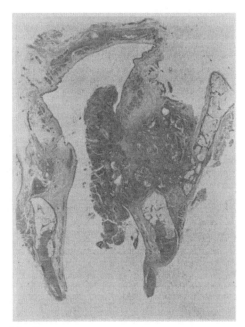

Fig. 2   **Fig. 3**

Fig. 2. Macroscopic view of a laryngeal tumor with involvement of all three compartments in cranio-caudal direction

Fig. 3. The microscopic view shows the same tumor as in Fig. 2. It appears that the piriform sinus is also involved, but the inferior level of the removed larynx seems free of tumor

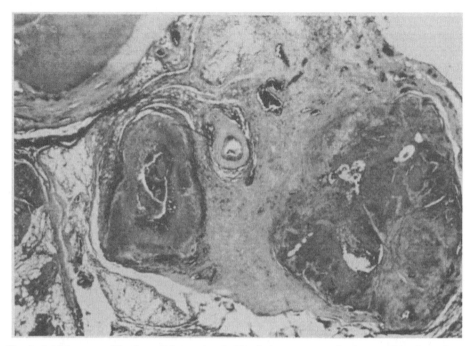

Fig. 4. A higher magnification of the section in Fig. 3 shows paratracheal tumor islands at the level of resection

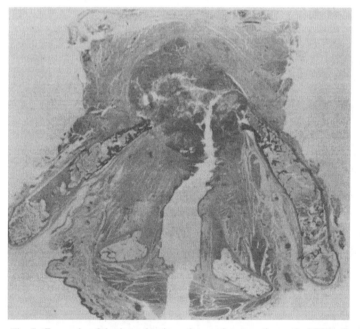

Fig. 5. Example of the introduction of a pretherapeutic symbol "S" = "spread". Bilateral vocal cord involvement (T_2), thyroid cartilage infiltration (S_1) and invasion of the preepiglottic space (S_2) without clinical symptoms. The enlarged classification would read $T_2\ S_{1-2}\ N_0\ M_0$

These statistical preferences could widely by utilized for a better preoperative classification of the disease, which would definitely improve the planning of surgery.

In the world congress of Oto-Rhino-Laryngology in 1981 at Budapest I suggested the introduction of a pretherapeutical index "S" (=spread) to the TNM-formula of tumour classification, based on the statistical probability of occult cancer invasion of the larynx. It should be added to the staging label in all cases with an incidence of masked proliferation higher than fifty percent of all examined cases. The experiences of various investigations should be evaluated by synopsis, in order to base the additional information for the individual case on a large representative sample.

A corresponding example is given by Fig. 5. The index "S" should serve as a warning to the surgeon, requiring increased attention, resulting, at least, in the meticulous scrutiny of the adjacent laryngeal regions. Care should be taken not to confine the excision to the macroscopically visible lesion, but to eradicate the disease by a generous resection based on the statistical probability of invisible tumour spread.

References

Harrison DFN (1970) Pathology of hypopharyngeal cancer in relation to surgical management. J Laryng Otol 84:349–365

Hommerich KW (1982) The micromorphology of the spread tendency of larynx and hypopharynx tumors and their importance for operative indications. In: Surján L, Bodó GY (eds) Borderline problems in otorhinolaryngology. Excerpta Medica, Amsterdam Oxford Princeton, pp 67–74

Hommerich KW, Sauer H, Weede W (1971) Zur Wachstumstendenz von Larynxtumoren. Arch klin exp Ohr Nas Kehlk Heilk 199:748–751

Kirchner JA (1969) One hundred laryngeal cancer studies by serial sections. Ann Otol Rhinol Laryngol 78:681–710

Kirchner JA (1977) Two hundred laryngeal cancers; patterns of growth and spread as seen in serial sections. Laryngoscope 87:474–482

Kleinsasser O, Madjd S (1969) Rückblick auf die Ergebnisse von 224 Totalexstirpationen des Kehlkopfes. Z Laryngol Rhinol 48:161–178

Leroux-Robert J (1936) Les epitheliomas Intra-Laryngeé. Formes Anatomo-Clinique. Voies Déstension, Doin, Paris

Menke M (1974) Ausbreitungstendenzen der glottischen Larynxkarzinome. Inaugural Dissertation, Berlin

Olofsson J, van Nostrand AWP (1973) Growth and spread of laryngeal and hypopharyngeal carcinoma. Acta Otolaryngol [Suppl] (Stockh) 308:1–84

Pesch HJ, Glass V, Stephan M et al. (1981) Zum Ossifikationsprinzip des Schildknorpels. Arch Otorhinolaryngol (NY) 231:829–830

Sparmann M (1980): Ausbreitungstendenzen der Hypopharynxkarzinome. Eine histomorphologische Studie. Inaugural Dissertation, Berlin

Strüwind R (1977): Ausbreitungstendenzen der subglottischen Larynxkarzinome. Eine histomorphologische Studie. Inaugural Dissertation, Berlin

Weede W (1974): Histologische Untersuchungen über die Wachstumstendenzen supraglottischer Kehlkopftumoren. Inaugural Dissertation, Berlin

Correlation Between Clinical and Histological Staging in Laryngeal Cancer

D. F. N. Harrison, London

Clinical staging of human cancer is widely accepted as an effective and acceptable means of predicting prognosis and comparing treatment modalities. Consequently, intrinsic and unknown errors in such classifications may be erroneously construed as supporting forms of therapy which infact may be less rather than more effective than expected. Unfortunately, it is not possible to measure the inherent accuracy of many classifications. The larynx is an exception, and this paper is devoted to a comparison between clinical and histological staging in 145 laryngectomised patients. This detailed and time consuming examination was carried out by myself during the years 1965–1975 as part of a more extensive personal research programme devoted to the natural history and surgical pathology of laryngeal and hypopharyngeal cancer. However, identifying the intrinsic, and possibly unavoidable errors in any specific classification system, is only one part of the clinical problem. These 145 patients were then followed up for a minimum of 5 years in order that the significance of these errors might be determined in relation to long term survival. Such an analysis has never been carried out for laryngeal cancer, nor in fact for any other site within the head and neck. Indeed, it is probable that the exercise will never be repeated since the cost and time involved is prohibitive.

The results of this project, presented for each of the main regions within the larynx, are of great interest and significance. They illustrate that despite errors as large as 50%, providing laryngeal surgery is radical – prognosis is largely related to whether the disease remains within the laryngeal framework. Histology is relevant, in that site for site undifferentiated neoplasms do worse than differentiated carcinoma; and the significance of regional lymph node metastases is generally accepted as always bad although difficult to relate accurately to the true extent of primary tumour.

To the statistician the numbers are small and woefully uncontrolled, the laryngologist however will appreciate the considerable in-built deficiencies of the existing systems of classification. In applying the UICC classification (the most commonly utilised internationally) for the purpose of comparing specific tumour incidence or success of therapy, this analysis illustrates the considerable errors which must distort final conclusions. It also confirms the difficulties of determining the true extent of laryngeal cancer two dimensionally and the potential dangers of conservation surgery!

This work is presented not as a guide book to the natural history and treatment of laryngeal cancer. It does however lay the surgical pathological foundations on which a realistic system of classification could be constructed and effective surgical excision performed.

C. Vertical Partial Resection of the Larynx

I. Surgical Techniques and Modifications of Vertical Partial Laryngectomy

History, Indications and Techniques of Vertical Partial Laryngectomy

J. LABAYLE, Paris

History and Evolution of Techniques

Vertical partial laryngectomy has a place between cordectomy for epitheliomas of the middle of the vocal cord and total laryngectomy for all other glottic and transglottic cancers.

All the modifications of vertical laryngectomy derive from three surgical principles and are linked to three names:
1. Saint Clair Thompson, who extended the indications for cordectomy by cutting an opening into the thyroid cartilage.
2. Hautant, who described hemilaryngectomy with excision of large portions of the thyroid cartilage and portions of the cricoid ring.
3. Gluck and Sörensen, who were the first to work out a true hemilaryngectomy, of which the wound closure, however, offered difficult problems.

All contemporary operations are based on these techniques, but aim to achieve fundamental improvements:
1. A better knowledge of cancer spread and, consequently, excision of the anterior commissure.
2. A reconstruction of the larynx to restore respiratory function while overcoming the problems of swallowing.
3. Improvement of phonation by creation of a new vocal cord.

Several authors have lent their names to surgical refinement of vertical hemilaryngectomy. It is impossible to cite them all, but they include: Tapia, Figi, Leroux-Robert, Mündnich, Denecke, Conley, Aubry, Norris, Piquet, Rethy, Bailey etc.

Indications and Contra-Indications for Vertical Laryngectomy

Indications

It is of the utmost importance to define precisely the indications for partial laryngectomy and to recognize the extension of the particular lesion before surgery. Appropriate candidates for vertical partial laryngectomy have a cancer of the vocal cord with invasion of the:

- Anterior commissure,
- laryngeal muscles,
- arytenoid,
- false cord,
- upper and lateral parts of the subglottis.

Contra-Indications

- Extension into the contralateral side of the thyroid cartilage, anteriorly or laterally.
- Extension into the contralateral soft tissues:
    a) through the anterior commissure or
    b) through the posterior commissure.
- Extension through the epiglottic cartilage.
- Extension below the cricoid ring.
- Dorsal extension into the piriform sinus.

Some Techniques of Vertical Partial Laryngectomy

Frontolateral Excision: Leroux-Robert

This is a vertical partial laryngectomy with excision of the anterior commissure by triangular resection of the thyroid cartilage (Fig. 1). Technical variants intended to avoid anterior webs and to gain a better voice include:
a) Vertical and parallel incisions to obtain a broader angle (Fig. 2).
b) Utilization of prostheses inserted into the glottis for two or three weeks (Denecke).
c) Sutures for precise adaptation of the remnants of the vocal cords.
d) Resection of anterior scar webs by laser.
e) Rethis operation with skin grafting.

Hemilaryngectomy with Arytenoidectomy and Reconstruction of the Pharyngo-Laryngeal Wall

Grafting by Skin Flaps. We only quote these techniques because they are almost never used, except, perhaps, Conley's technique who used the transposition of a cervical skin flap for the reconstruction of a new vocal cord. Rethi's modification is illustrated by the sketch in Fig. 3. The techniques of Aubry-Rouget and Aubry-Labayle are shown by Figs. 4 and 5.

Mucous Membrane and Cartilaginous Grafting
Kambic's Operation. Kambic bisects the preserved epiglottis, and swings on part down to reconstruct a wall at the site of the removed hemilarynx. It is a useful procedure, but its indications are rare.
Operation of Bouche and Freche. This technique uses the preserved epiglottis as a whole. It is mobilized from its upper connections, and is turned down to replace the excised hemilarynx (Fig. 6).

Surgical Techniques and Modifications of Vertical Partial Laryngectomy

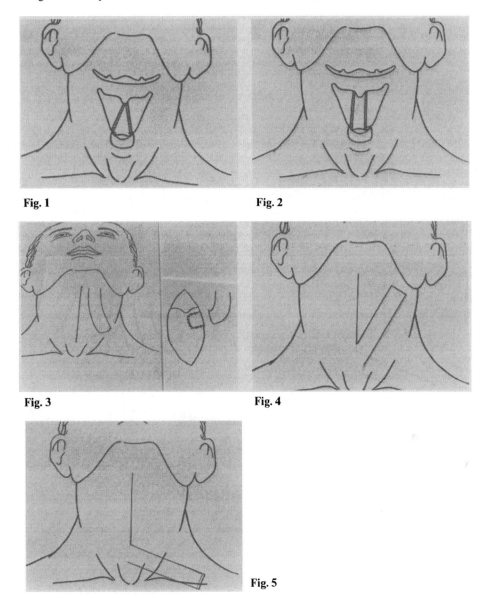

Fig. 1

Fig. 2

Fig. 3

Fig. 4

Fig. 5

Rotation of Mucous Membrane from the Piriform Sinus for Reconstruction of a Lateral Laryngo-Pharyngeal Wall. It is, in my opinion, the best operation following hemilaryngectomy. An appropriate flap of the mucosa is cut from the piriform sinus (Figs. 7 and 8), and is rotated into the remaining hemilarynx to line the resulting cavity. This principle of plastic reconstruction was inaugurated by Denecke and Som, among others.

Sometimes, swallowing becomes difficult, and a secondary dysphagia with aspiration may result. This problem can be solved by the following technique either at the same time or at a second stage.

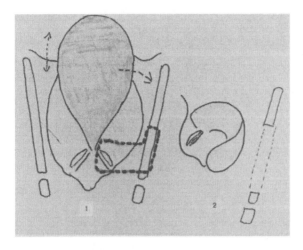

Fig. 6

This operation includes:
- the use of a piece of thyroid cartilage transposed to the posterior wall,
- rotation of mucosa from the upper side of the cricoid,
- insertion of cartilage to replace the missing arytenoid,
- suturing muscles and mucosa to cover the cartilage graft.

This method is very easy and gives very good results.

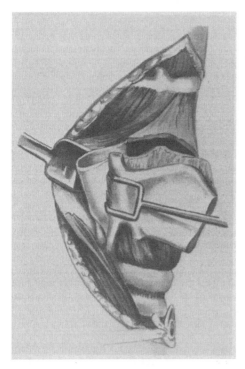

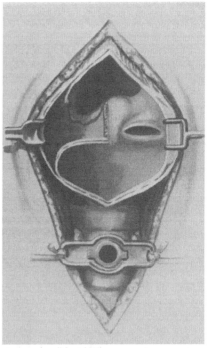

Fig. 7   Fig. 8

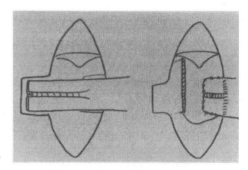

Fig. 9

Techniques for Reconstruction of the Vocal Cord for Restoration of Voice

When we use skin as a rotation flap, this can be achieved by Conley's method which was mentioned before. We prefer Ganz's operation: he folded the skin flap before suturing it to the appropriate site (Fig. 9).

When we use a mucosal graft for glottic reconstruction Senechal's technique is preferred. He recommended free grafting of the helix root.

Also Bouche's technique should be mentioned using the upper epiglottis as a free graft.

Bailey and Rodriguez-Adragos have obtained good results by muscular interposition (Fig. 10), a simple and easy operation consisting of interposition of a free thyroid cartilage graft from the same side and suturing sterno-cleido-mastoid muscle over the thyroid cartilage. Naturally this method is only used when the thyroid cartilage is not involved by the tumor.

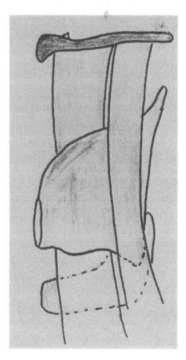

Fig. 10

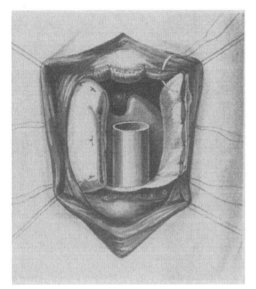
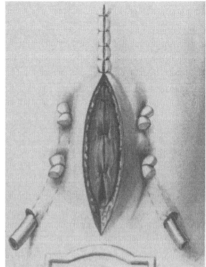

Fig. 11 Fig. 12

Stenting the Larynx

- Is not really necessary in every case.
- Must not be used for more than three weeks.
- Is of use especially in grafts of free skin or mucosa.
  Two techniques may be recommended:
a) *Mikulicz.* The "Mikulicz tamponade" is used for a short period of time The bag is made of a dry "biogauze". A ribbon gauze of 1 cm breadth is folded into the cavity. The ribbon gauze and bag are fixed by two thick nylonthreads. These threads are marked so that the thread that holds the ribbon gauze can be taken out first.
b) *Silastic tube.* Care should be taken to fix the tube, either by fixation to the stent (Fig. 11)

or by transcutaneous sutures (Fig. 12).

To give an impression of the place of vertical hemilaryngectomy in surgery for cancer of the larynx, two tables of our statistics are presented. In Table 1 the number

Table 1. Number of operations between 1965 and 1979

Laryngectomies total	950
Horizontal and reconstructive (the latter only from 1970)	164

Table 2. Cordectomies and vertical partial laryngectomies

Cordectomies	84
Vertical hemilaryngectomies	42

of operations between 1965 and 1979 is given. Table 2 shows the figures for cordectomies and vertical partial laryngectomies.

Conclusions

Vertical hemi-laryngectomy is a good operation because it is a functional operation. It is not traumatic and it is useful for persons of reduced general conditions and for old people. But we have to regard the limited indications. We must be more oncologists than surgeons. Operations with preservation of the voice are especially useful for some professions such as doctors, judges, advocates etc. The additional help of phoniatric training after all these operations should not be forgotten.

For postoperative stenosis, bone grafting using iliac bone is the best technique. In extension of tumor into the upper and contralateral compartments our operation of "crico-hyoido-pexy" appears to be preferable and gives better results.

The Role of Laryngoplasty in Vertical Partial Laryngectomies

H. J. DENECKE, Heidelberg

In a high percentage of the cases of laryngeal carcinoma, total extirpation of the larynx can be replaced by one of the partial laryngectomies. This requires that the tumor resection is carried out under magnification and that the defects in the larynx are afterwards repaired by reconstructive measures. The safety of the patient has greatest priority, i.e. the tumors must be resected far into the healthy tissue and their tendency to growth must be taken into account. This can be achieved even in extensive carcinomas by magnification surgery with head light and binocular loupe or with surgical microscope when the tumor has not grown beyond certain limits which are specified below.

Relatively large raw areas in the larynx are left behind after tumor resection in many cases. Without resurfacing, these lead to an appreciable functional impairment or even loss of function of the larynx by subsequent scar contraction. It is therefore to be recommended that partial laryngectomies, especially the more extensive ones, are always accompanied by reconstruction of the defects, i.e. by laryngoplasties. Epithelialized tissue such as skin or mucosa is of course most suitable for resurfacing the raw areas.

Since basic rules of radical tumor resection must be observed in each case, whereas healthy parts of the larnyx must be carefully preserved for later reconstruction, partial laryngectomies can be carried out only on the basis of the operation procedures outlined briefly below both with regard to resection and in particular with regard to reconstruction. The procedure in the individual case must be determined by the respective extent of the tumor as found at operation. The main

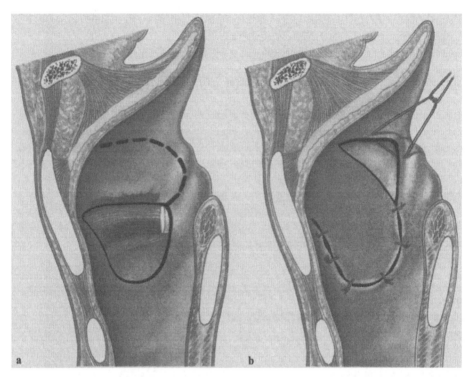

Fig. 1a, b. Forming a ventrally based rotation flap of mucous membrane from the ventricle (ventriculus laryngis Morgagni) and the false vocal cord for resurfacing larger superficial defects on the vocal cord (Denecke). **a** The broken line shows the flap marked out. Below is the defect over the vocal cord with the partially preserved M. vocalis and the site of detachment from the arytenoid cartilage. **b** The mucosal flap is sutured into the defect on the vocal cord. The donor site is closed by suturing with relief of tension at the base of the flap. From Denecke (1980)

problem is not the resection of the tumor with or without sacrifice of parts of the laryngeal skeleton, but the reconstruction of the larynx for its three functions: air passage, deglutition and phonation.

In larger superficial defects in the region of the glottis, pedicle flaps of the laryngeal mucosa from the immediate vicinity of the defects can be used for resurfacing (Figs. 1–3). Depending on the position and the extent of the defect, these flaps can be taken from the supraglottic or the subglottic region and can be based anteriorly or posteriorly (Denecke). They are mobilized, rotated into the defect and sutured to its margins without tension. The donor site is afterwards closed by sutures in such a way that there is a relaxation at the base of the flap.

In superficial defects of the posterior laryngeal wall such as are left behind after resection of superficially growing carcinomas of this region, it is especially important to resurface the raw area to maintain the mobility of the arytenoid cartilages. This can be achieved by pedicle mucosal flaps from the adjacent posterior wall of the airway (Denecke). It may become necessary to obtain the flap not only from the larynx but also from the posterior wall of the trachea (Fig. 4). The donor site should

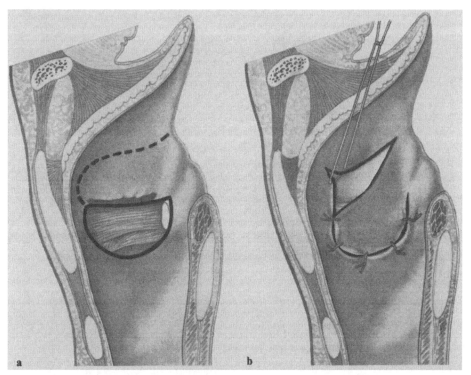

Fig. 2a, b. Forming a dorsally based rotation flap of mucous membrane from the ventricle (Morgagni) and the false vocal cord for resurfacing larger superficial defects on the vocal cord (Denecke). **a** The broken line shows the flap marked out. Below, there is the defect over the vocal cord with the partially preserved M. vocalis and the site of detachment from the arytenoid cartilage. **b** The mucosal flap is sutured over the defect on the vocal cord. The donor site is closed by suturing with relief of tension at the base of the flap. From Denecke (1980)

not exceed 50% of the width of the posterior wall of the airway, since otherwise it cannot be covered by mobilisation of the adjacent mucosa.

For various reasons, use of free grafts of split skin, full thickness skin or mucosa has not proven effective in the long term to resurface defects in the laryngeal region. On the one hand, the grafts do not heal in as well as pedicle flaps in an area which is in constant movement due to breathing, deglutition and coughing. On the other hand it must be borne in mind that grafts which have already healed in are endangered during postoperative radiotherapy and may become necrotic. In the region where the defect is not perfectly covered with skin or mucosa, a more or less intensive development of granulation tissue occurs leading to scars which subsequently disturb laryngeal function.

In deep-spreading carcinomas of the vocal cord which necessitate resection of the muscle (cordectomy) or in carcinomas which have invaded the Morgagni ventricle or the subglottic region, the defects after excision into healthy tissue cannot be covered and filled from the interior of the larynx. In these cases, a hair-free pedicle flap consisting of skin and subcutaneous tissue must then be used. It is brought in

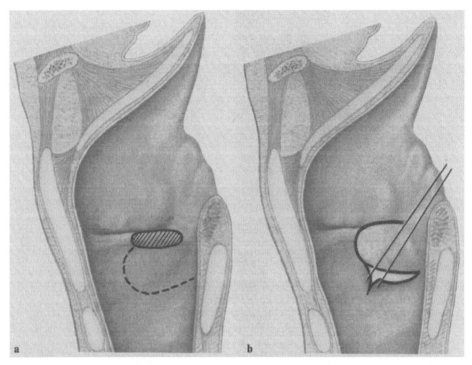

Fig. 3a, b. Fashioning the rotation flap of mucous membrane from the subglottic space for covering superficial defects on the vocal cord (Denecke). **a** For resurfacing a defect in the posterior part of the vocal cord (*hatched area*) a dorsally based, subglottic flap of mucous membrane (*broken line*) is used. **b** The flap is laid over the vocal cord defect. The donor site is drawn together so that the tension at the base of the flap is reduced. The flap is then fixed with sutures in its new position over the defect. From Denecke (1980)

from the neck in the vicinity of the laryngostome and sutured to the edges of the defect (Fig. 5). When the vocal process also had to be removed in tumor resection because the tumor had grown dorsally into the vicinity of this structure, the flap must be respectively larger (Fig. 6). The same applies to the cases in which the false vocal cord has also to be resected.

Since after being turned into the larynx the pedicle of the flap is located between the incision edges at the thyroid cartilage, it is advisable to resect a strip of cartilage to establish the blood circulation in the flap (Figs. 5, 7, 8). In this way, not only is a compression of the pedicle prevented in the postoperative phase, but there is also a better alignment between the incision edge on the thyroid cartilage and the more or less deep defect in the region of the vocal cord. Glottal closure for phonation and deglutition is appreciably improved after healing (Denecke).

If a bilateral vocal cord carcinoma is present with involvement of the anterior commissure, then a corresponding procedure is applied both in tumor resection and in resurfacing of the bilateral defects. This procedure is also possible when both vocal cords are invaded by the tumor from the anterior commissure up to the arytenoid cartilage. The resection defects are afterwards subjected to laryngoplasty.

Surgical Techniques and Modifications of Vertical Partial Laryngectomy

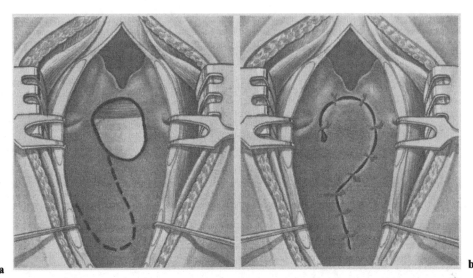

Fig. 4a, b. Situation after resection of a superficially spreading carcinoma of the posterior wall of the larynx. Closure of the defect with a rotation flap of mucous membrane from the posterior wall of the air passages. **a** In the base of the superficial defect (*inked-in horizontal lines*) the lamina of the cricoid cartilage and the transverse arytenoid muscle can be identified. Caudal to the defect a flap of mucous membrane will be cut from the posterior wall of the air passages (*broken line*). **b** The flap is rotated upwards and sutured into the defect and after mobilising the surrounding mucous membrane, the donor site is sutured (Denecke). From Denecke (1980)

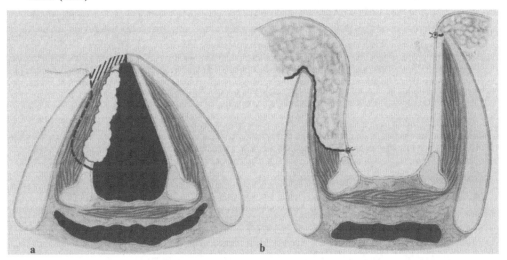

Fig. 5a, b. Excision and reconstruction of the vocal cord by a full-thickness rotation skin flap. Transverse section. **a** The broken line shows the excision of the tumor, up to healthy tissue. The hatched area shows the resection of the margin of the thyroid cartilage. This makes possible a better alignment between the incision edge on the thyroid cartilage and the defect in the vocal cord, as well as a better insertion of the pedicle flap. **b** The pedicle skin flap is laid in position and sutured. The outer perichondrium of the thyroid cartilage is turned in over the line of resection of the cartilage. On the opposite side, the skin which is to epithelialize the laryngostome is stitched to the mucous membrane of the vocal cord and to the perichondrium of the thyroid cartilage. From Denecke (1980)

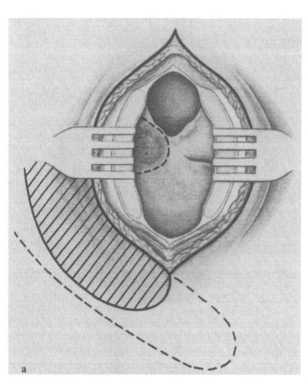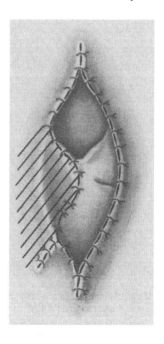

Fig. 6a, b. Cordectomy and resection of part of the arytenoid cartilage. The covering of the remaining portion of the arytenoid cartilage is particularly important for preserving its mobility. The pedicle full-thickness skin flap must be cut correspondingly larger. **a** The broken line in the larynx shows the line of excision around the tumor, into healthy tissue. The hatched area shows the donor site for the flap, which one can elongate in the direction of the broken line, according to requirement. **b** The flap is stitched in place, right up to the posterior wall. The laryngostome is completely epithelialized. From Denecke (1980)

Depending on the extent and depth of the defects, either pedicle flaps from the vicinity of the laryngostome can be used on both sides (Fig. 7) or the larger defect on one side is covered with a pedicle skin flap whereas a pedicle mucosal flap is used to resurface the superficial defect on the opposite side (Fig. 8).

After completion of the operation in the larynx, the question arises as to whether the larynx can be primarily closed or whether it is better to carry out an open postoperative treatment. According to the experience of the author, primary closure should only be carried out when small carcinomas have been excised, when no resurfacing of the defect was necessary and when the danger of postoperative bleeding can be excluded with certainty. In all larger defects and a correspondingly extensive reconstruction, open postoperative treatment with secondary closure is to be preferred for reasons of safety and for better fixation of the flaps. This enables the insertion of an intralaryngeal dressing (Fig. 9) in which the larynx lumen is filled with a Mikulicz tampon and the trachea cannula is wound around with gauze strips. This dressing prevents postoperative bleeding and hematomas after extensive resections

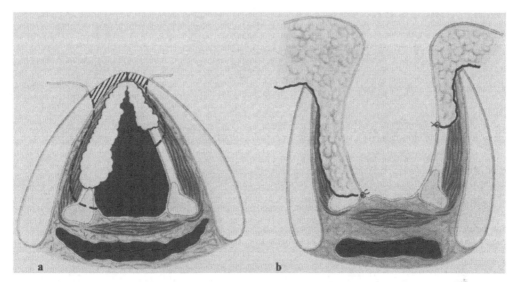

Fig. 7a, b. Resection of a bilateral deeply infiltrating carcinoma of the vocal cord with involvement of the anterior commissure, and reconstruction of the vocal cords. Transverse section. **a** Resection of the bilateral tumor, to healthy tissue (*broken lines*). On the left the carcinoma has reached the arytenoid cartilage. For this reason a part of this cartilage has to be resected. A resection of the border of the thyroid cartilage is performed on both sides (*hatched areas*) which, because of the extent of the tumor, is correspondingly larger on the left than on the right. Moreover the external perichondrium is preserved. **b** The reconstruction of the resected parts of the vocal cords is performed with bilateral pedicle full-thickness skin flaps, on account of the depth of the defects. On the left this flap reaches over the defect in the arytenoid cartilage and is sutured without tension. On the right some subcutaneous fat was excised from the skin flap to adapt it to the vocal cord. The mobilized perichondrium covers the resected surface of the thyroid cartilage bilaterally. From Denecke (1980)

and protects the lower airways against wound secretion, saliva and food going down the wrong way. In addition, it fixes the flaps sutured into the larynx. Depending on the position and size of these flaps and the length of the laryngostome, the cannula is inserted into the caudal part of the laryngostome or into a tracheostome formed for this purpose.

The intralaryngeal dressing can be removed after four to six days. Up to then, the histological findings have been finally verified especially with regard to the boundaries of the tumor resection. Secondary resections which may be required are then still possible through the open laryngostome.

When mucosal flaps from the interior of the larynx were used for the laryngoplasty and an epithelialized laryngostome was not formed, and when the laryngeal edema has subsided sufficiently, the larynx can be directly closed on removal of the intralaryngeal dressing by suture and a compression bandage. When pedicle flaps from the skin of the neck were used for laryngoplasty and an epithelialized laryngostome was formed, then surgical closure of the laryngostome is necessary. This operation can only be carried out when the flaps have healed in securely in the region of their new base in the larynx and when they tolerate severance of their pedicle without disturbance of nutrition. Experience shows that this is the case about 10 to 14 days after the primary operation.

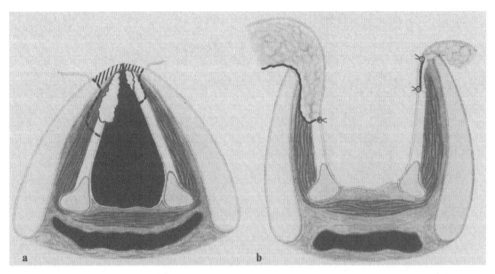

Fig. 8a, b. Resection of a carcinoma of the vocal cords with involvement of the anterior commissure, and reconstruction of the vocal cord defects. Transverse section. **a** After resection of the growth to healthy tissue (*broken lines*) there follows a resection of the border of the thyroid cartilage bilaterally (*hatched areas*) with preservation of the external perichondrium. **b** On the left side of the larynx the filling in and covering of the deeply extending defect is done with a pedicle full-thickness skin flap. On the right, the smaller superficial defect is covered by a pedicle flap of mucous membrane which is stitched into place in the defect. In the region of the anterior commissure the adjoining skin of the neck is sutured to the flap and to the mobilized perichondrium. From Denecke (1980)

If surgery of laryngeal carcinomas is carried out on the guidelines outlined briefly above, total extirpation of the larynx can be avoided in a relatively large number of cases and partial laryngectomy can be carried out with good functional results. The indication for partial laryngectomy is limited by certain tumor localizations. There is thus a contraindication when both crico-arytenoid joints are infiltrated by the tumor, since relearning of deglutition is then practically impossible despite reconstructive measures. When only one crico-arytenoid joint is affected, hemilaryngeal resection with its modifications and with laryngoplasty is to be considered. Carcinomas which have perforated the thyroid cartilage or have infiltrated the entire cricoid arch are likewise a contraindication against partial laryngectomy. It is better to carry out total extirpation in these cases, since the paratracheal lymph nodes are mostly also affected in tumors of this extent. The age of the patient also plays a certain role in the indication for partial laryngectomy with reconstruction. When deglutition is impaired postoperatively after extensive resections, younger, intellectually adaptable patients learn the altered swallowing technique more easily than older patients. Though an additional crico-pharyngeal myotomy can improve deglutition, one should be rather cautious with the indication for partial laryngectomy in old or prematurely aged patients and extensive tumors. The indication for partial laryngectomy after radiotherapy is discussed elsewhere in this book.

In a film, the long-term results of this surgery are demonstrated. The patients were filmed 15 to 20 years after partial laryngectomy. In these patients, total ex-

Surgical Techniques and Modifications of Vertical Partial Laryngectomy

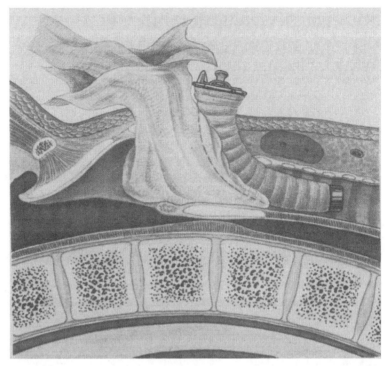

Fig. 9. Intralaryngeal dressing. After operations on the larynx an intralaryngeal dressing is inserted to protect the lower air passages from blood and exudate, which may run down, and from swallowing of saliva and food. The dressing also fixes the flaps in position during the postoperative phase. It consists of a Mikulicz tampon and a tracheal cannula wrapped around with strips of gauze. From Denecke (1980)

tirpation had been recommended by other physicians and also by the author. Since they refused this operation, extensive vertical or horizontal partial laryngectomies were carried out depending on the site and extent of the tumor. The larynx was afterwards reconstructed by appropriate pedicle flaps. Thanks to this reconstructive surgery, scar contraction or sickle formation with restricted laryngeal function did not occur despite the large defects. The film shows a good mobility of the arytenoid region and of the reconstructed vocal cords in all patients. Deglutition and air passage are normal. The voice is in some cases good, in some cases hoarse or husky. – The film was recorded more than ten years ago by means of indirect laryngoscopy.

Reference

Denecke HJ (1980) Die oto-rhino-laryngologischen Operationen im Mund- und Halsbereich. In: Allgemeine und spezielle Operationslehre, Bd. V, 3. Springer, Berlin Heidelberg New York

Selection of Treatment for In Situ and Early Invasive Carcinoma of the Glottis: Surgical Techniques and Modifications

H. BRYAN NEEL III, Rochester (Minnesota)

Squamous cell carcinoma of the larynx is the most frequent cancer of the upper air and food passages. Glottic cancers, those arising on the true vocal folds, constitute about 75% of all laryngeal cancers at the Mayo Clinic.

Three treatment options exist for early (stage I) glottic cancer: (1) transoral removal at laryngoscopy, (2) resection by laryngofissure and cordectomy, sometimes with a portion of the thyroid cartilage ("partial vertical laryngectomy"), and (3) external beam radiation. Each form of treatment has its place, and none exists to the exclusion of the others.

Transoral Cordectomy

Transoral removal by electrocautery or carbon dioxide laser is appropriate for very early stage I tumors that can be *completely* exposed at laryngoscopy and comfortably excised through the laryngoscope. The decision to remove the tumor at the time of direct laryngoscopy depends on the preoperative assessment, the discussion of options with the patient, the exposure that can be obtained at laryngoscopy, and the clinical appearance of the tumor. Tumors suitable for transoral excision must be limited to the true vocal cords; they should *not* extend above or below the cords or to the anterior or posterior commissure. Most in situ cancers of the vocal cord or cords can be treated by some form of transoral removal.

My associates (DeSanto et al. 1977; Lillie and DeSanto 1973) reported on 98 patients treated transorally; five of these patients had local recurrences, which were retreated transorally. No patient died of cancer, and one patient had a laryngectomy 8 years later. With transoral removal, the operative morbidity and cost were minimal. Usually, 1 day of hospitalization was needed. No patients required tracheotomies. Voice quality was altered minimally, and some voices returned to normal.

Laryngofissure and Partial Vertical Laryngectomy

Larger tumors on mobile vocal cords can be surgically removed by way of a laryngofissure and cordectomy. The involved vocal cord must be mobile, and the tumor should not extend beyond the anterior one-third of the opposite cord or posteriorly beyond the vocal process of the arytenoid. The lesion should also not extend beyond the obvious portion of the vocal cord into the subglottis or into the ventricle or false cord. Lillie and Devine (1959) suggested that tumor extension across the anterior commissure was a contraindication to the operation. Most surgeons no longer adhere to that suggestion, but 2 of 15 of our patients with tumors at the anterior commissure had recurrences. A tumor at the anterior commissure, an ill-defined area that abuts the supraglottis and the subglottis, may extend into these areas and into the anterior thyroid cartilage. Whenever the tumor approaches or involves the anterior commissure, a strip of overlying thyroid cartilage should be included en bloc with the tumor to afford adequate clearance of the tumor anteriorly. Also, the surgical pathologist should assist the surgeon by providing immediate frozen section histopathologic information on a minute-to-minute basis.

We have not found useful the so-called hemilaryngectomy operation, in which about half the thyroid cartilage is removed with the underlying mucosal structures and tumor. During the course of the laryngofissure, however, we remove a strip of thyroid cartilage with the underlying tumor in about 25% of our patients; this procedure is sometimes called "partial vertical laryngectomy".

The voice is altered permanently; however, not all of our patients demand or require a perfect voice. Most are reassured to know that the tumor has been removed. The operation is safe, predictable, and effective (Neel et al. 1980). It is the standard by which other forms of therapy should be compared. In a total of 182 laryngofissures and cordectomies reported by Neel and associates, three patients had local recurrences and three patients (2%) died of their cancer. Three patients required laryngectomies later, and two of these were among those who died. This cure rate, with preservation of glottic voice, is well above 90%.

Surgical Technique. With the patient under general endotracheal anesthesia, the laryngoscope is introduced, the larynx is examined, and a specimen is removed for immediate histopathologic examination. When the diagnosis of cancer is confirmed by frozen section, a tracheotomy is made through a low transverse incision just above the sternal notch. A portion of the second or third tracheal ring is removed, and general anesthesia is continued by this route. Generally, a transverse incision is made across the middle portion of the thyroid cartilage in a skin crease to expose the thyroid cartilage. In the ideal situation, once the thyroid cartilage is exposed, a midline vertical incision is made through the thyroid cartilage to the interior of the larynx. The internal perichondrium is not transected until the cricothyroid membrane is incised vertically in the midline; this allows *direct visualization* of the interior surfaces of the true vocal cords and the anterior commissure before the internal perichondrium and mucous membranes of the larynx are broached. After the larynx is opened, incisions are made below the true vocal cord and above or through the false cord, parallel to these structures. It may be necessary to excise only the true cord if the tumor is small and superficial. This wedge of tissue is grasped at the midline and elevated from the internal surface of the thyroid cartilage. A curved, right-angled Panzer scissors is used to cut through the vocal process of the arytenoid to release the specimen from the larynx posteriorly.

There were variations in technique: In 54 (30%) of the patients, Broyles' tendon and a small portion of the opposite vocal cord were included with the tumor-bearing cord to ensure adequate clearance of the tumor anteriorly as the larynx was opened. In 45 (25%) of the patients, two saw cuts were made so that a strip of thyroid cartilage a few millimeters wide was left attached to the specimen, a maneuver that afforded wider clearance at the anterior commissure. In two patients, one of whom had a recurrence, the tumor was primarily anterior at the anterior extremes of the true cords and the anterior commissure; in these two, a strip of midline cartilage and the anterior portions of both true cords were removed. In one patient, the tumor extended onto the arytenoid cartilage, so that the entire arytenoid was removed with the specimen.

The mucous membrane of the uninvolved cord may undergo so-called smoker's changes appearing as "leukoplakia", which can contain small foci of cellular atypia or in situ cancer or both. The abnormal membrane should be removed, and the edges of the healthy membrane should be approximated with fine absorbable sutures.

It is important to determine at laryngoscopic examination whether the invasive tumor is contiguous, that is, involves both cords in a horseshoe configuration; such tumors usually are diffuse and superficial and are better treated by external irradiation.

In summary, with use of specific principles in selecting one of these forms of treatment, approximately 25% of our patients with early glottic cancer receive external fractionated irradiation, 20% receive transoral treatment, and the remainder undergo laryngofissure or some form of partial vertical laryngectomy. In many instances, the exact choice is made by the patient after careful review of the options.

References

DeSanto LW, Devine KD, Lillie JC (1977) Cancers of the larynx: Glottic cancer. Surg Clin North Am 57:611–620
Lillie JC, DeSanto LW (1973) Transoral surgery of early cordal carcinoma. Trans Am Acad Ophthalmol Otolaryngol 77:92–96
Lillie JC, Devine KD (1959) Laryngofissure: Indications and technique. Arch Otolaryngol 69:589–593
Neel HB III, Devine KD, DeSanto LW (1980) Laryngofissure and cordectomy for early cordal carcinoma: Outcome in 182 patients. Otolaryngol Head Neck Surg 88:79–84

Partial Glottic Laryngectomy (Moser's Modification)

J. WILCKE, Erfurt

As early as the beginning of the 1960's Moser had performed a method of partial laryngectomy, which was named after him. Meanwhile, I have operated on more than 70 patients applying his method in Leipzig, and, later, between 1971 and 1981, I operated on 137 patients in Erfurt by Moser's technique in addition to preserving techniques. The technique of this partial laryngectomy includes a generous resection of the tumor, and resection of the cartilage with its perichondrium in the tumor region.

We could not always adhere to the safety zone of one centimeter.

After a laryngofissure the tumor of the larynx is clearly visible (Fig. 1). Subsequently, on the diseased side, both the vocal cord and the vestibular ligament are

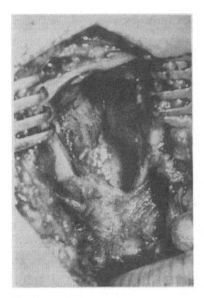

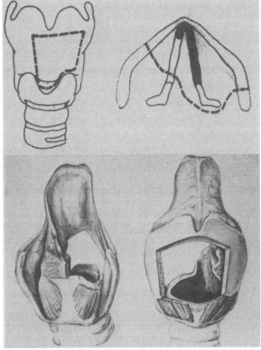

Fig. 1. Exposure of a carcinoma of the right vocal cord by laryngofissure

Fig. 2. Schematic drawing of the resection comprising the thyroid cartilage, vocal cord with arytenoid and vestibular ligament as well as the cartilage (lamina of the thyroid cartilage covered by the vocal cord and vestibular ligament)

Fig. 3. Schematic drawing of the remaining laryngeal superstructure after extensive vertical partial laryngectomy for glottic cancer involving the anterior commissure

resected en bloc together with the neighbouring cartilage. This may also be done electrosurgically. There will always be a frame maintained by the upper and lower edge of the thyroid cartilage.

In our experience it is the preservation of this framework which helps to diminish postoperative laryngeal stenoses which might be due to scar tissue formation in the operating area, and to collapse of the external soft tissues into the larynx. Over the period of 20 years, during which we have applied this method, post-operative formation of stenoses was extremely rare, although we never performed artificial epitheliasation of the laryngeal wound by grafting. It must be emphasized, however, that in addition to the resection of the larynx on the affected side the adjacent arytenoid cartilage, and at least the frontal third of the contralateral vocal cord and vestibular ligament were removed also by resecting the overlying part of the thyroid cartilage (Fig. 2).

After the resection, a Mikulicz tamponade in a rubber cap, is inserted into the preserved laryngeal lumen, secured both through the oral aperture and through the tracheostomy. The transected thyroid cartilage portions are then refixed in the midline. The patient is fed through a feeding tube for some days, the tamponade is left in situ for 8 to 10 days, and the tracheostomy tube is removed after 2 to 3 weeks.

With vertical partial laryngectomy for T_1 tumors, and even for tumors involving the anterior commissure (Fig. 3), we were able to achieve a 5-year cure of 89 percent, which corresponds to the results obtained by Jackson, Blady, Norris and Robbin in a total of 695 cases.

References

Arslan M (1957) Résultats de la Chirurgie du cancer du larynx à la Clinique ORL de Padoue pendant la période 1936–1956. J Fr Otorhinolaryngol 6:861
Moser F (1967) Glottische Horizontalresektion und ihre Indikation. Wiss Zschr Univ Leipzig 16:711
Portmann G (1962) Traité de technique opératoire oto-rhinolaryngologique. Masson, Paris
Jackson ChL, Blady J, Norris M, Robbin R (1956) Cancer of the larynx. Study based on twenty-five years experience. Arch Otolaryngol 64:435

Experiences with Vertical Partial Laryngectomy with Special Reference to Laryngeal Reconstruction by Sternohyoid Fascia

Z. KRAJINA and F. KOSOKOVIC, Zagreb

Between 1955 and 1960 at the Department of Otorhinolaryngology, University of Zagreb, vertical partial laryngectomy was performed for small glottic tumors. The endolaryngeal defect was covered by Thiersch grafts, but the functional results were disappointing. After 1960 the hypopharyngeal mucosa was used in smaller vertical procedures. Again we were not satisfied by the reconstructed larynx. Since 1969 the use of either the superficial or medial cervical fascia was introduced, while in recent years we have combined both layers of fascia for the reconstruction of the inner laryngeal surface. There is always material enough to cover even large defects. This is essential for the prevention of stenosis and disturbed respiration. The fascia has also proven to be resistant to infections and to maceration by saliva.

Indications

While in earlier years only T_1 and T_2 tumors were submitted to partial laryngectomy, during recent years T_3 tumors were also treated by this method. Vertical partial laryngectomy may be performed if a tumor is unilateral or involves all three compartments of the larynx. Combined vertical and horizontal laryngectomy may be carried out if the tumor has infiltrated the epiglottic laryngeal surface and one side of the larynx. The indications for vertical and frontolateral partial resections were:

1. unilateral tumor involving one, two or three compartments but not the laryngeal skeleton. If the vocal cord was fixed, the resection included the subglottic compartment to the lower edge of the cricoid.
2. Tumors involving the anterior commissure with possible resection of not more than the anterior third of the contralateral vocal cord.

Combined and sub-total partial laryngectomies were performed on supraglottic tumors spreading to the glottis and subglottis of one side. The anterior commissure and one arytenoid may be involved.

Unilateral mobile lymph nodes without perinodular infiltration were no contraindication to partial laryngectomy, while histologically positive bilateral metastases required total laryngectomy or pharyngolaryngectomy.

In addition to the tumor's size and localization the patient's general condition and age are of importance for the selection of surgery. In older people we prefer total laryngectomy because of a higher incidence of complications and infection. Also chronic alcoholism is a contraindication.

Preoperative irradiation (20–30 gy) is administered during three days to laryngo-pharyngeal tumors and to undifferentiated tumors with marked cell mitoses. Operation follows on the fourth day. There was no increased hemorrhage. Adjuvant chemotherapy was rarely applied to partial laryngectomies.

Surgical Technique

The skin incision was made in a "half-U" shape. The superficial and medial fascia together are cut by a U incision and elevated up to the hyoid bone. The prelaryngeal muscles are severed along the inferior edge of the hyoid bone and moved aside. The perichondrium of the thyroid cartilage is mobilized and preserved for reconstruction. Only after the larynx has been opened on the preserved median or paramedian side of the thyroid cartilage and direct observation of the lesion has become possible will the extent of the resection be decided. Biopsies are taken from the edges of the defect for histological analysis. The combined fascial flap is then sutured to the hypopharyngeal mucosa and to the edges of the remaining larynx.

Before closing the wound we construct a fold in the fascia serving as vocal cord substitute. This helps voice production by the healthy vocal cord. The replaced prelaryngeal muscles are fixed by chromic catgut to the fascia, and to the hyoid bone. This will reinforce the new laryngeal wall.

If the arytenoid cartilage had to be removed a bulk of the surrounding mucosa is formed in its place. This detail is important for good deglutition.

The patient needs a tracheostomy for about one week. He begins to swallow solid food on the third postoperative day. After combined partial laryngectomy a nasogastric feeding tube is left in for 8 to 10 days. From our experience with bilateral section of the superior laryngeal nerves we recommend sacrificing the nerves if necessary. This would not increase the incidence of disordered deglutition.

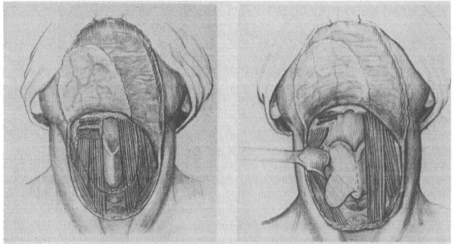

Fig. 1

Fig. 2

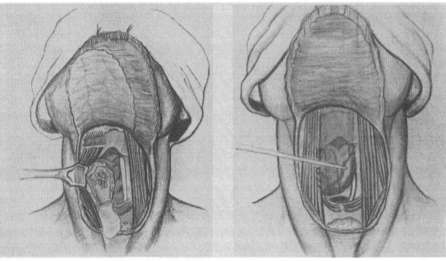

Fig. 3

Fig. 4

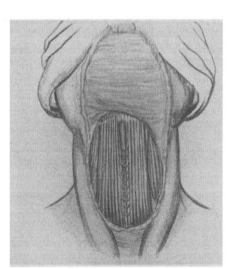

Fig. 5

Fig. 1. Dissection of the superficial and medial cervical fascia. "Half-U" skin incision. The pedicled fascial flap is lifted up to the hyoid bone

Fig. 2. Preparation of the thyroid perichondrium and incision of the sternohyoid muscles along the inferior edge of the hyoid bone

Fig. 3. Removal of the thyroid lamina together with the tumor

Fig. 4. Closure of the laryngeal defect with the fascial flap. It is sutured to the mucosa of the hypopharynx and to the edges of the rest larynx

Fig. 5. Suture of the sternohyoid muscles in the mid line. Construction of the external layer of the remodelled larynx

Material and Clinical Results

From January 1, 1970, to June 30, 1975 eighty-six vertical and frontolateral, and 46 combined partial laryngectomies were performed according to the method described above. Table 1 shows the 5-year survival rates for the different T-N-stages of 65 vertical partial laryngectomies. Fifty of 65 patients (77%) were without local recurrence or metastasis after five years. Twelve patients had received preoperative irradiation.

Table 1. Stages and 5-years survival rates of 65 patients with glottic carcinoma submitted to vertical partial laryngectomy (January 1, 1972 – June 30, 1975)

Tumors	Patients	Without recurrence or metastasis after five years
$T_1N_0M_0$	4	4
$T_2N_0M_0$	30	26
$T_3N_0M_0$	20	15
$T_4N_0M_0$	3	1
$T_1N_1M_0$	1	1
$T_2N_1M_0$	1	1
$T_3N_1M_0$	3	1
$T_2N_3M_0$	1	0
$T_3N_3M_0$	2	1
	65	50

Five years survival rate = 77%
12 patients irradiated = 19%

Table 2. Stages and 5-years survival rates of 34 patients with carcinoma of the larynx submitted to combined vertical and horizontal partial laryngectomy (January 1, 1972 – June 30, 1975)

Tumors	Patients	Without recurrence or metastasis after five years
$T_2N_0M_0$	7	5
$T_3N_0M_0$	11	7
$T_2N_1M_0$	3	1
$T_3N_1M_0$	6	2
$T_3N_2M_0$	5	3
$T_4N_2M_0$	1	1
$T_3N_3M_0$	1	0
	34	19

Five years survival rate = 56%
19 patients irradiated = 56%

Table 2 gives the data for 34 combined horizontal plus vertical partial laryngectomies, of whom 19 had received preoperative irradiation. Nineteen of the 34 patients (56%) were free of local recurrence or metastasis after five years.

Only one patient with a vertical and three patients with a combined partial laryngectomy suffered from a postoperative laryngeal stenosis. One patient with a vertical and four with combined partial laryngectomies experienced difficulties with swallowing and had to wear a feeding tube for two months. Voice production was satisfactory in 92 percent of our cases.

Conclusion

We believe that surgery takes priority in the treatment of laryngeal carcinomas. Relatively good survival rates with preservation of phonatory function can be obtained by reconstructive partial resections of the larynx, if they are properly chosen. Pre- and postoperative radiotherapy in combination with surgery is indicated for some tumor localizations and for anaplastic carcinomas. The application of a double layer flap of the superficial and medial cervical fascias has definite advantages for the reconstruction of the larynx.

The Use of Cervical Fascia After Vertical Resection of the Larynx

D. Collo, Mainz

Following vertical partial laryngectomy defects of the larynx and hypopharynx may result which, if not treated by plastic surgery, would cause considerable functional disturbances. It is therefore advisable to close extensive defects by a flap (Denecke 1980; Leroux-Robert 1959; Ogura and Dedo 1965). While multi-staged reconstruction procedures are often unavoidable after vertical partial resection of the larynx, we prefer a safe, one-stage reconstruction technique on the remaining larynx section which was described by Krajina and Kosokovic (1976). For coverage of the defect we use superficial cervical fascia.

The superficial cervical fascia reaches superiorly from the outer surface of the mastoid process, and the mandible, inferiorly to the clavicle and presternum (Fig. 1). While in the lateral area the cervical fascia is thin and in parts perforated, in the medial cervical region it connects both anterior edges of the sternocleidomastoid muscles and constitutes a firm, closed layer. Above the larynx it is often fused with the medial cervical fascia. This fascial duplicature is well suited as material for defect coverage after larynx and pharynx resections.

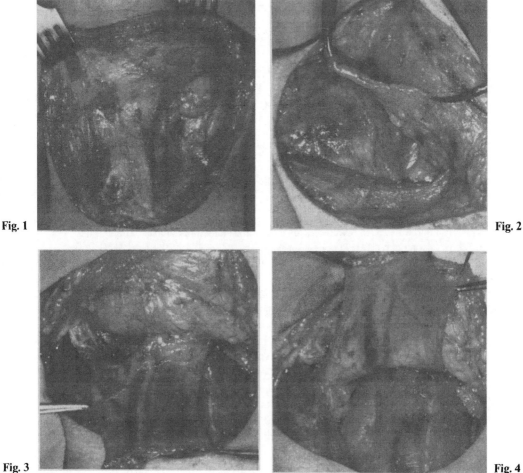

Fig. 1. The superficial neck fascia after incision of the skin and the platysma
Fig. 2. At the anterior edge of the sternocleidomastoid muscle the incised neck fascia
Fig. 3. The cranially pedicled flap of the fascia
Fig. 4. The fascia flap is cut up to the level of the hyoid bone

Technique

After a low tracheotomy, an apron-shaped skin flap is cut and, after incision of the platysma, developed superiorly.

At the anterior edge of the sternocleidomastoid muscle, there is an area, where the cervical fascia becomes thicker and can be lifted, incised in an apron shape and developed superiorly as a pedicled flap (Fig. 2).

Depending on the size of the laryngeal defect, this fascial flap can be tailored as large as desired, possibly up to the level of the hyoid bone (Figs. 3, 4).

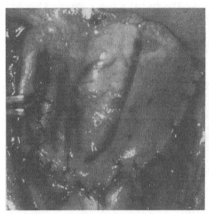
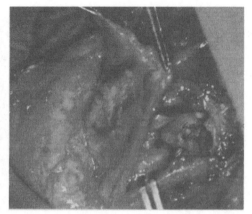

Fig. 5 Fig. 6

Fig. 5. The tumor has been resected. The fascial flap is folded into defect of the larynx

Fig. 6. The fascial flap is sutured to the remaining thyreoid, hyoid and the lateral musculature

The approach to the larynx depends on the location of the tumor; it may be a thyreotomy, a laryngofissure or a pharyngotomy. The tumor resection should be done generously and, if necessary, under a surgical microscope. The surgical specimen has to be marked geometrically.

In contrast to other operative techniques, the external and internal perichondrium may be resected, depending on the size and localization of the tumor, because it is not needed for reconstruction of the larynx.

After tumor resection laryngoplasty is performed: The fascial flap with its superior pedicle is folded into the defect and fixed with 4/0 Vicryl sutures beginning at the upper lateral edge of the excision, after trimming it to the size of the defect in order to avoid graft rejection (Fig. 5).

After closure of the lateral section, a vocal cord substitute is formed by fascial duplication under a mucosal covering, which opposes the healthy vocal cord. This fascial projection imitates the resected vocal cord and acts as a support for the still functioning vocal cord of the contralateral side.

Closure of the inferior and opposite edge of excision follows. To prevent neck and facial skin emphysema, deep sutures should be used to fix the fascial pedicle to the tissue below.

The fascial flap is then sutured to the remaining thyroid, hyoid and lateral musculature (Fig. 6). In this manner the laryngeal lumen remains open after a hemilaryngectomy, so that neither shrinkage nor strain occurs. Even after extended tumor resections, collapse of the larynx can be avoided by this technique. Primary wound closure is accomplished. Internal tamponade therefore becomes unnecessary.

Figure 7 shows a picture of a patient 2½ years after hemilaryngectomy. The resected vocal cord was reformed by fascial duplication and the larynx lumen is open.

In the past 4 years we have performed 79 partial resections of the larynx and pharynx using this technique. Hemilaryngectomy was done in 45 patients, horizontal in 12 and combined horizontal-vertical laryngectomy in 22. 4 patients developed

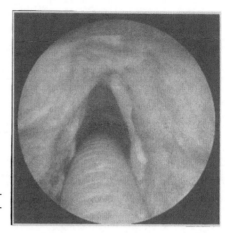

Fig. 7. Situation 2½ years after hemilaryngectomy. The resected vocal cord has reformed by fascial duplication, the larynx lumen is open

local recurrences, 3 had distant metastasis, while in 6 patients a secondary tumor developed which was fully independent of the carcinoma of the larynx (Table 2).

Decannulation was possible in 61 patients (77%), while it could not be done in 4 patients because of bronchial tumor, and in 2 patients because of pulmonary complications (Table 3).

Postoperative impairment of wound healing was observed in 2 patients, temporary skin emphysema occurred three times due to insufficient muscular fixation of the cranial pedicled fascial flap.

Table 1. Partial resections of the larynx 1979 – 1982 (n = 79)

Hemilaryngectomy	45
Horizontal laryngectomy	12
Horizontal-vertical laryngectomy	22

Table 2. Results after partial resection 1979 – 1982 (n = 79)

Local recurrence	4 (5.0%)
Secondary tumor	6 (7.5%)
Distant metastasis	3 (4.0%)

Table 3. Decannulation after partial laryngectomy 1979 – 1982 (n = 79)

I. Decannulation	61 (77%)
II. No Decannulation	18 (23%)
a) Secondary tumor	4
b) Pulmonary complication	2
c) Distant metastasis	2
d) Extended resection	10

Although we have only 4 years of experience with this operative technique, it can be said that closure of defects after partial larynx and pharynx resections can be accomplished more safely and easily than before, and two-staged laryngoplasties can be avoided.

References

Denecke HJ (1980) Die oto-rhinolaryngologischen Operationen im Mund- und Halsbereich. Springer, Berlin Heidelberg New York

Krajina Z, Kosokovic F (1976) Unsere Resultate bei partiellen vertikalen Laryngektomien. Laryng 55:460–463

Leroux-Robert J (1959) Etude statistique de 644 cas de cancers du larynx et de l'hypopharynx traités par chirurgie depuis plus cinq ans. Ann Otolaryngol Chir Cervicofac 76:533

Ogura JH, Dedo HH (1965) Glottis reconstruction following subtotal glottic-supraglottis laryngectomy. Laryngoscope 75:865

A Vascular Pedicled Flap of the Thyroid Gland and Its Application in Vertical Partial Laryngectomy

E. Mozolewski, P. Maj, P. Wdowiak, K. Jach, and C. Tarnowska, Szczecin

In cases of extended fronto-lateral resections of the larynx or of hemilaryngectomy a vascular pedicled flap from the thyroid gland, with the ipsilateral superior thyreoideal artery as the nourishing vessel, was used for reconstruction of the lateral laryngeal wall.

This method offers several advantages:

1. Excellent vitality of the flap with little or no tendency to shrink.
2. The pedicled flap may be tailored in larger sizes and greater in volume than regional mucosa flaps. Therefore, every size of defect may be covered in a one-stage intervention. This helps the surgeon to radically resect even those lesions with uncertain oncologic borders in an appropriate security distance.
3. The three-dimensional repair of the lateral laryngeal wall by a voluminous pedicled flap of the thyroid gland provides a certain kind of substition of both the vocal cord and an eventually missing arytenoid cartilage.
4. The immediate closure of the surgical defect in hemilaryngectomy prevents postoperative hemorrhage and shortens the time of disablement considerably.

The biological behaviour of the vascular pedicled thyroid gland flap was investigated by angiography, scintigraphy and histological examination. On the basis of these data the vitality of the flap is strong enough to serve as a much versatile tool for reconstructive purposes. The described technique was applied in cases of extended fronto-lateral resections (2 cases), in fronto-lateral partial laryngectomy with excision of the arytenoid cartilage (3 cases), and in hemilaryngectomy (8 cases). The absence of local tissue break down and of oncological complications has to be emphasized.

Extended Frontolateral Partial Laryngectomy

C. NAUMANN, Würzburg

In stage T_2 tumors of the vocal cord, microscopic examination of the larynx often shows an extension to the vocal process of the arytenoid cartilage. In fronto-lateral partial laryngectomy by Leroux-Robert's technique (1957) resection of the anterior commissure offers no problem, but this method appears not to be radical enough to encompass posterior invasion. In tumors having reached the vocal process (and being verified as a carcinoma) we prefer an extended frontolateral partial laryngectomy. Resection of the vocal cord is extended into the ventricle and a half or one centimeter below the vocal cord – depending on the tumor extension. Posteriorly the resection may be extended about half a centimeter by removing the arytenoid cartilage. The first figure shows the borders of resection in extended fronto-lateral resection. The specimen shows that the arytenoid cartilage of the affected side of the larynx is resected together with a triangle from the thyroid cartilage. In the center we can see that the tumor (stage $T_2N_0M_0$) has already reached the vocal process (Fig. 2b). This surgical technique should be reserved for cases with retained mobility of the involved vocal cord. Any impairment of mobility, being suspicious of

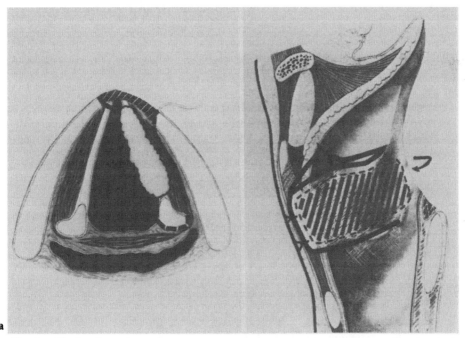

Fig. 1. **a** The borders of resection in a case of extended frontolateral resection. Posteriorly the resection included the arytenoid cartilage. **b** The mucosal flap from the former aryepiglottic fold and from the upper part of the piriform sinus (*arrow*) is fixed to the anterior commissure by two sutures and to the lateral laryngeal wall by fibrin tissue adhesive

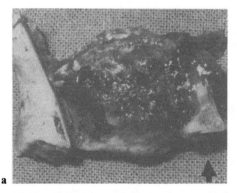 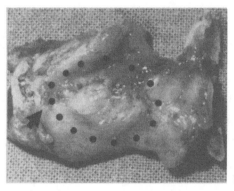

Fig. 2a. Surgical specimen seen from an external view. The arytenoid cartilage (*arrow*) was resected together with a triangle from the thyroid cartilage. **b** Surgical specimen seen from the interior side. The tumor (*pointed*) had already spread to the vocal process of the arytenoid cartilage (*arrow*)

tumor infiltration of the inner laryngeal musculature, contraindicates the classical method, according to Leroux-Robert (1957) as well as the extended frontolateral laryngectomy.

The resulting defect of the lateral laryngeal wall may be covered by mucosa. For substitution of the removed arytenoid cartilage a dorsal mucosal flap from the ventricle, described by Denecke in 1970/1980, may be rotated dorsally. The mucosa from the former aryepiglottic fold and from the upper part of the ipsilateral piriform sinus may be mobilized to cover the whole wound including the anterior commissure. The mucosal flap is fixed to the anterior commissure by two or three sutures and to the lateral laryngeal wall by fibrin tissue adhesive (Fig. 1b). By this method a cavity between the lateral laryngeal wall and the covering mucosa is avoided. Beside a complete epithelisation of the larynx, resistance is provided for the contralateral vocal cord during phonation.

Almost complete glottic closure could be shown by endoscopy. The quality of the postoperative voice was good and any difficulty in swallowing normally disappears within a few days.

References

Denecke HJ (1970) Plastische Chirurgie am Larynx nach partieller Laryngektomie. Arch Ohr-Nas-Kehlk-Heilk 196:327–332

Denecke HJ (1980) Die oto-rhino-laryngologischen Operationen im Mund- und Halsbereich. Springer, Berlin Heidelberg New York, p 227–263

Leroux-Robert J (1957) La chirurgie conservatrice par laryngofissure ou laryngectomie partielle dans le cancer du larynx. Ann Otolaryngol Chir Cervicofac 74:40–74

Vascular Pedicle Flap of the Thyroid Gland in the So-Called 3/4-Laryngectomy

E. Mozolewski, P. Maj, P. Wdowiak, K. Jach, and C. Tarnowska, Szczecin

A 3/4 laryngectomy was performed in 50 of 322 partial laryngectomies, carried out between 1971–1981, without radiotherapy of any form. Until 1980 this operation was done in cases of T_1 and T_2 without limitation of mobility of the vocal cord, with reconstruction of the excised vocal cord by Ogura's method or Biller's modification. Since 1980 this operation was applied also in stage T_{2-3} supraglottic carcinoma. Extension of indications in our clinic resulted from application of the vascular pedicled thyroid flap for repair of the larynx. Reconstruction of the larynx after small or large excisions, ranging up to a 3/4 laryngectomy was achieved by this technique. The crude survival rate of patients with follow-up of more than 3 years was 65%. With the thyroid flap technique the functional results for phonation and deglutition were much better than with previously applied techniques.

In conclusion, the so-called 3/4-laryngectomy presents a valuable method of treatment of far advanced cancer of the larynx. The application of the vascular pedicle flap of the thyroid gland in this surgery:
a) Allows a reliable repair of the laryngeal remnant.
b) In comparison with other methods of reconstruction the thyroid gland flap seems to offer better conditions for securing good respiration, swallowing and good phonation.

Surgical Technique in Frontolateral Laryngectomy and Cordectomy

P. Federspil, Homburg

The modification of the Hautant method of hemilaryngectomy by Leroux-Robert is to be regarded as a most essential advance in larynx surgery to which many patients owe their residual larynx or even their life.

The original technique, however, could be slightly improved by a modified approach. We punch out the lower margin of both thyroid cartilages very carefully up to about 5 mm (Fig. 1). After opening the cricothyroid ligament we can see the vocal cords from below, that is from a supracricoideal aspect (Figs. 1 and 2). It is useful to wear a Denecke forehead lamp in order to see the tumor without sacrificing the internal perichondrium and, then, to perform a controlled excision. After marking the borders of the tumor, we can detach the internal perichondrium of the anterior thyroid area, and open the larynx further medially if we are not obliged to cut out a broad strip of the thyroid cartilage.

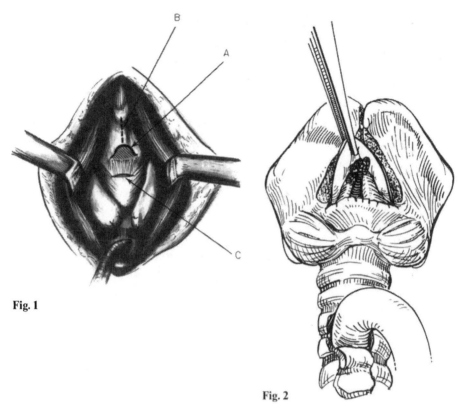

Fig. 1. Approach to the larynx for vertical partial resection. *A,* Subperichondrial excision of thyroid cartilage; *B,* Incision of the outer layer of the thyroid cartilage; *C,* Horizontal incision of the cricothyroid membrane

Fig. 2. Intraoperative exploration of tumour extension. From an inferior incision of the cricothyroid membrane the glottis can be seen from below

This approach – the first without complete opening of the larynx – can also be chosen for cordectomy.

The surgical procedure is facilitated by using a thin intubation tube or tracheotomy in case the tumor proves unsuitable for this procedure. If we do not use fibrin glue, we superimpose the laryngeal grafts of oral mucosa by a Mikulicz tamponade or a stent and, therefore, need a tracheotomy.

A median skin incision prolonged for the tracheotomy appears to be ideal in all those cases in which removal of the cervical lymph nodes does not seem necessary. In this context we have to emphasize that the above mentioned prolonged median skin incision guarantees an optimal view while significantly lessening the risk of infectious complications by securing an optimal inferior drainage. We do not favour the preservation of a skin bridge between the tracheotomy and the opening of the larynx as various authors have recommended.

Transoral Microsurgical CO_2-Laser Resection of Laryngeal Carcinoma

W. STEINER, Erlangen

Anaesthesia for Microlaryngoscopy [1]

With a few exceptions, endoscopic surgery for laryngeal carcinoma is performed under intubation anaesthesia.

For this purpose, we use the Mallinckrodt ventilation tube with a low-pressure cuff which, during laser surgery, is protected with small moist gauze compresses.

Anaesthesia is induced with a barbiturate (Thiopental, Methohexital) and maintained with an oxygen/nitrous oxide mixture, intermittent injection of barbiturate and/or enflurane (Ethrane) ventilation.

Relaxation: For short interventions succinyldicholine 1–2 mg/kg body weight (Suxamethonium); for longer interventions nortoxiferine (Alloferin) or pancuronium bromide (Pancuronium, Pavulon). In high-risk patients: Modified neuroleptanalgesia with diazepam (Valium), flunitrazepam (Rohypnol, Fentanyl).

In rare cases, we employ the jet ventilation system without intubation. Alternatively, for ventilation, an injector jet integrated within the laryngoscope tube can be used, or a flexible injector tube may be placed in the trachea. A technical variation is the Injectoflex endotracheal tube manufactured by Rüsch.

Anesthesia in Jet Ventilation

Premedication: Atropine and Thalamonal (combination of dehydrobenzperidol and Fentanyl base) for reflex suppression. Prior oxygen ventilation 4–5 min. Induction and maintenance with large doses of a barbiturate possibly Diazepam, Fentanyl.

Relaxation. Succinyldicholidine 1.5–2 mg/kg body weight in individual doses. For longer interventions: non-depolarising relaxants (nortoxiferine or pancuronium bromide).

Equipment

Various sizes and shapes of laryngoscopes for direct inspection and surgery of the larynx using the operation microscope (OPMI I/Zeiss) are available (Storz/Wolf).

Accessories: Chest support, supporting bridge, light sources, light transmitting cable, Jet Ventilation unit Riwomat (Wolf) in conjunction with N_2O-blender; En-

---

[1] *Acknowledgement.* I should like to thank Dr. Götz (Department of Anesthesiology, University Erlangen-Nürnberg) for his cooperation

doscopy trolley including photo-cine-light source, Riwomat, Air insufflator (to prevent fogging), suction pump.

Laser unit:
CO_2 Sharplan Laser (1979–1982)
NIIC CO_2 Surgical Laser Model – 500 Z Cooper Medical (1983)
Varipulse Technique, high peak power over very short period of time.

Advantages:
Clean cut – no carbonisation
better control of the depth of cut
less necrosis of surrounding tissue

Special Laryngoscopes

Laser-Tube with a wider proximal end, built-in suction and insufflation tubes (Wolf).

Weerda Distending Laryngoscope (Storz) and MV-Laryngo-Pharyngoscope (Wolf); the latter has a matt finish of the blades for reducing glare.

By inserting the laryngoscope beneath the tube and opening the distending blades, an even better view of the operating field, especially in the supraglottic region and the posterior laryngeal region, can be obtained. In addition, the greater action radius facilitates the manipulation of instruments.

Special instruments such as a tumour-grasping forceps and a protector for the vocal cords and subglottis (also with a black matt finish preventing light reflection) and a suction tube opening for simultaneous aspiration of smoke, facilitate the use of the laser[1].

For the electro-coagulation of small bleeding vessels, we employ small slightly curved, insulated forceps.

After introducing the laryngoscope over the upper jaw fitted with a rubber dental protector, the face is covered with moistened gauze around the laryngoscope to protect the patient from burns caused by laser light accidentally straying outside the tube. The staff in the operating room must wear plain-glass spectacles.

Laser Application

Depending upon the localization and spread of the tumour, we employ a power setting of between 5 and 20 watts for cutting (partial cordectomy, epiglottectomy). At the continuous setting, too deep a (punctiform) penetration into the tissue is avoided by making small back-and-forth movements with the manipulator. Thanks to the paucity or absence of bleeding during cutting, the layers of tissue can be dissected, step by step, under microscopic magnification, and the resection monitored in a convenient way that is not as readily possible with any other conventional surgical technique. The advantage of the new pulsed CO_2 laser is the low carbonization ef-

---

1 Manufacturer: R. Wolf, Knittlingen, West-Germany

fect on the tissue. The narrower coagulation range and the reduced heat effect on the surrounding tissue are favourable both for healing and for the histological work-up.

Surgical Procedure

A prerequisite for transoral tumour surgery of the larynx is the complete exposure of the tumour. In patients with a markedly prognathic upper jaw or other local obstacles to an optimal view of the endolarynx, this problem can often be overcome by the lateral introduction of small-diameter laryngoscopes while simultaneously applying pressure to the larynx from the outside. In 2% of the cases, however, we had to abandon the endoscopic intervention and revert to an external surgical approach. On no account should the transoral procedure be forced.

As a first step the extent of the tumour is determined by changing the position of the laryngoscope and using the suction tube and small grasping forceps as aids.

The following procedure can be recommended: Exposure of the laryngeal epiglottis in the case of supraglottic tumours by introducing a laryngoscope with distending blades; one blade may be placed against the vallecula, the other on the tube in the endolarynx. With the aid of the blade-distending capability, the margin of the epiglottis, the laryngeal epiglottal surface and the aryepiglottic fold can be exposed. This also applies to the posterior region of the larynx, in particular the interarytenoid region with the subglottis where, by introducing the laryngoscope beneath the tube and additionally opening the blades, vision can be markedly improved.

In order to accurately establish the spread of a vocal cord process in the direction of the ventricle, it usually suffices to push aside the vestibular fold with the laryngoscope tube introduced somewhat obliquely. In individual cases, it has proved necessary to coagulate the anterior margin of the false vocal cord to permit the tumour of the ventricle to be reliably removed under microscopic vision.

The post-therapeutic course has shown that this sacrifice of the false vocal cord margin can be performed without reservation, since there is no risk of defective healing and possible voice impairment. In individual cases of very extensive tumours with spread into the ventricle and to the thyroid cartilage, thinning down the vestibular fold can help to improve the inspection of the resection site during follow-up examination.

In our experience, the additional use of an angled telescope for the assessment of tumours with subglottic spread, is only rarely necessary. It has proved useful first to resect the tumour in the posterior, lateral and anterior regions, and then continue in the caudal direction. For this purpose, the laryngoscope (if necessary one with a smaller diameter) is introduced into or through the glottis and the area of resection well displayed, which often requires oblique introduction. So far, it has always been possible to remove the tumour, even when it extends close to the superior border of the cricoid, under microscopic control, with a (macroscopic) margin of healthy tissue.

With the aid of nitrogen insufflated during cutting or coagulation with the laser, and continuous suction via special tubes integrated within the laryngoscope, smoke is removed from the laryngoscope tube as soon as it develops.

Tumour Resection

The resection of a circumscribed carcinoma localized to the middle of a freely mobile vocal cord presents no difficulties; as a rule, partial cordectomy is the suitable procedure. The tumour can be removed with a safety margin of approximately 3 mm in all directions, so that the pathologist examining the resected material is able to decide whether the tumour has been completely removed or not. If it is not possible to obtain resected material in which serial sectioning makes it possible accurately to assess all the cut margins, we subsequently obtain marginal specimens of tissue which, however, in the glottic region at least, depending on the site and size of the lesion, are usually only random samples.

If a cordectomy is required to treat a more extensive tumour, this, too, usually presents no technical problems. If necessary, the resection is carried right up to the thyroid cartilage. Small bleeding vessels in the anterior subglottic and dorsolateral regions must be treated by additional electrocoagulation. We have not seen any reactionary haemorrhage after partial or complete and extended cordectomy, which is usually carried out on an outpatient basis.

A technical problem can be posed by the tumour in the posterior region of the larynx extending into the subglottis.

In contrast, the carcinoma at or close to the epiglottic margin can be resected just as reliably and readily as the circumscribed vestibular fold carcinoma. The resection may be a problem in the angle between the false vocal cord and the epiglottis, and also in the region of the epiglottic tubercle, since even with the use of the adjustable laryngoscope endolaryngeal removal of the tumour can be difficult on account of the tangential cutting direction. In such cases, it is better to carry out either a partial or a complete epiglottectomy through the vallecula, or a classical horizontal partial resection.

The limits of endolaryngeal laser-microsurgery are reached when the tumour extends to the thyroid or cricoid cartilage or has invaded it. This applies to vocal cord carcinomas that extend into the anterior commissure and into the subglottis, to carcinomas that originate in the anterior commissure, and also to supraglottic tumours with deep infiltration. The decision as to whether thyroid cartilage also has to be resected is usually taken only during, or after, surgery, on the basis of the histological examination of the resected material. In such cases, which are fortunately rare, a transcervical operation with cartilage resection, is subsequently performed. An invasion of the cartilage of the epiglottis is less of a problem since the cartilage can be completely removed, and any invaded soft tissue in the pre-epiglottic region likewise. If necessary, the resection is extended to the posterior surface of the hyoid bone, and to the thyroid cartilage.

Prevention of Scar Formation

Attention should be drawn to the possibility of avoiding adhesions by carrying out local aftercare. If the extent of the tumour growth required a resection involving the anterior commissure of the anterior glottis, in the post-operative phase we paint the resected area twice a week with a special solution (comprising alphachymotrase, cortisone and gentamycin) until healing is complete. A curved cotton wool carrier a pledget of cotton wool soaked with the special solution described by Huzly is introduced between the vocal cords into the anterior commissure under magnifying endoscopic vision, after spray anaesthesia of the endolarynx: Vigorous painting of the wound is then performed to deliberately disturb healing – recognized by fibrin exudate and incipient formation of granulation tissue. This delaying of the healing process is performed with the intention of giving the healthy surrounding mucosa a chance to grow into the epithelial defect. Without this local treatment, adhesions would rapidly occur due to the formation of cicatricial tissue, taking the form of a "web", in the anterior glottis. Although not always successful, this treatment, employed in numerous patients subjected to extensive resections to treat papillomatosis or carcinoma, has helped avoid the severe adhesions in the anterior glottis, that can lead to impairment of the voice, and even of the breathing.

References

Kleinsasser O (1968/1976) Mikrolaryngoskopie und endolaryngeale Mikrochirurgie. Schattauer, Stuttgart

Weerda H, Pedersen P, Wehmer H, Braune H (1979) Ein neues Laryngoskop für die endolaryngeale Mikrochirurgie. Arch Otorhinolaryngol (NY) 225:103

II. Posttherapeutic Histology and Microstaging in Vertical Partial Laryngectomy

Vertical Partial Resections of the Larynx – Posttherapeutic Histology, Microstaging

J. A. KIRCHNER, New Haven (Connecticut)

Vertical partial laryngectomy (V.P.L.) is usually performed for T_2 glottic lesions that are too large to be resected endoscopically by laser, or by cordectomy. T_3 glottic lesions are not usually suitable for V.P.L. because of the danger of cutting across submucosal cancer at the lower edge of the resection (Fig. 1).

Selected cases, however, may be amenable to vertical partial laryngectomy, providing that subglottic extension does not exceed 8–9 mm in the anterior or midlarynx. Posteriorly, the margin of safety is much less because the proximity of the cricoid rostrum renders this structure vulnerable to invasion, and because resection of the arytenoid and adjacent cricoid may result in aspiration postoperatively (Fig. 2).

Surgical specimens that have been studied by serial section have provided the following information:

T_1. Early glottic tumors, rarely removed by vertical partial laryngectomy, reveal that in the presence of a fully mobile vocal cord, the tumor remains superficial to the conus elasticus (Fig. 3).

T_2. Impaired mobility may be due to several causes:
1. Bulky tumor (Fig. 4).
2. Moderate degrees of invasion of the thyro-arytenoid muscle by tumor.
3. Extension of tumor along the superior surface of the vocal cord (Fig. 5).

T_3. Vocal cord fixation is most often due to infiltration of the thyro-arytenoid muscle by tumor (Kirchner and Som 1971). Less often, it can be due to one of the following:
1. Spread of tumor along the superior surface of the true cord extending to the thyroid cartilage. This binds the vocal cord to the thyroid cartilage without actually replacing the thyro-arytenoid muscle. In this case, the ventricle is not obliterated. Exophytic tumors which are less infiltrating sometimes exhibit this type of growth.
2. Subglottic extension, especially posteriorly, may fix the v.c. to the underlying cricoid rostrum (Fig. 2).
3. Radiation fibrosis with residual tumor. Continued fixation after radiation therapy has not been observed in the absence of residual cancer.

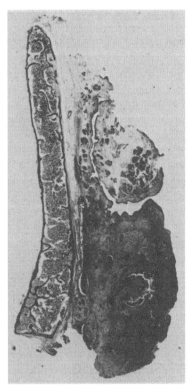 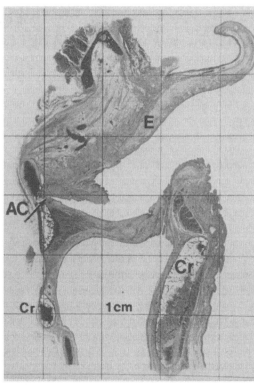

Fig. 1 **Fig. 2**

Fig. 1. Glottic cancer incompletely removed by vertical partial laryngectomy. Cancer at the lower edge of resection is the most frequent cause of recurrence with this operation

Fig. 2. Sagittal section of normal adult larynx (1 cm grid). The distance between the glottis and the upper edge of the cricoid is much greater in the anterior larynx than in the posterior. Subglottic extension of cancer is, therefore, more easily resected in the anterior part of the larynx, since there is less likelihood of invasion into the cricoid cartilage

Fig. 3. Hemilaryngectomy specimen, sectioned coronally. Mobile vocal cord. T_1 glottic lesions do not invade deeper than the conus elasticus (*CE*). *VB*, Ventricular band

Fig. 4. Hemilaryngectomy specimen, T_2 glottic lesion showing adequate inferior margin. Limitation of motion in this type of lesion is due merely to the bulk of the tumor, not to deep invasion

Fig. 5. T_2 glottic lesion removed by vertical partial laryngectomy. Impaired mobility in this type of lesion is often due to extension of tumor along the superior surface of the true cord. There is no invasion of the thyro-arytenoid muscle

Fig. 6. Glottic cancer extending downward below the edge of the thyroid cartilage. This type of lesion tends to escape the larynx via the crico-thyroid membrane, and it often invades the lower edge of the thyroid cartilage, as shown here. Further downward extension often results in invasion of the upper part of the cricoid ring

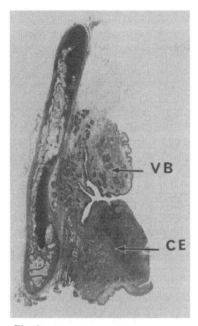

Fig. 3

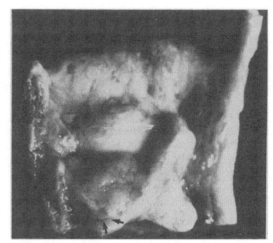

Fig. 4

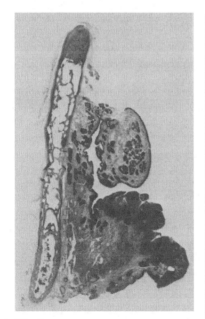

Fig. 5

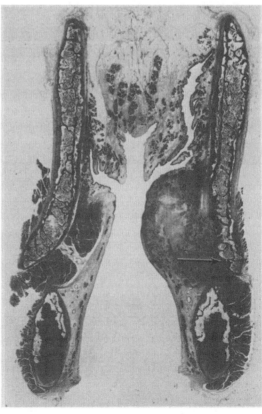

Fig. 6

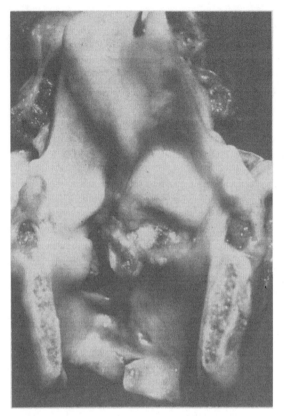 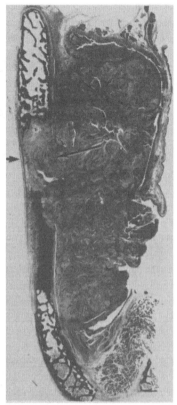

Fig. 7 **Fig. 8**

Fig. 7. Unusual pattern of spread for glottic cancer, extending upward under an intact ventricular band

Fig. 8. Coronal section of specimen shown in Fig. 7, illustrating invasion of the thyroid ala at arrow. Elevation of external perichondrium in this type of lesion risks exposing cancer. Upward extension of cancer from a vocal cord should therefore alert the surgeon to the probability of invasion of the thyroid ala

4. Infiltration of the cricoarytenoid joint may limit the movement of the vocal cord, but this is invariably associated with extensive invasion of the thyro-arytenoid muscle.

T_4. Cancer extending beyond the inferior edge of the thyroid cartilage may invade the framework at this level. With more extensive spread, it may destroy the upper portion of the cricoid cartilage (Fig. 6). Although T_4 lesions are obviously not candidates for vertical partial laryngectomy, the danger is that the tumor's extent may be underestimated, and an attempt made to resect it by partial, rather than total laryngectomy (Pillsbury and Kirchner 1979).

Less often, glottic cancer may extend upward under an intact ventricular band. In the single such case that we encountered, a vertical partial laryngectomy had been started, but a soft spot was discovered in the thyroid ala as the external perichondrium was being elevated. A total laryngectomy was therefore performed. Histological study revealed extension of cancer into the thyroid ala. The external perichondrium was still intact, and it is possible that the lesion could have been resected by partial laryngectomy (Figs. 7, 8).

This type of spread is rare in our experience. Except for this single case, glottic cancer has invaded the thyroid ala only when its inferior margin has extended below the edge of the thyroid cartilage, i.e., approximately 1 cm below the glottis in the anterior and mid-larynx. Extension beyond this limit should be treated by total laryngectomy because the margin of the tumor in such cases is indistinct.

References

Kirchner JA, Som ML (1971) Clinical significance of fixed vocal cord. Laryngoscope 81:1029–1044

Pillsbury HRC, Kirchner JA (1979) Clinical vs histopathologic staging in laryngeal cancer. Arch Otolaryngol 105:157–159

Glottic Carcinoma – with Special Reference to Tumors Involving the Anterior Commissure and Subglottis. Posttherapeutic Histology

J. OLOFSSON, Linköping

Glottic carcinoma may extend to or arise from or in the neighborhood of the anterior commissure (Figs. 1 and 2), which is defined as the anterior midline between the vocal cords measuring only 2–3 mm in height (van Nostrand 1974). There is only a thin layer of submucosa and a fibrous cord – "the anterior commissure tendon" – that separates the mucosa from the underlying cartilage in the anterior commissure area, which may explain the increased risk for cartilage invasion compared to that for tumors on the vocal cords where muscles and perichondrium intervene.

The anterior midline is the most frequent location for invasion of the laryngeal framework (Ogura 1955; Olofsson and van Nostrand 1973). When the framework is invaded it is the ossified part of the cartilage that is invaded most frequently. Local bone destruction by osteoclasts active at the margin of the tumor seems to precede the tumor invasion (Carter and Tanner 1979). The vascularization of the ossified portions of the cartilage plays an important role, too. The unvascularized cartilage has, on the other hand, a great resistance to tumor invasion (Olszewski 1976; Guerrier and Andrea 1977).

The carcinomas may spread outside the larynx through the cartilage or by extension subglottically with escape through the cricothyroid membrane sometimes using preformed vascular channels (Fig. 3). Tumors growing lateral to the conus elasticus may extend through the cricothyroid triangle – bounded by the cricothyroid membrane, the thyroid cartilage and the medial edge of the cricothyroid muscle.

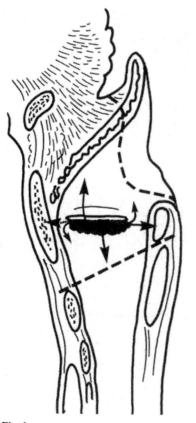

Fig. 1

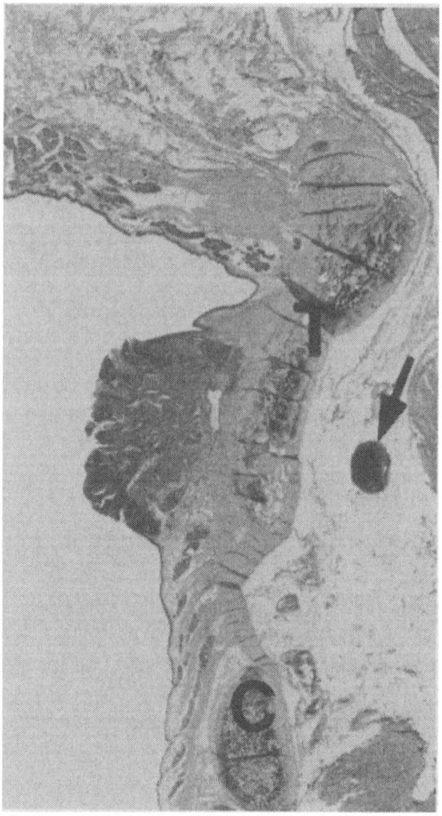

Fig. 2

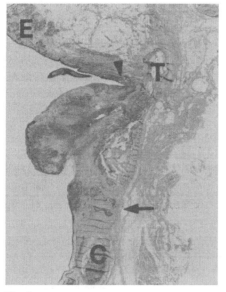

Fig. 3

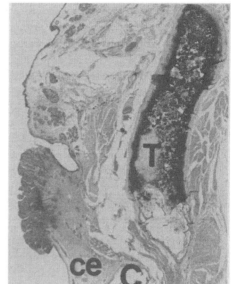

Fig. 4

The patients with carcinomas involving the anterior commissure must be carefully selected for partial laryngectomy especially after previous radiotherapy. Computed tomography may add information concerning cartilage invasion and spread outside the larynx. The final assessment has to be performed at the time of operation.

Strict definitions are a prerequisite for correct classification of sub- and supraglottic extension of glottic carcinoma. The criteria laid down in Toronto (van Nostrand 1974) imply that the undersurface of the vocal cords covering the conus elasticus is included in the subglottis. When looking at serial sections it is easy to see that the conus elasticus acts as a barrier to tumor spread. Superficial spread may, however, occur (Fig. 4).

The distance between the free edge of the vocal cords and the upper border of the cricoid cartilage has importance for the decision whether partial laryngectomy is feasible or not. The distance is much greater anteriorly than posteriorly below the vocal process (Fig. 1). Subglottic extension posteriorly means an increased risk for invasion of the upper border of the cricoid cartilage.

When the vocal cord muscles are invaded the tumor may extend along the muscle bundles anteriorly or posteriorly and reach the area lateral to the arytenoid cartilage, where the tumor comes close to the mucosa of the piriform sinus. Invasion of the posterior cricoarytenoid muscle may occur. Tumor spread lateral to the arytenoid cartilage with widening of the thyroarytenoid space is difficult to diagnose with conventional clinical and radiographic methods but may be assessed by computed tomography.

Fixation of the vocal cord indicates deep invasion and at least invasion of the thyroarytenoid muscle. Vocal cord fixation, especially when the posterior part of the cord is involved may be due to invasion of the arytenoid or cricoid cartilages or the cricoarytenoid joint. Perineural invasion may be another etiologic factor to a paralyzed cord but is seen mainly in major carcinomas. Fixation means a high risk of cartilage invasion and spread of tumor outside the larynx through the cartilage or the cricothyroid spaces (Olofsson et al. 1973; Olofsson and van Nostrand 1973). Limited mobility is often not a contraindication for partial surgery. Fixation of the vocal cord should, however, in most cases be considered a contraindication. Kirchner (1974) does not consider fixation a contraindication for partial laryngectomy "if

---

Fig. 1. Glottic carcinoma – modes of extension. Note the distance from the edge of the vocal cord down to the upper border of the cricoid cartilage (*lower dotted line*)

Fig. 2. Sagittal section through the anterior midline showing a localized carcinoma involving the anterior commissure and extending subglottically but with no invasion of the thyroid cartilage (*T*). Such a tumor can be resected by partial laryngectomy using an anterior commissure technique. Arrow marks a prelaryngeal lymph node. *C*, Cricoid cartilage

Fig. 3. Sagittal section through the anterior midline. A glottic carcinoma with sub- and slight supraglottic (*arrowhead*) extension. This tumor invades the thyroid cartilage (*T*) and extends through the cricothyroid membrane using vascular channels (*arrow*). Postirradiation specimen. *C*, Cricoid cartilage; *E*, Epiglottis

Fig. 4. Coronal section at the midline of the vocal cord. Glottic carcinoma with subglottic extension but no deep invasion. Note the distance down to the upper border of the cricoid cartilage (*C*). *CE*, Conus elasticus; *T*, Thyroid cartilage

the lower edge of the growth is less than one cm below the free edge of the vocal cord in the membranous portion". Computed tomography may increase the safety in selection of patients for partial laryngectomy, but further evaluation of the role of computed tomography in the diagnosis of laryngeal cancer is necessary.

References

Carter RL, Tanner NSB (1979) Local invasion by laryngeal carcinoma – the importance of focal (metaplastic) ossification within laryngeal cartilage. Clin Otolaryngol 4:283–290
Guerrier Y, Andrea M (1977) La vascularisation des cartilages du larynx. Son importance clinique (1). Ann Otolaryngol Chir Cerviofac 94:273–289
Kirchner JA (1974) Growth and spread of laryngeal cancer as related to partial laryngectomy. Can J Otolaryngol 3:460–465
van Nostrand AWP (1974) Classification, anatomy, growth, and spread of laryngeal cancer. Can J Otolaryngol 3:408–411
Ogura JH (1955) Surgical pathology of cancer of the larynx. Laryngoscope 65:867–926
Olofsson J, Lord IJ, van Nostrand AWP (1973) Vocal cord fixation in laryngeal carcinoma. Acta Otolaryngol (Stockh) 75:496–510
Olofsson J, van Nostrand AWP (1973) Growth and spread of laryngeal and hypopharyngeal carcinoma with reflections on the effect of preoperative irradiation. Acta Otolaryngol [Suppl] (Stockh) 308:1–84
Olszewski E (1976) Vascularization of ossified cartilage and the spread of cancer in the larynx. Arch Otolaryngol 102:200–203

Histomorphological Behaviour of the Tumour Growth in the Glottic Region

K. W. HOMMERICH, Berlin

With respect to their different growth patterns glottic carcinomas may be subdivided into three groups according to their sites of origin from the three thirds of the vocal cords.

In tumours of the *anterior third* (anterior commissure included) the main direction of invasion is ventral (see arrows in Fig. 1). The thyroid cartilage was infiltrated anteriorly in more than one half of the cases in our material (Table 1). The ossification process of the larynx framework, which begins at the age of sixteen and

Table 1. Percentages of involvement of the adjacent structures by tumours of the glottic area (n = 35)

Localization	Spread	%
Anterior third (10)	Involvement of thyroid skeleton (6)	60
Middle third (20)	Lateral-cranial extension (15)	75
Posterior third (5)	Arytenoid cartilage involvement (3)	60
	Morgagni's ventricle involvement (4)	80

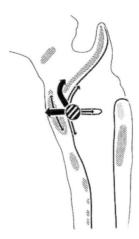

Fig. 1. Note the main direction of the tumour growth into the anterior third of the vocal cord in ventral direction (*big arrows*)

Glottic tumors anterior third

reaches its maximum at about the age of fifty, enhances tumour infiltration into the cartilage (Müller 1966; Pesch 1981). In our material there were some cases of anterior glottic cancers with invasion of the anterior commissure. All of them had entered the thyroid cartilage through its area of ossification (Fig. 2).

In tumours of the *middle third* of the vocal cord the main spread was in a lateral direction. In contrast to the established behaviour of the tumours arising from the

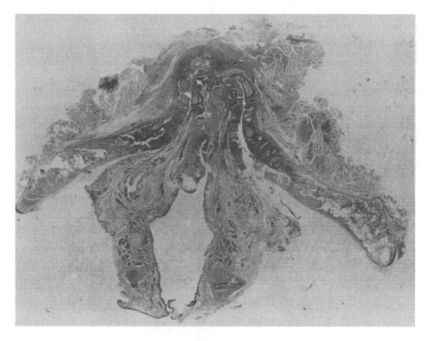

Fig. 2. Glottic tumour from the anterior third of the vocal cord. The horizontal section shows the wide infiltration zone in the ossified thyreoid cartilage (case 366, slide 25)

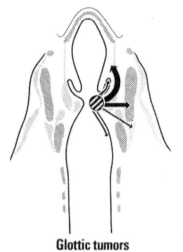

Glottic tumors middle third

Fig. 3. The big arrow shows the main aggressive extension of this tumour group beside minor growth tendencies (*small arrows*)

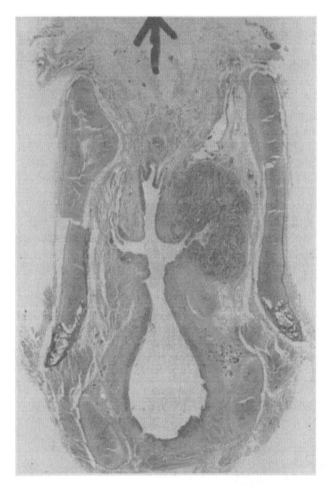

Fig. 4. Glottic tumour, arising from the middle third of the vocal cord. The involvement of the vestibular fold by a tumour originating from the left true vocal cord, without superficial lesion of the false vocal cord (case 343, slide 149)

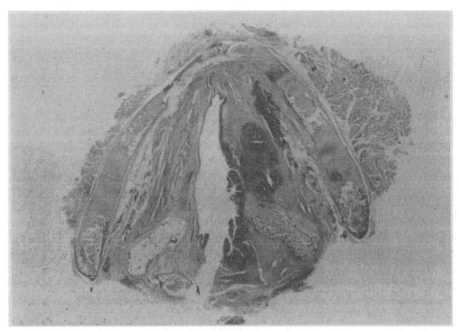

Fig. 5. Glottic tumour of posterior origin: The involvement of the arytenoid cartilage is one of the critical growth patterns. They sometimes grow without functional symptomes of hoarseness (case 216, slide 93)

anterior third we found an invasion of the thyroid cartilage in only 20% (Menke 1974). Mostly (see Table 1) the cartilage was spared by the tumour which spread superiorly without alteration of the epithelium and the false cord relief (Figs. 3–4).

It seems that the lateral portion of the thyroid cartilage resists the tumour growth and deflects the primarily horizontal direction of invasion upward. Spurs of the lesion may enter the ventricular fold from this lateral position. This pattern of detour infiltration may deceive the examining laryngologist because it is hidden by the unaffected surface of the ventricular fold (Fig. 4). In 75 percent of our 20 carcinomas originating from the middle third of the vocal cord this kind of upward lateral invasion was detected by serial section.

With carcinomas arising from the *posterior third* of the vocal cord, both involvement of the arytenoid cartilage by encircling tumour growth (Fig. 5), and penetration of Morgagni's ventricle were predominant (Table 1). While the arytenoid was involved in 60 percent of these cases, infiltration of Morgagni's ventricle was observed in 80 percent. The invasion of the subglottic level is the result of either an inner, superficial, mostly visible tumour growth or of an outer postcricoid, easily overlooked tumour spread. Another danger of occult inferior cancer proliferation is infiltration of the crico-tracheal ligament, which enhances the invasion of both the paratracheal space and the thyroid gland (Fig. 6).

For all these reasons this group of posterior glottic carcinomas which easily spread out to the subglottic region, has the worst prognosis of all groups of glottic cancer.

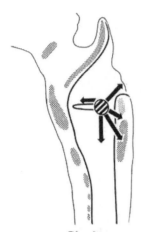

Glottic tumors posterior third Fig. 6. In posterior glottic carcinomas the behaviour resembles that of subglottic tumours. The tendency to inferior tumour spread is remarkable

According to our experience, which resembles that of Kirchner (1969, 1977) and Olofsson (1973), glottic cancer can only be regarded as a tumour of good prognosis, if the surgeon considers the above mentioned peculiarities of its growth tendencies, and adheres to appropriately radical techniques of resection.

References

Kirchner JA (1969) One hundred laryngeal cancers studied by serial sections. Ann Otol Rhinol Laryngol 78:681–710
Kirchner JA (1977) Two hundred laryngeal cancers; patterns of growth and spread as seen in serial sections. Laryngoscope 87:474–482
Menke M (1974) Ausbreitungstendenzen der glottischen Larynxkarzinome. Inaugural Dissertation Berlin
Olofsson J (1973) Growth and spread of laryngeal and hypopharyngeal carcinoma. Acta Otolaryngol [Suppl] (Stockh) 308
Pesch HJ, Glass V, Stephan M et al. (1981) Zum Ossifikationsprinzip des Schildknorpels. Arch Otorhinolaryngol (NY) 231:829–830
Müller E (1966) Über den Befall des Gerüstes beim inneren Kehlkopfkarzinom. Z Laryngol Rhinol 45:512–523

Posttherapeutic Histopathology of Laryngeal Carcinoma

L. H. WEILAND, Rochester (Minnesota)

The specimen received in the pathology laboratory includes vocal cord mucosa from a vocal cord *stripping* or a near total laryngectomy and all sorts of partial vertical

(Fig. 1) and horizontal resections in between. The specimen already has a microscopically confirmed diagnosis of malignancy. The specimen may or may not have been previously treated with surgical radiation or other forms of treatment in the recent or remote past. Regardless of the circumstances the most immediate and urgent obligation of the pathologist is to determine if the cancer extends to the margins of the excision.

To perform this important function the examining pathologist must be able to orient the specimen in relationship to the larynx and the patient from which it was taken (Fig. 2). It is most helpful if the laryngologist provides this orientation with appropriate markings on the specimen and perhaps with an accompanying diagram. This also allows the surgeon to mark those margins of excision about which he is most concerned.

The most acceptable way to examine the margins is to make microscopic sections parallel and as closely to the surgical margin as possible (Fig. 3). The specimens taken for microscopic sections should be thin since even millimeters of tumor free clearance might be considered adequate in some of the very strategic anatomic

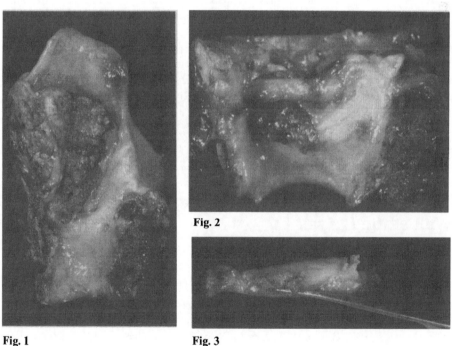

Fig. 1   Fig. 3

Fig. 1. Subtotal *vertical* laryngectomy. The large exophytic carcinoma extends from the glottis and occupies much of the epiglottis. Microscopic sections from the surgical margin to the left of the tumor and from the preepiglottic space should be immediately examined

Fig. 2. Partial laryngectomy. Orientation of the specimen requires a knowledge of laryngeal anatomy. Tumor on the right vocal cord, the anterior commissure, false vocal cord and arytenoid prominence are obvious in this specimen

Fig. 3. Right cordectomy specimen including the anterior commissure. Margins are examined microscopically by taking sections parallel to the surgical margin of excision sites. These margins should include the deep (underside) portion of the specimen as well as from the mucosal and submucosal tissues. It is occasionally necessary for the surgeon to obtain additional biopsies from the "bed" from which the larger specimen was taken, especially if there is concern about the completeness of tumor resection.

Ideally, the resected specimen should be examined immediately and with rapid frozen sections. Thus, the critical information can be conveyed to the surgeon so that decisions can be made intraoperatively and the surgical procedure altered if necessary.

In addition to determining if the margins of resection contain tumor the specimen is also examined for the presence, type, and extent of the tumor and the tissue reaction to the tumor. This provides an opportunity for accurate pathological staging of the carcinoma. This information can also be obtained by frozen section techniques but it is not essential. Paraffin imbedded sections are always necessary to provide a permanent second of the case.

The examination of the surgical margins, the tumor and the entire specimen is more difficult if the tumor has had previous treatment. If the specimen has been removed with coagulative techniques the artifacts produced in the tissue can make recognition of the tumor in the margins quite difficult.

This importance may be somewhat reduced since the zone of coagulation necrosis left in the excision bed undoubtedly detroys tumor cells that might not have been removed. Previous radiation of the tumor usually produces fibrosis in the tissues. This may make gross examination of the specimen difficult; it may make it impossible for the surgeon to determine the limits of the tumor. Microscopic examination is indispensible; it should generally create no difficulty in determining if the fibrosis is created by the tumor or by radiation.

Squamous Cell Carcinomas of the Anterior Wall of the Larynx

E. MEYER-BREITING, Frankfurt

Early subglottic spread and high tendency to penetrate through the framework were described as typical behaviour of carcinomas at the anterior commissure of the cords (Broyles 1943; Ogura 1955; Leroux-Robert 1957; Kirchner 1970; Olofsson et al. 1972; Tucker 1973; Bridger 1974). From 1966 to 1972 more than five hundred glottic carcinomas were treated and histologically investigated in the Department of Otorhinolaryngology of the University of Frankfurt. The following questions should be answered by the histological examination of this material:
1. Which anatomical structures influence the behaviour of anterior commissure carcinomas?
2. Where and how often could involvement of the laryngeal framework by glottic carcinomas be found, and which sites of tumor favour this invasion?

3. Which consequences result for our attitude to conservative surgery of early glottic cancer?

From 1966 to 1982, 406 early glottic carcinomas were treated by *conservative surgery* with the following indications:

For T_{1a}:
  Endolaryngeal vocal cord stripping,
  Thyrotomy with vocal cord excision including the vocal cord muscle

For T_{1b}:
  Thyrotomy with vocal cord excision including greater parts of the endolaryngeal soft tissue,
  Frontolateral hemilaryngectomy (Leroux-Robert, Tapia),
  Hemilaryngectomy (Som, Ogura)

For T_2 with small extension into neighbouring regions:
  surgery as described for T_{1b}

For T_2 with greater extension into neighbouring regions:
  Hemilaryngectomy (Som, Ogura)
  Hemilaryngectomy including parts of the cricoid cartilage (Gluck-Soerensen, Hautant)

For T_3 with no suspicion of involvement of the posterior wall:
  surgery as described for T_2 (this indication was rare)

100 other T_3 and T_4 carcinomas involving the glottic region underwent total laryngectomy.

Formerly our *histological examination* of the partial laryngeal specimen was performed by vertically sectioning into 5 to 8 parts and preparing single slides of each part. Since 1977 each specimen has been prepared by serial vertical sectioning according to the coronal sections of the whole larynx.

The spread of *vocal cord cancer* is essentially determined by anatomic conditions. The area in which most of residual tumors and recurrences could be observed was the anterior wall near to the anterior commissure, followed by the vocal process

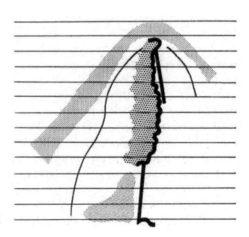

Fig. 1

Table 1. Incidence of residual tumors and recurrences after conservative surgery of the larynx performed in the Department of ENT of the University Hospital Frankfurt am Main 1966 – 1982

		Local recurrences of glottic cancer localizations					
		Sub-glottic	Anterior wall	Supra-glottic	Contra-lateral	Posterior wall	Multi-loculated
Conservative surgery (n)							
Thyrotomy with chordectomy	(143)	1	5	4	3	1	1
Extended chordectomy	(44)	–	5	1	3	4	2
Hemilaryngectomies							
Leroux-Robert, Tapia	(63)	6	1	3	2	2	–
Som, Ogura	(81)	1	2	–	2	–	1
Hautant	(44)	4	4	1	1	1	–
Gluck-Soerensen	(20)	2	3	–	3	–	–
Total		14	20	9	14	8	4

(Table 1). The tight connective tissue structures of the vocal ligaments and thyreoepiglottic ligament at the anterior commissure represent a barrier to most squamous cell carcinomas. After crossing this area to the sub- or supraglottic regions with their loosely structured submucosa containing glands and fat tissue, tumor extension in all directions becomes possible. The lymphatic drainage of the vocal cord region is very poor and has no connections to the contralateral side. Toward the anterior commissure Reinke space is smaller than in the middle third of the vocal cords. From here a cancer can reach the neighbouring regions and their lymphatic vessels earlier than from other parts of the vocal cords. A midline barrier exists only in a small part of the anterior commissure with a diameter between 2 and 4 mm. Above and below this part carcinomas can easily spread to both sides. This explains why residual tumors often remain in the anterior wall after conservative surgery, especially after the extended hemilaryngectomies of Gluck-Soerensen and Hautant with their resection line neighbouring the midline (Meyer-Breiting and v. Ilberg 1981).

Penetration through the laryngeal framework remains in most cases unrecognized. Clinical evidence of involved laryngeal framework was apparent in all 18 cases of T_4 carcinomas. However, nearly 50% of all 91 clinical T_3 tumors and 5% of 115 T_2 carcinomas also showed an involved laryngeal framework. The areas of penetration were the ossified part of the lower anterior third of the thyroid cartilage partly including the cricothyroid membrane. Only a few isolated penetrations of the cricothyroid membrane were observed. Lateral penetration took place mainly in the ventral region of the lower paraglottic space mostly combined with a simultaneous penetration of the anterior wall. Only 12 of 406 cases, who underwent conservative surgery, showed involvement of the laryngeal framework, mostly originating from the anterior subglottic wall and the ventral part of the lower paraglottic space. Nevertheless the conservative surgery including excision of parts of the thyroid cartilage brought better results in T_{1b} and T_2 tumors than soft tissue resection only. According to Kirchner (1975) we could not observe any isolated tumor penetration through the thyroid cartilage adjacent to the anterior commissure.

Since we started histologically controlled surgery we have not observed any cases of local recurrences. Since 1977 we reduced our use of the techniques of Gluck-Soerensen and Hautant to seven of 157 conservative procedures. Based on a restriction of indication for conservative surgery – e.g. glottic cancers with a subglottic extension of less than 10 mm – we could see only one case with an involved thyroid cartilage. Our experiences allow the following conclusions:

1. Glottic carcinomas of the anterior laryngeal wall have a high tendency to involve the neighbouring sub- and supraglottic spaces and to spread out in all directions. The loosely structured submucosa of these spaces facilitates a proliferation without evidence on the mucosal surface.

2. Involvement of the laryngeal framework was most frequent in the lower ventral part of thyroid cartilage. Carcinomas with clinical signs of deep infiltration (T_3 and T_4) histologically show an involved thyroid cartilage in over 50%, whereas superficial cancer (T_1 and T_2) in only less than 1.5%. The infiltration of the subglottic anterior wall is essential for cancer-penetration through the lower part of the cartilage and of the cricothyroid membrane.

3. The described morphological behaviour of squamous cell carcinomas of the anterior laryngeal wall should stimulate us to confine certain methods of partial laryngectomy to limited indications. The control of conservative surgery of early glottic cancer by serially sectioning the surgical specimen is an essential contribution to the definite improvement of results.

References

Bridger GP (1974) Mucous gland involvement in cancer at the commissure. Can J Otolaryngol 3:507–511
Broyles EN (1943) The anterior commissure tendon. Ann Otol Rhinol Laryngol 52:342–345
Kirchner JA (1970) Cancer at the anterior commissure of the larynx. Arch Otolaryngol 91:524–525
Kirchner JA (1975) Staging as seen in serial sections. Laryngoscope 85:1816–1821
Leroux-Robert J (1957) La chirurgie conservatrice par laryngofissure ou laryngectomie partielle dans les cancers du larynx (Resultats de 150 cas personnels avec recul de plus 5 ans). Ann Otolaryngol Chir Cerviofac 74:40–74
Meyer-Breiting E, v Ilberg C (1981) Behandlungsergebnisse der Chirurgie früher Stimmbandkarzinome. HNO 29:41–46
Ogura JH (1955) Surgical pathology of cancer of the larynx. Laryngoscope 65:867–926
Olofsson J, Williams GT, Rider WD, Bryce DP (1972) Anterior commissure carcinoma. Arch Otolaryngol 95:230–239
Tucker GF (1973) The anterior commissure revisited. Ann Otol Rhinol Laryngol 82:625–636

III. Oncological and Functional Results as the Basis of Surgical Indications

Vertical Partial Laryngectomy – Results

Y. GUERRIER and N. JAZOULI, Montpellier

The results for cancer of the glottis are given in the following paragraphs in terms of 3 years- and 5 years survival rates. Aside from the oncological outcome the functional results will also be reported.

Material

This investigation was based on the evaluation of the hospital charts of patients undergoing vertical partial laryngectomy (V.P.L.) between January 1, 1970, and December 31, 1981. During this period
774 total laryngectomies, and
950 partial laryngectomies or pharyngectomies were carried out.
among whom 292 were vertical partial laryngectomies for cancer of the glottis. Other partial laryngectomies were for cancer of the epilarynx. The data show that V.P.L. represented 30.73% of all partial laryngectomies and 16.8% of all laryngectomies.

Clinical Data

Distribution of Sex. The distribution of sex revealed the classical preponderance of men: Only 16 out of 292 patients were women, that is 4.8 percent.

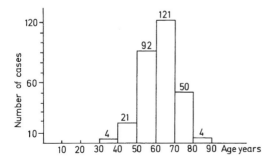

Fig. 1. Distribution of age among 292 patients undergoing vertical partial laryngectomy for glottic cancer

Distribution of Age. The distribution of age of our patients, undergoing V.P.L., is given in Fig. 1. The average was 62 years. Glottic cancer in people of less than 40 years of age was rare.

Symptoms and Signs. The presenting symptoms were practically always hoarseness and progressive dysphonia of relatively short onset, on average five months before the first consultation.

Indirect laryngoscopy by itself always established the diagnosis of glottic cancer. The extension of the tumor was recognized by additional direct laryngoscopy and by radiological studies. After histopathological confirmation of the malignancy the indication for V.P.L. could be established in a rigid therapeutical concept.

Analysis of Different Vertical Partial Laryngectomies

102 cordectomies were performed for cancer of one mobile vocal cord, neither involving the anterior commissure nor the vocal process of the arytenoid cartilage (stage T_{1a}).

12 bilateral cordectomies, using the right-angle larynx prosthesis (Guerrier and Pillet) were carried out on patients with limited cancer of both mobile vocal cords, frequently arising from a degenerating mucosa showing the signs of chronic laryngitis (stage T_{1b}).

140 fronto-lateral resections were done for lesions reaching or crossing the anterior commissure with retained mobility of the involved vocal cord (stage T_2). It should be emphasized, however, that this surgical technique was never used for tumors arising from the anterior commissure with invasion of either the subglottis or the epiglottis.

21 hemiglottectomies were done for cancer of a mobile vocal cord, with extension to the arytenoid cartilage, but not to the anterior commissure.

17 hemilaryngectomies by Hautant's method were performed for cancer of the vocal cord with partial reduction of mobility and slight subglottic extension, the anterior commissure and the arytenoid being still intact (stage T_2).

Table 1. Resumé of the type of operation

Type of V.P.L.	Number of cases	%
Cordectomy	102	34.9
Bilateral cordectomy	12	4.1
Fronto-lateral resection	140	47.9
Hemiglottectomy	21	7.1
Hemilaryngectomy (Hautant)	17	5.8

Post-operative radiotherapy was added in 34 patients (15%):
 11 cordectomies
  2 bilateral cordectomies
 20 fronto-lateral resections
  1 hemi-laryngectomy

Crude Survival Rates

Our results will be tabulated as crude uncorrected survival rates. All patients lost for follow-up or dying of intercurrent diseases will be included as fatal oncological outcome. With these presuppositions our 3 years survival rates are listed below for 208 cases, treated before January 1, 1979. The 5 year survival data include 157 cases, whose treatment was started before January 1, 1977. Those patients operated upon between January 1979 and December 1981 will not be considered:
Crude 3 year Survival: 154/208 = 74.03%
Crude 5 year Survival: 89/157 = 56.68%
These figures will be analysed in detail by the following tables 2 and 3, always expressed as crude survival rates.

There was a striking decrease of survival between the third and fifth postoperative year after V.P.L. This can be interpreted as due to intercurrent fatal diseases. From the data it can be seen that the 3-year and 5-year survival rates after cordectomy for T_{1a} cancer of the glottis are significantly higher than those for frontolateral resections in T_2 cases.

Table 2. Crude 3 years survival rates after V.P.L. (operated before 1. 1. 1979)

Type of V.P.L.	Number of cases	%
Cordectomy	59/ 70	84.2
Bilateral cordectomy	6/ 8	75.0
Fronto-lateral resection	71/105	67.6
Hemiglottectomy	7/ 12	58.3
Hemilaryngectomy (Hautant)	10/ 13	76.9

Table 3. Crude 5 years survival rates after V.P.L. (operated before 1. 1. 1977)

Type of V.P.L.	Number of cases	%
Cordectomy	42/57	73.5
Bilateral cordectomy	1/ 5	20.0
Fronto-lateral resection	37/75	49.3
Hemiglottectomy	4/ 8	50.0
Hemilaryngectomy (Hautant)	4/ 9	44.4

Oncological Evaluation of the Different Vertical Partial Laryngectomies

Among our 102 cordectomies for T_{1a} glottic cancer there were 8 local recurrences with 2 deaths. They appeared after about 3 years in 6, and after 8 years in the other 2 patients.

Out of 140 fronto-lateral resections we observed
18 local recurrences
3 lymph node metastases, and
3 cases of local recurrence with positive lymphatic nodes.

Nine patients of these 24 cases died from their cancer. There was no doubt that a more radical operation, e.g. crico-hyo-epiglottopexy (Mayer-Piquet), would have been superior.

There was only one local recurrence among our 12 bilateral cordectomies. 3 local recurrences were observed after hemiglottectomy (21 cases), and 3 others after hemilaryngectomy (17 cases). Table 4 resumes these data.

Table 4. Frequency of local and regional lymph node recurrences after V.P.L.

Type of V.P.L.	Recurrence local	lymph nodes	%
Cordectomy (102)	8	0	7.84
Bilateral cordectomy (12)	1	0	8.33
Fronto-lateral resection (140)	18	3	17.1
Hemiglottectomy (21)	3	0	14.3
Hemilaryngectomy (17)	3	0	17.6
Total		39	13.3

Table 5. Localization of metastases and second primary malignancies in 292 cases of glottic carcinoma

Metastases (number of cases)		Second primary tumor (number of cases)	
Lung	10	Posterior pharyngeal wall	1
Liver	1	Tongue	1
Cerebrum	1	Submaxillary gland	1
Bone	1	Stomach	2
		Tonsil	1
		Esophagus	4
		Rectum	1
4.4%		3.76%	

Death: 33 cases = 11.30%

Failures

The role of distant metastases and of the occurrence of a second primary tumor for the frequency of failures is illustrated by the following data from our material:
- 12 patients died from distant metastases. The most frequent site was the lung. Other sites were the liver, cerebrum, bones, and sometimes several localizations were present at the same time (table 5).
- 6 patients developed a second primary malignancy.
- 3 patients died from biliary cirrhosis.

Functional Results

The functional result with regard to speech may be limited by the occurrence of scar tissue, granulomas or by glottic incompetence. The quality of the postoperative voice, usually ranging from medium to excellent, can, on the other hand, be improved considerably by speech therapy, if the patient is cooperative.

Anterior synechia due to scar tissue formation was observed in 40 patients (6 cordectomies, 4 bilateral cordectomies, 27 fronto-lateral resections, and 3 hemiglottectomies), after a postoperative interval of 1 to 5 years (maximum at 2 years).

Glottic granulomas with scar formation were detected in 14 patients (5 cordectomies, 1 bilateral cordectomy, 7 fronto-lateral resections, 1 hemiglottectomy), after 6 months on average (ranging from 3 months to 2 years). The commonest sites were the anterior commissure, which was excised in fronto-lateral resections, or at the anterior third of the new vocal cord. They generally disappear spontaneously. Surgical removal was necessary in 4 cases. These lesions are important as they may represent recurrence.

Only one glottic incompetence was observed, following an extended cordectomy. In conclusion, the functional results of the operations described above were strikingly satisfactory.

References

Fini Storchi O, Rucci L, Agostini V (1981) Sull'Indicazione Dello Laringectomia Fronto-Laterale. Valutazione Critica Del Decorso Di 49 cas. Acta Otorhinol Ital 1:95–99

Guerrier Y (1977) Traité de Technique Chirurgicale O.R.L. et Cervico-Faciale, Tome III. Pharynx et Larynx. Masson

Laccourreye H, Bentter P, Bodard M, Brasnu D, Donnadreri S, Dore L, Neuveu MH (1981) Anesthésie, trachéotomie dans la chirurgie partielle verticale du larynx. Ann Otolaryngol Chir Cervicofac 98:581–585

Luboinski B, Schwaab G (1981) Cancer du larynx. Encycl. Méd. Chir., Paris, O.R.L., 207 10 A[10] et A[20], 12

Pinel J, Cachin Y, Laccourreye J (1980) Cancers du larynx. Arnette

Piquet JJ, Desaulty A, Madelain M, Verplanken M, Bailliard F (1981) Le traitement des épithéliomas de la corde vocale. Rev Laryngol Otol Rhinol (Bord) 102:9–10

Indications for Surgery or Radiotherapy for Glottic Cancer and Their Oncological Results

J.-J. PIQUET, Lille

Dealing with the indications for surgery or radiotherapy for laryngeal cancer, two propositions can be formulated with regard to oncological and functional results:
1. Post-operative radiotherapy is not indicated after a partial vertical laryngectomy, because the surgical resection must be extensive enough to cure the carcinoma.
2. If the tumor is too large to allow a partial vertical laryngectomy, pre-operative radiotherapy does not change the surgical indication.

Thus we must choose between surgery or radiotherapy and not between the two in association. In my experience surgery or radiotherapy must be proposed for different types of patients: We must consider age, general condition and the local extension of the tumor. The extent must be investigated carefully by indirect laryngoscopy, radiography, tomography and chiefly by microlaryngoscopy. Microlaryngoscopy, with a telescope in particular, allows one to inspect the floor of the ventricle and the subglottic area. The palpation of the vocal cord with the tip of the suction cannula can demonstrate deep infiltration.

Only after this endoscopy can the tumor be staged according to the UICC classification.

The T_{1a} Tumor

The T_{1a} tumor can be divided in two groups:
- A small tumor confined to the middle third of the vocal cord with good mobility. If the patient is young, a cordectomy is proposed (Fig. 1).
- A small tumor of the middle third of the cord with a dysplastic lesion in the glottic area (Fig. 2). If the mobility is good and the patient is over fifty, radiotherapy is proposed.

The cure rate for each technique is good and our 3-years results were 15/17 (88%) by cordectomy and 21/25 (84%) by radiotherapy. The percentage of failure was the same: 12% with radiotherapy and 17% with surgery.

The T_{1b} Tumor

The T_{1b} tumor can also be divided in two groups:
- A tumor of both vocal cords without deep infiltration of the anterior commissure: these patients are treated by irradiation (Fig. 3).
- Tumor of the anterior commissure with deep infiltration should be treated by partial resection with reconstruction or total laryngectomy (Fig. 4).

Oncological and Functional Results as the Basis of Surgical Indications 151

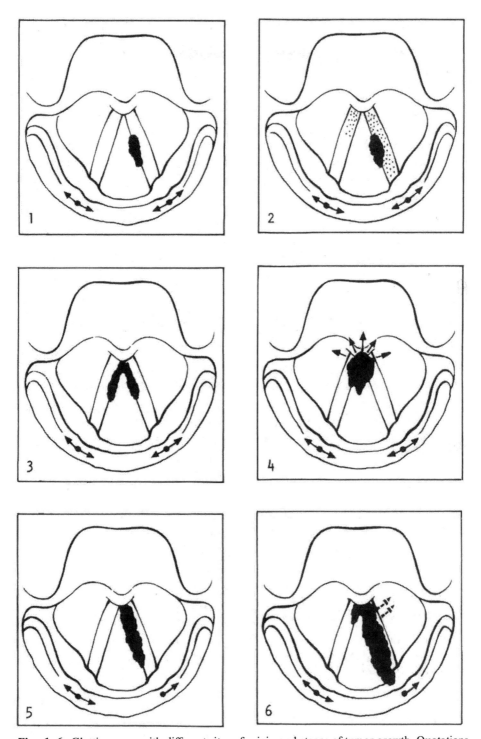

Figs. 1–6. Glottic cancer with different sites of origin and stages of tumor growth. Quotations in the text

T₂ Tumors

The most important fact is that the mobility of the vocal cord is impaired without fixation. The arytenoid is free of tumor and mobile. We can also divide this group into two sub-groups:

The small T_2 (i.e. the tumor arises from the anterior two thirds of the vocal cord): a fronto-lateral laryngectomy must be considered. This operation is possible with good results when there is no deep infiltration of the ventricle (Fig. 5). Our 3-years results were good with 36/42 (86%) surviving and only 2 failures (5%).

The extended T_2 tumor. The tumor extends from the anterior commissure to the vocal process of the arytenoid, with minimal invasion of the floor of the ventricle, or of the subglottic area by less than 1 cm, the arytenoid is mobile but the anterior third of the cord is deeply infiltrated and fixed (Fig. 6).

The major risk is deep infiltration of the tumor to the thyroid cartilage. A subtotal laryngectomy with crico-hyoidepexy must be performed.

The 3-years results of the subtotal laryngectomy are better than the results of vertical laryngectomy for the same lesion, as we can see in the table 1. The percentage of survival increases from 63% to 78% and the percentage of failure falls from 26% to 6%.

The extended T_2 vocal tumor is the appropriate indication for the subtotal laryngectomy.

Table 1. Patients with T_2 vocal cord tumor. 3 years results with partial laryngectomy or subtotal laryngectomy

Surgery	Living		Failure	
Partial vertical				
1959 – 1967	68/108	(63%)	14/52	(26%)
1968 – 1978	11/ 12		3/12	(25%)
Subtotal surgery				
1970–1978	38/ 49	(78%)	3/49	(6%)

Phonatory Function Following Unilateral Laser Cordectomy

Z. Krajina, Zagreb

Six male patients with different duration of postoperative follow-up (6 months to 2 years) were selected in our retrospective study. All of them had undergone laser cordectomy.

Indirect laryngoscopy demonstrated that in all cases a new fold resembling the normal vocal fold closely had formed spontaneously on the operated side. Adduction of the both folds seemed to be sufficient. Stroboscopy revealed that in 6 cases, both folds were vibrating during phonation. The vibration of both folds was synchronous and in phase, but the amplitude of the vibrations of the newly created fold was shorter.

Frontal phonatory tomography confirmed the presence of the new fold having practically the same configuration and thickness as the healthy vocal fold. Acoustic analysis showed that fundamental frequency, extent of harmonically distributed acoustic energy and the degree of hoarseness varied although morphological and stroboscopic findings were practically uniform in all six cases. In all six cases glottal periodicity was completely preserved. The mechanism of new fold development could be attributed to the well known Bernoulli phenomen. Since the healing process of the laryngeal mucosa after laser cordectomy took place without marked scar formation, the spontaneous formation of a new prominent vocal fold had to be attributed to a negative pressure at the glottic level, sucking substitute connective tissue into the glottic cleft.

Oncological and Functional Results After Vertical Partial Laryngectomy

E. Mozolewski, P. Maj, P. Wdowiak, K. Jach, C. Tarnowska, and M. Wasilewska, Szczecin

322 partial laryngectomies without radiotherapy of any form were performed between 1971–1981 (52% of all operated cases of laryngeal carcinoma). Thirty-two percent of all partial resections were vertical partial laryngectomies (103 cases). Among them 57% were limited procedures (cordectomy, fronto-lateral resection). 43% were extended partial laryngectomies (Gluck-Soerensen, Sedlacek, Meyer-Piquet and others). In 13 cases our method of repair, using a vascular pedicled thyroid flap, was applied. Crude 3-year survival, including 2% second-stage salvage total laryngectomies, was 90%.

The functional results, especially after the extended vertical laryngectomies, performed with the thyroid pedicled flap technique, were in all respects better than with others.

Conclusions

1. Oncological results in the group of vertical laryngectomies were satisfactory, except in the T_2 group in which failures were more frequent. This fact seems to be mainly due to preoperative underestimation of the invasion of the cancer into the thyreoarytenoid muscle.

2. The easy repair after extended resection of the larynx with thyroid gland pedicled flap technique and other techniques may allow a more radical partial resection of the larynx in cases with doubtful spread in this region.

3. The better the oncological results the more attention should be paid to the functional results. It seems that in the extended resections a due respect is not yet paid to the mild to moderate degrees of aspiration and poor quality of voice. In this respect also the threedimensional reconstruction with the thyroid gland pedicled flap technique seems to offer some advantages over other methods.

Laryngofissure and Partial Vertical Laryngectomy for Early Cordal Carcinoma: Outcome in 182 Patients

H. BRYAN NEEL III, Rochester (Minnesota)

From 1962 to 1974, 182 patients with early squamous cell carcinoma of the true vocal cord were treated by laryngofissure and cordectomy at the Mayo Clinic (Neel et al. 1980). The indications for the operation are as follows: The involved vocal cord must be mobile, and the tumor should not extend beyond the anterior one-third of the opposite cord or posteriorly beyond the vocal process of the arytenoid. Also, the tumor should not extend beyond the obvious portion of the vocal cord into the subglottis or into the ventricle or false cord. Any attempt to overstep these indications reduces the patient's chance for recovery.

All 182 tumors were squamous cell carcinomas: 149 were invasive, 12 were in situ, and 21 were both invasive and in situ. One hundred sixty-two involved one true vocal cord, 15 involved one true cord on the anterior commissure, 2 involved the anterior extremes of both true cords and the anterior commissure, 1 involved one true cord and the arytenoid, and 2 involved both true cords (not contiguous).

Two patients had tumor extension into the ipsilateral false cord, and three had extension into the subglottis; in these five, the tumor was otherwise limited to the true cord. One patient in each of these two categories eventually died of the disease. In one of the patients with subglottic extension, the surgeon noted that the cricoid perichondrium was included with the specimen; the patient had a recurrence and ultimately died. In these instances, an attempt had been made to overstep the specific indications for the operation.

In 45 (25%) of the patients, a strip of thyroid cartilage a few millimeters wide was removed with the specimen to afford wider clearance at the anterior extreme of the vocal cord or cords. In two patients, one of whom had a recurrence, the tumor was primarily an anterior commissure tumor; in these two, a strip of midline cartilage and the anterior portions of both true cords were removed.

Two patients had irradiation therapy before the laryngofissure, so that the laryngofissure was carried out for recurrent or residual carcinoma. One of these patients has survived without recurrence, and the other underwent a laryngectomy subsequently and has done well.

Follow-up

The median duration of follow-up was 6 years: 42 (23%) patients were followed up for more than 8 years; 53 (29%), between 6 and 8 years; 54 (30%), between 3 and 6 years; 25 (14%), between 1 and 3 years; and 8 (4%), less than 1 year.

Cancer Recurrence and Survival

Seven (4%) patients had recurrences: three, in the larynx only; one, in the larynx and neck; and three, in the neck only. Of the four patients with laryngeal recurrences, two were alive and well at follow-up; both had laryngectomies, one preceded by irradiation. One patient died as a consequence of distant metastases after a laryngectomy preceded by irradiation, and one died of regional and distant cancer after irradiation, thyroidectomy, and excision of tumor from the tracheoesophageal tissues.

Three patients had metastases to the neck, although the larynx was free of cancer. One patient with ipsilateral neck metastasis and one patient with contralateral neck metastasis were successfully treated by radical neck dissection. The third patient, who had metastasis to the neck and axillary nodes treated by irradiation, died as a consequence of distant metastases.

The Kaplan-Meier analysis was used to estimate the probability of survival as a function of the interval that elapsed from the time of surgical treatment. Based on our data, the probability of surviving 15 years without a recurrence is 0.9537, or in excess of 95%. The "expected" survival for comparison represents the survival of a group of 182 subjects of the same age and sex and is based on the life tables for the west north-central United States white population. Survival of the study patients is virtually identical to that of the "expected" population.

In summary, three (2%) of the 182 patients died of laryngeal cancer: two from distant metastases and one from regional and distant metastases.

A detailed analysis of the patients with recurrences has been published (Neel et al. 1980).

Reference

Neel HB III, Devine KD, DeSanto LW (1980) Laryngofissure and cordectomy for early cordal carcinoma: Outcome in 182 patients. Otolaryngol Head Neck Surg 88:79–84

Vertical Partial Resection. Oncological and Functional Results

L. TRAISSAC, Bordeaux

Introduction: Epidemiology

Our experience is mainly in cordectomies and fronto-lateral hemilaryngectomies of the Leroux-Robert type. These operations have been codified and the carcinological and functional results have been known for a long time to be quite satisfactory.

Unfortunately, this is only a small area in the domaine of operations for cancers of the larynx. Of 408 cases of cancers of the larynx, only 120 affected the vocal cords:
55% were confined to the vocal cords themselves,
42% affected the vocal cords and the anterior commissure, and
3% arose from the anterior commissure alone.
The problem of node metastasis differs according to whether or not the lesion involves the anterior commissure. In any case it is quite rare (c. 2%).

Even if the sub-digastric node is invaded in the classical manner, there may also exist an invasion of the pre-cricothyroid (or delphian) node, the state of which can only be determined during surgery. Fortunately, its presence is not a sign of invasion which is only found in 10% of cases. However, this does change the prognosis due to the possibility of invasion of the mediastinal nodes.

The stages were as follows:
24% Stage I $(T_1N_0M_0)$
37% Stage II $(T_2N_0M_0)$
38% Stage III $(T_3-T_4N_0M_0)$ or all $TN_1-N_2M_0$)
1% Stage IV (all TN_3)
Partial vertical surgery is used for only some of the lesions in stages I and II (77 cases out of 120 where the lesion began on the glottis).

Choice of Treatment

Four types of surgery need to be distinguished.

Cordectomy

For very limited lesions on mobile vocal cords we have chosen simple cordectomy.
The problem lies in defining the extension to (Fig. 1):
the anterior commissure,
the floor of the Morgagni ventricle,
the lower surface of the cord (front tomography),
the posterior commissure.

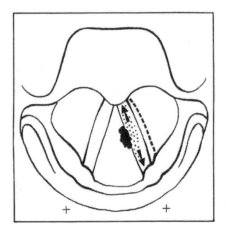 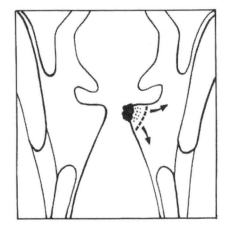

Fig. 1. Simple cordectomy. →, problems of extension; - - - limits of extension

Surgical intervention is often compared with cobalttherapy which produces similar results. However, with the latter treatment, the patient must be followed up regularly. Also, whereas local recurrence almost never appears following good cordectomy, this cannot be said for cobalttherapy.

This is probably due to the cases with hyperkeratosis or chronic laryngitis where irradiation is only partially successful. For this reason our choice of treatment is most often surgery. The age and general state of health of the patient, which play an important part in the choice of other more complex operations, are rarely of importance when considering cordectomy due to its simplicity.

Extended Cordectomy or Hemi-Glottectomy (Fig. 2)

This procedure requires complete freedom of the anterior commissure, of the lower surface of the vocal cords and the posterior commissure.

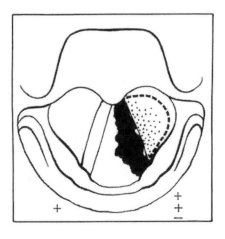 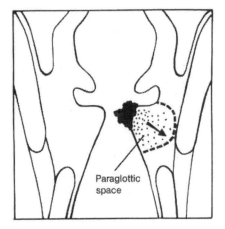

Fig. 2. Enlarged cordectomy. - - -, Internal subperichondral excision

The problem lies in the invasion of the floor of the ventricle. The vocal cord must have retained at least partial mobility. Also, the problem of the invasion of the paraglottal space is difficult to resolve. Frontal tomography is helpful in these cases, as excision under the internal sub-perichondrium must be carried out with a wide margin.

Fronto-Lateral (Leroux-Robert) (Fig. 3)

This operation has, for a long time, proved its worth. Here again, the lesion must be limited to the vocal cord, but the anterior commissure is often involved without in fact being invaded.

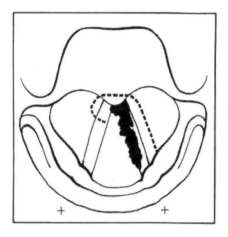

Fig. 3. Fronto-lateral cordectomy. - - -, limit of excision

If this is the case, this procedure can be used, but the other vocal cord must only have been invaded at its anterior attachment. The mobility of the vocal cord is, of course, preserved.

Enlarged Fronto-Lateral

Recommendation of this procedure poses the same problems as extended cordectomy (i.e., invasion of the floor of the ventricle and of the paraglottic space), but in this case the anterior commissure has been invaded.

This is the extreme limit for partial surgery of vocal cords. Fortunately, over the past few years it has been possible to change tactics in mid-operation, if necessary, and to transform a partial operation of the vocal cord into a wider excision (the translaryngeal glottic operation of Calearo or Tucker or even the crico-hyo-epiglottopexy (C.H.E.P.) described by Piquet and Majer).

Surgical Techniques

Vertical partial operations on the larynx have the reputation of being rapid and easy and therefore have a tendency to tempt beginners more than would a more ex-

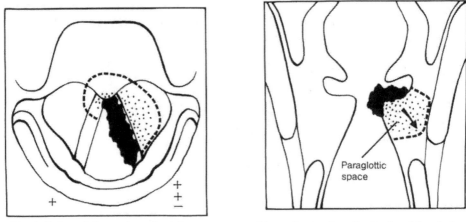

Fig. 4. Enlarged fronto-lateral cordectomy. →, problem of extension; limit of excision (subperichondral excision)

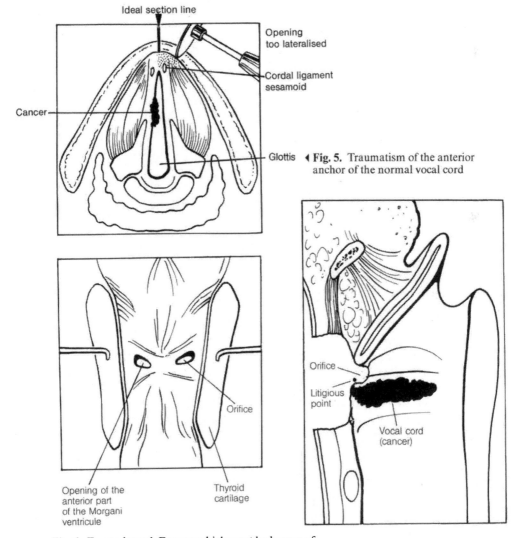

◀ **Fig. 5.** Traumatism of the anterior anchor of the normal vocal cord

Fig. 6. Fronto-lateral. Danger which must be known of

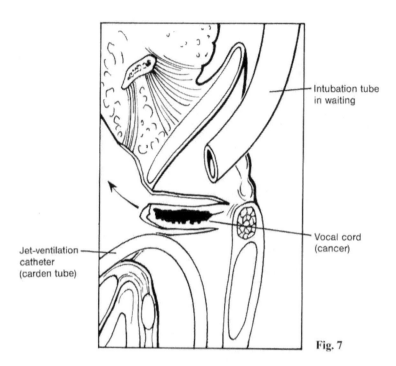

Fig. 7

tensive operation. It must therefore be stressed that this apparent simplicity hides many pitfalls.

We have covered the problems involved in the choice of operation but there are also quite a few technical problems:

the invasion of the precricothyroid node,

opening the larynx at the right place:

Avoidance of injury to the other vocal cord (simple cordectomy) to obtain the best possible vocal result (Fig. 5).

Giving the widest possible berth to the anterior commissure (fronto-lateral) particularly in the upper part where the opening of the anterior part of the ventricle is almost constant and is often made too near the anterior commissural lesion (Fig. 6).

absolutely complete excision.

It is necessary to have a clear field of vision. Some carry out a routine tracheotomy so as not to be obstructed by an intubation tube. This tube, they maintain, has the inconvenience of "traumatising" the lesion during intubation.

This point of view is obviously quite theoretical and ignores the indubitable psychological and pulmonary inconveniences of tracheotomy.

We have avoided this difficulty by intubing the patient with a tracheal probe of reduced diameter and by replacing it, during excision, with a jet-ventilation catheter introduced through the thyrotomy. The tracheal probe is left at the vestibule to be reintroduced into the trachea ready for the reconstruction phase (Fig. 7).

The problems of excision still remain. To achieve a wide margin it is necessary to assess, quite carefully, the periphery of the lesion. One must be capable of changing technique, if necessary, rather than sticking to insufficient surgery. The acid test is pathological examination of the excised specimen which may well cause unpleasant surprises.

The ideal would be to carry out biopsies of the periphery of the excision, during the operation, and to have pathological examination performed immediately.

Unfortunately, this is not always possible in practice. Some propose the use of a magnifying glass or even a surgical microscope. In reality the naked eye is sufficient as long as the surgeon has a clear vision of his field and knows where to look for difficulties.

Carcinological and Functional Results

The 5 years prognosis of partial vertical operations has been known for a long time to be excellent.

Cordectomies

Carcinological Results. The figure of 90–95% 5 years success rate is usually put forward.

The 5–10% failure rate is still difficult to analyse as it usually coincides with exceptional factors:
  no initial control of the cancer,
  node recurrence,
  cordectomy after irradiation (although this procedure is questionable),
  a second tumour, particularly of the lung.

Functional Results. These results vary from patient to patient depending on scar formation and whether the patient stops smoking. Many technical points need to be specified:

1. If the cord has been detached anteriorly and the ligamentous-sesamoid articulation has not been respected, the recreated vocal cord will be particularly rigid.

This is why some recommend the conservation of the small anterior sesamoid cartilage of the cordal ligament (Fig. 5).

2. Reattachment of the base of the epiglottis at the time of reconstruction seems to be an important element in vocal recovery (Fig. 8).

3. Reconstruction of the cricothyroid membrane is also quite important.

In certain cases one cannot avoid the formation of a granuloma on the excision scar. This usually disappears in time but delays vocal recovery for a few weeks.

4. Some advocate certain cordal reconstructions:
  a lowering of the roof of the ventricle,
  a tendon graft (intermediary of the omo-hyoid muscle) or a cartilage graft from the helix (Sénéchal).

The reliability of all these procedures is far from being absolute. To lengthen an operation with this aim in mind seems to us somewhat unnecessary.

5. Post-operative vocal reeducation is, in our opinion, of much greater importance.

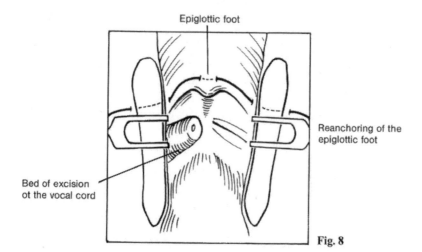

Fig. 8

The argument of post-operative vocal deterioration has been used in the choice of radiation treatment. This does not take into account the inevitable sequelae of radiotherapy which cause a significant post-irradiation dysphonia.

In general, the functional results are quite satisfactory. Breathing and swallowing remain unaffected.

Fronto-Lateral Laryngectomy

Carcinological Results. The 5 year success rate is significantly lower for cordectomy, i.e. 75%.

The approach to invasion of the anterior commissure poses a different problem to that of cordectomies because of lymphatic spread.

The respect of excision limits is more delicate. Postoperative follow-up has to be even more strict than after cordectomy.

Experience shows that salvage surgery (usually total laryngectomy) allows satisfactory survival in the case of a relapse.

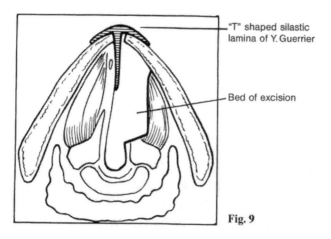

Fig. 9

Functional Results. These too are less satisfactory. An anterior fibrosis affects the anterior section of the remaining vocal cord, forming a sometimes extensive web. In this case even re-education cannot improve the dysphonia. Certain devices have been proposed to avoid this problem, e.g. the interpositioning, in particular, a "T" shaped silastic lamina which needs to be extracted later (Fig. 9).

The advantage of such a device is not obvious due to the need for further intervention. It would seem to be more logical to use an internal tubular mould. In fact, the problem is still to be resolved, but even if the voice is affected, in most cases it is still socially acceptable.

Conclusion

The carcinological and functional results of partial vertical laryngectomies are satisfactory, but it is pertinent to insist on:
1. the necessity to pay careful attention to the definition of the extent of the lesion,
2. the scrupulous respect of the carcinological rules concerning the excision of tumours, which is not always a simple matter.

Endoscopic Therapy of Early Laryngeal Cancer. Indications and Results

W. STEINER, Erlangen

Since 1975 preference has been given to the microlaryngoscopic treatment of early laryngeal cancer, provided that an endoscopic exposure of the lesion is possible to such an extent that the excision can be performed with a margin of healthy tissue under microscopic control.

We believe that the kind of approach, transcervical or endoscopic, and the mode of resection, either surgical laser or scalpel, is of minor importance compared with a reliable histomorphologic examination of the excised specimen in order to guarantee oncological safety for the patient.

Management of Carcinoma In Situ, T_1 and T_2 Tumours (Fig. 1)

When endoscopy of the larynx with the magnifying laryngoscope reveals circumscribed leukoplakia, hyperplasia or papilloma, with cytological findings of Papanicolaou types I to III, the lesion is completely removed by excisional biopsy.

The smaller a lesion of unknown biological status, the less its excision by surgical laser is indicated, because accurate histological determination of whether the resection has been performed with a margin of healthy tissue, is difficult with a surrounding zone of carbonization, which can easily mask the tissue structure of a very small specimen. Microknives are therefore used for the excision of small lesions.

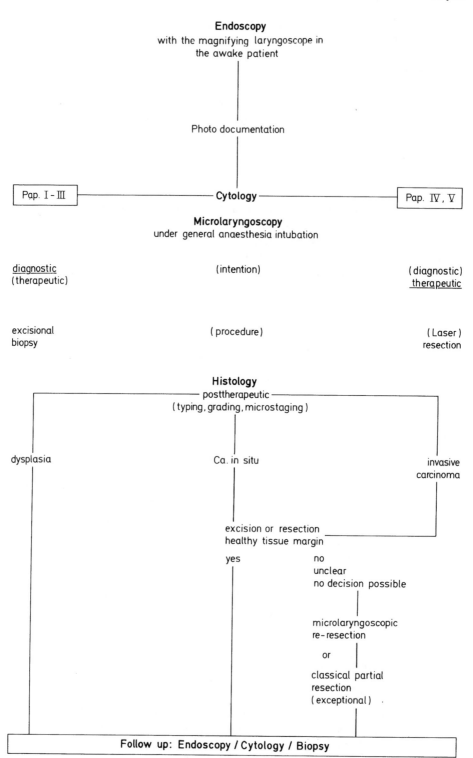

Fig. 1. Concept of endoscopic diagnosis and treatment of early laryngeal cancer

If magnifying laryngoscopy has revealed a clinical stage T_1 or T_2 laryngeal tumour, and swab cytology shows Papanicolaou types IV or V, a curative microsurgical resection with the CO_2 laser is indicated, irrespective of the localization of the lesion. The patient has to be instructed, however, that additional surgery might become necessary if the meticulous histological examination of the excised specimen shows that the lesion has not been removed with a margin of healthy tissue. Postsurgical grading, typing, and microstaging, therefore, will determine the further steps.

Repeated endoscopic resections are indicated
a) for reasons of safety, when excision has been performed on the assumption of a benign or precancerous lesion, but histology reveals carcinoma in situ or invasive carcinoma
b) when it is very probable or even certain that the tumour has not been removed with a margin of healthy tissue
c) in the case of an unusual or unfavourable healing process, the occurrence of suspicious granulations or atypical cicatrization.

Indications, Borderline Indications, Contraindications

Carcinoma in situ and circumscribed T_1 or T_2 tumours (UICC classification) of the freely mobile vocal cord(s) which do not extend to the anterior commissure, have not invaded the vocal process, and which show no (or only slight) subglottic and/or supraglottic spread, represent the ideal indications for curative transoral microlaryngoscopic resections (Fig. 2).

With this technique, the above-mentioned tumours can readily be resected with a histologically assessable margin that permits the pathologist to determine whether removal has been effected with a margin of healthy tissue or not. This also applies to T_1 tumours of the supraglottis, provided they show no infiltrative growth ($T_1 = pT_1$). Particularly amenable to a transoral resection are the carcinomas located at or close

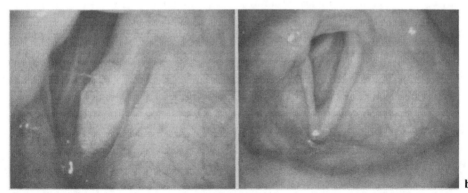

Fig. 2a, b. Vocal cord carcinoma, left, ($pT_2N_0M_X$), 70-year-old male. **a** Pre-therapeutic magnifying laryngoscopic finding. **b** Three years after transoral magnifying laser resection, no sign of local recurrence

to the epiglottic margin which can be resected with a margin of healthy tissue and the histological scrutiny with a high degree of reliability.

More difficult is the pre-treatment determination of tumour spread in the region of the epiglottic tubercle, and in the angle between the vestibular fold and the epiglottis. It is known that tumours that appear small on gross inspection may, in fact, have penetrated into the pre-epiglottic space ($T_1 = pT_{3/4}$) (see also the article by Kirchner on page 69, and that of Olofsson on page 79).

Although, in these cases, a transoral (extended) epiglottectomy can be performed with the laser, in which the pre-epiglottic soft tissues invaded by the tumour can also be removed, it is difficult to verify histologically that the tumour has indeed been removed with a margin of healthy tissue.

Even taking multiple marginal biopsy specimens, which, of course, can only be random samples, fails to reliably establish complete removal of the tumour.

If such cases are to be treated curatively by surgery alone, preference must be given to a classical horizontal partial resection during which the entire pre-epiglottic space, together with parts of the thyroid cartilage, can also be resected. Whenever the tumour grows in the direction of, or close to, the cartilage (thyroid cartilage – anterior commissure, ventricle – cricoid, arytenoid cartilage), the limitations of the transoral laser surgical procedure have been reached. Although the perichondrium and the underlying cartilage can be coagulated with the laser, in such cases it is difficult to evaluate the resected material for reliable tumour removal. Here, the open operation with resection of the cartilage offers greater oncological safety. This procedure is indicated primarily when the pre-therapeutic diagnostic work-up, for example with computerized tomography, has clearly demonstrated a relevant spread of the lesion, and, secondarily, when during or following microlaryngoscopic laser resection, the histological work-up of the resected material reveals the true extent of the tumour, or leaves doubt as to the completeness of its removal.

For these reasons, both the Boston Group (Strong, Vaughan and Jako), who have been treating early laryngeal cancers transorally with the laser beam since the beginning of the nineteen-seventies, and the Rochester (Mayo Clinic) Group (DeSanto et al., see the article by Neel on page 104), who have been using the microlaryngoscopic approach without the laser, apply very strict criteria and limit such treatment to circumscribed carcinoma in situ and T_1 tumours of the glottis. It is on this basis that they have achieved excellent oncological results, which are in close agreement with those we have obtained in carcinoma in situ and microcarcinoma since 1975 (Steiner 1979, 1982).

In our opinion, the only absolute contraindication to curative transoral tumour resection as the single form of therapy, is the T_3 lesion with fixed vocal cord.

Material and Results

Since 1975 177 patients with early laryngeal cancer (carcinoma in situ, T_1 or T_2 tumour) have been treated by microlaryngoscopy at our hospital – mostly by myself – with curative intent.

This article reports on the 145 patients treated between 1975 and 1981. The follow-up period extended to December 31, 1982.

Based on the UICC classification, 60 patients had a carcinoma in situ, 43 presented with a T_1 tumour and 42 had a T_2 tumour with unrestricted vocal cord mobility.

The ages of the 136 male and 9 female patients ranged from 15 to 82, the average age being 64.

80% of the patients were smokers at the time of treatment, 12% had given up smoking and 8% were non-smokers.

In roughly two-thirds of the patients only one vocal cord was affected; in about 10% the process was localized to the posterior glottis, mainly in the area of the vocal process.

In 40 patients endoscopic treatment had been preceded years before by some other form of therapy, usually for laryngeal dysplasia (22). 16 patients (12%) had already undergone partial resection or radiotherapy for a carcinoma in situ or invasive laryngeal cancer (Table 1). Almost every fifth patient with carcinoma in situ or

Table 1. Diagnosis and primary therapeutic modalities prior to endoscopic treatment in 145 patients with early laryngeal cancer (1975 – 1981)

Laryngeal cancer (pT_{is}; pT_1; pT_2)
Endoscopic treatment (n = 145)
Primary therapy prior to endoscopic treatment (n = 40)

	Diagnosis: Dysplasia	Carcinoma in situ	Carcinoma
Primary therapy			
Endoscopy	19	–	–
Vertical partial resection	3	2	10
		12%	
Radiotherapy	–	1	5

Table 2. Histological analysis of 62 re-resections oriented at tumour stages in 145 patients with early laryngeal cancer treated by microlaryngoscopy between 1975 and 1981

Laryngeal cancer (pT_{is}; pT_1; pT_2)
Endoscopic treatment (n = 145)
Endoscopic Re-resection (n = 62)

	pt_{is} 26	pT_1 20	pT_2 16
Histology			
Dysplasia	19	15	14
Carcinoma in situ	7	2	–
Carcinoma	–	3	2

a T_1 tumour, and every tenth patient with a T_2 laryngeal tumour had been previously biopsied elsewhere.

In 62 patients (about 40%) a re-resection was performed. In 77% of the specimens obtained at re-resection, no histological evidence of carcinoma was found, but only benign proliferations, or at most dysplastic changes of the laryngeal mucosa (Table 2).

In almost every fourth patient, however, re-resection proved useful, since a carcinoma in situ or residual carcinoma was removed.

Oncological Results

For the whole group of 145 patients subjected to endoscopic treatment, the post-therapeutic period of observation has averaged
60 months for the carcinoma in situ
51 months for the T_1 and
30 months for the T_2 tumour patients.

About 10% had either local recurrent lesions or a new cancer, ipsilateral or contralateral (Table 3).

With the exception of three patients, who needed extralaryngeal surgery – classic vertical partial resection – all the others had such small lesions that it was possible to treat them either once or several times exclusively by microlaryngoscopy. Up to December 31, 1982 no other treatment (radiotherapy, laryngectomy or neck dissection) had become necessary. No patient has died of his tumour.

13 patients died of myocardial infarction, stroke, a second malignancy in the bronchial, gastrointestinal or urogenital tract, or in an accident.

The possibility of treating advanced laryngeal carcinomas, normally requiring laryngectomy, by a curative combination of transoral laser surgery and radiotherapy with a full tumour dose will be described elsewhere (Steiner, Sauer, in preparation).

Also described in the same place will be the palliative use of laser surgery in very old patients with a hopeless prognosis, in whom a laryngeal carcinoma is causing

Table 3. Recurrent disease, treatment and death in 145 patients with early laryngeal cancer treated by microlaryngoscopy, broken down by tumor stages

Laryngeal cancer (pT_{is}; pT_1; pT_2)
Endoscopic treatment (n = 145)
Follow-up

	pT_{is}	pT_1	pT_2
Local recurrence	6	4	4
Therapy			
Endoscopy	6	2	3
Class. partial resection	–	2	1
Death not due to laryngeal cancer	5	2	3
Lost to follow-up	3	2	1

respiratory distress. For these cases such a procedure spares the patient a tracheotomy and improves the quality of the (short) life span still remaining to him.

Conclusions

The transoral microsurgical (laser) treatment of early laryngeal cancers is very precise and oncologically safe.

With this reliable approach the patient is stressed only minimally, – the intervention can usually be performed on an outpatient basis, is complication-free, and recovery is quick.

The functional results are very good.

The prerequisites are
a) accurate pre-therapeutic evaluation and photodocumentation of the tumour extent and laryngeal function with a magnifying laryngoscope
b) the microlaryngoscopic representation in a relaxed, intubated patient must always guarantee resection under visual control of the macroscopic tumour boundaries. If the view of the area is poor, and representation of the tumour inadequate, endoscopy should be abandoned in favour of laryngofissure
c) experience on the part of the therapist in performing microlaryngoscopy, laryngeal surgery and laser surgery
d) close cooperation with the pathologist to ensure an accurate histomorphological work-up of the resected material including the margins to permit assessment of tumour spread and ensure resection with a margin of healthy tissue
e) regular, short-term endoscopic postoperative checks with photographic documentation and possibly a cytological swab. Systematic cytological-bioptic clarification, and removal of proliferations irrespective of their clinical aspect
f) patient advice and counseling to ensure appreciation of the need for therapy and aftercare, and to obtain an agreement to stop smoking and accept measures designed to clear up the upper airway.

References

Burian K, Höfler H (1979) Zur mikrochirurgischen Therapie von Stimmbandkarzinomen mit dem CO_2-Laser. Laryngol Rhinol Otol (Stuttg) 58:551

DeSanto LW (1982) Current concepts in otolaryngology: The options in early laryngeal carcinoma. N Engl J Med 306:910

Jako G, Vaughan CW, Strong MS, Polanyi TG (1978) Surgical management of malignant tumours of the aero-digestive tract with CO_2 laser microsurgery of malignant tumours of the vocal cords. Int Adv Surg Oncol 1:265

Steiner W, Pesch H-J (1977) Vor- und Frühstadien des Kehlkopfkarzinoms. Prospektive endoskopisch-histologische Untersuchungen. Verh Dtsch Ges Pathol 61:364

Steiner W (1979) Vergleichende Beurteilung endoskopischer Diagnostik- und Therapieverfahren beim Kehlkopfkrebs und seinen Vorstadien. Habilitationsschrift, Erlangen

Steiner W, Jaumann MP, Pesch H-J (1981) Endoskopische Therapie von Krebsfrühstadien im Larynx – vorläufige Ergebnisse. Arch Otorhinolaryngol (Berlin) 231:637

Steiner W (1982) Aspects of Clinical Differential Diagnosis and Therapy of Early Laryngeal Cancer (Microcarcinoma). In: Burghardt E, Holzer E (eds) W. B. Saunders Company Ltd., London Philadelphia Toronto, p 495

Strong MS (1975) Laser Excision of Carcinoma of the Larynx. Laryngoscope 85:1286
Strong MS, Jako GJ (1972) Laser Surgery in the Larynx – Early clinical experience with continuous CO_2 laser. Ann Oto Rhino Laryngol 81:791
Vaughan CW (1978) Transoral Laryngeal Surgery using the Carbon Dioxide Laser. Laboratory Experiments and Clinical Experience. Laryngoscope 88:1399

Oncological Results of Vertical Partial Laryngectomy

W. STEINER, Erlangen

Laryngofissure and Cordectomy
Frontolateral Partial Resection (Leroux-Robert)

Between 1973 and 1977, 109 patients with glottic cancer were treated by cordectomy via thyreotomy or by a Leroux-Robert frontolateral partial resection; 59 presented with a pT_1 tumour, 50 with a pT_2 tumour involving one or both vocal cords. With few exceptions, surgery was always carried out under local anaesthesia, without tracheotomy. In two cases a secondary tracheotomy had to be performed because of postoperative bleeding or subcutaneous emphysema.

Follow-up to December 31, 1982

78 (72%) patients are still alive, which means that all of them have survived for 5 years or more.

69 of the survivors showed no evidence of disease. 5 patients with local recurrence, and 2 with late neck metastasis, were salvaged by surgery, and 2 with a second primary – 1 in the oropharynx, 1 in the stomach – were also treated successfully.

31 (28%) patients had died by December 31, 1982. Causes of death were cardiac or pulmonary disease, stroke, etc. (25), postoperative pulmonary embolism (2), suicide (1), second primary in the oropharynx (1), and lung (2).

Local Recurrence

8 (7%) patients developed a recurrent laryngeal tumour. An analysis of their clinical histories revealed that their recurrent or new cancers were predominantly ipsilateral (5), and developed at an interval of between 7 and 72 months (average 32 months) after primary surgery. The survival time of this group of patients varied from 31 to 86 months. Two of the eight non-survivors died of postoperative complications. One patient who developed a cancer of the prostate seven years after successful laryngeal surgery, committed suicide. Five patients are still alive.

Treatment of the recurrences (r Tis:2/r $T_{1/2}$:6) was as follows: microlaryngoscopic resection (3), partial vertical resection (Hautant) (2), and total laryngectomy (3).

Discussion

A number of parameters – different staging systems, various surgical techniques and nomenclatures (what might be termed an extended cordectomy by one surgeon is a hemilaryngectomy to another) – make a comparison with the results reported by other authors difficult. In the case of glottic carcinoma, the international literature quotes figures for permanent healing of between 70% and 95% for surgery or radiotherapy (review of the literature in Schwab and zum Winkel 1975; Bohndorf and Höcker 1976). These reports show that the results achieved by surgery alone are somewhat more favourable than those obtained by radiotherapy alone.

Our results with radiotherapy were even poorer than those reported in the literature (Steiner 1979). However, the more favourable chances of survival must, to some extent, be paid for by functional disorders resulting from scarring in the region of the anterior commissure, especially in patients subjected to partial resection after Leroux-Robert – more rarely after cordectomy.

In conclusion it may be said that our oncological results obtained with classical vertical partial resection for T_1 and T_2 lesions of the glottis in 109 patients (1973–1977) are completely satisfactory. They correlate well with other reports (Neel, page 104).

If we consider that the local recurrences or new cancers that developed in 7% of our patients were managed successfully by salvage surgery (with the exception of two patients who died of postoperative complications), and that in only 3 cases laryngectomy had to be performed, our preference for surgery over radiotherapy appears justified. No patient died of his laryngeal carcinoma or of a regional metastasis.

Since 1977, most patients with a T_1 or T_2 tumour of the mobile vocal cord have been subjected to transoral microsurgery – since 1979 using the CO_2 laser – at our clinic. (See also the article by Steiner on page 163.)

Frontolateral Partial Resection (Hautant) Defect Closure with Whole-Skin or Split-Skin Grafts

Of the 14 patients treated by Hautant's modification between 1973 and 1977, 5 had a pT_2 and 9 a pT_3 tumour.

Follow-up to December 31, 1982

Of the 6 survivors, 3 had no evidence of disease, 2 a local recurrence and 1 had a late neck metastasis.

Of the 8 non-survivors 4 died of tumour-unrelated causes. The 4 remaining patients who died of tumour-related causes, all had local recurrent disease, which was treated by palliative radiotherapy (1) or by total laryngectomy (3). In the latter 3 patients death was due to the stomal recurrence, hypopharyngeal carcinoma and oesophagus carcinoma, respectively. The survival time of the patients who died of tumour-related causes ranged from 13 to 55 months.

In view of the small number of cases, an evaluation is difficult. The percentage of recurrences (n = 6) requiring radical surgery (laryngectomy) on account of the size of lesion, is high.

It is known that covering the defect with a skin graft makes early detection of local residual or recurrent tumour difficult (only rarely successful).

The conclusion that may be drawn from all this is that the indication for this type of intervention is very limited – "advanced" T_2 at the vocal cord with mobility slightly restricted.

Therefore in recent years we have performed a hemilaryngectomy (Gluck-Soerensen) in the case of unilateral T_3 carcinoma (fixed vocal cord). For a critical analysis of the oncological results, however, it must be considered that patients subjected to primary laryngectomy for the same tumour stages, die primarily or secondarily from their cancer with almost equal frequency.

Hemilaryngectomy and Laryngoplasty (Gluck-Soerensen)

Of the 16 patients treated by hemilaryngectomy between 1973 and 1980 6 had an "advanced" pT_2 and 8 a pT_3 tumour.

Follow-up to December 31, 1982

Of the 11 survivors, 10 had no evidence of disease, while 1 developed a late neck metastasis.

Of the 5 non-survivors, 2 deaths were tumour-related. Their local recurrences were treated by laryngectomy and radiotherapy, and death was due to a second carcinoma in the trachea in 1 case, and pulmonary metastasis in the other.

For the two patients in this group who died of tumour-related causes, the same applies as in the case of the "Hautant group". The patients are relatively young and the basic biological-immunological situation is apparently particularly unfavourable. All laryngeal surgeons will be acquainted with such cancers which, despite aggressive treatment with radical surgery and irradiation, simply do not respond, and end in the death of the patient.

The patients died of the uncontrollable primary tumours in the upper aerodigestive tract or, secondarily, of massive regional or distant metastatic disease.

Basically, our efforts are aimed at preserving parts of the larynx in the case of unilateral tumour growth including T_3 tumours, by performing hemilaryngectomy or "three-quarter"-laryngectomy for tumour spread to the contralateral side of the larynx, and at ensuring full rehabilitation (with no tracheostomy) of the patient by reconstructive measures. Here it is only the advanced age of the patient which sets limits to reconstructive surgery in several sessions.

In the case of T_3 carcinoma at least a regional functional neck dissection should always be carried out – prophylactic if nodes are not palpable (see Steiner, page 253).

References

Bohndorf W, Höcker G (1976) Würzburger Therapieergebnisse beim Larynxkarzinom. Strahlentherapie 151:132

Denecke HJ (1980) Die oto-rhino-laryngologischen Operationen im Mund- und Halsbereich, Bd. V/Teil 3. Springer, Berlin Heidelberg New York
Gluck Th, Soerensen J (1932) Die Exstirpation und Resektion des Kehlkopfs. In: Katz L, Blumenfeld F (eds), Handbuch der speziellen Chirurgie des Ohres und der oberen Luftwege, Bd. IV. Kabitzsch, Leipzig
Leroux-Robert J (1957) La chirurgie conservatrice dans le cancer du larynx. Ann Otolaryngol Chir Cervicofac 74:40
Naumann HH (1972) Kopf- und Hals-Chirurgie, Bd. 1. Thieme, Stuttgart
Neel HB III, Devine KD, DeSanto LW (1980) Laryngofissure and cordectomy for early cordal carcinoma: Outcome in 182 patients. Otolarnygol. Head Neck Surg 88:79
Schwab W, zum Winkel K (1975) Möglichkeiten der Strahlentherapie in der Hals-, Nasen- und Ohrenheilkunde. Thieme, Stuttgart
Steiner W (1979) Vergleichende Beurteilung endoskopischer Diagnostik- und Therapieverfahren beim Kehlkopfkrebs und seinen Vorstadien. Habilitationsschrift, Erlangen
Steiner W (1982) Chirurgie des Larynxkarzinoms. Munch Med Wochenschr 124:198

Indications for Moser's Glottic Partial Resection

J. WILKE, Erfurt

Provided that there are no contraindications of age, general condition or internal disease surgical treatment of vocal cord carcinoma is our method of choice, and is preferred to radiotherapy.

While in earlier years glottectomy using Moser's technique was reserved for T_{1a} tumors of the glottis, we have extended this indication also to stage T_{1b} carcinomas with slight involvement of both the anterior commissure and the contralateral vocal cord. Also extension of the tumor to the arytenoid cartilage does not exclude glottectomy, provided the affected cord is still mobile. Palpable enlarged ipsilateral lymph nodes with suspicion of metastatic spread do not permit a partial resection of the larynx.

Also subglottic tumor invasion precludes the patient from this kind of surgery: There are no indications for T_2 tumor stages because of an expected high incidence of recurrences. This restriction can be substantiated by the topographic relationships: From the subglottic region tumor invasion will easily reach the arytenoid cartilage, the cricoid cartilage and the inferior parts of the thyroid cartilage. It is from here that tumor perichondritis will start and lead to cancerous penetration of the laryngeal skeleton (Zöllner).

A second site of predilection of tumor invasion of the cartilage superstructure is the anterior commissure, from where the thyroid alae are easily accessible for the carcinoma. This condition, however, was rare in our material of the Department of Oto-Rhino-Laryngology at the University of Leipzig. The possibility of unforeseen tumor extension should always be kept in mind, and the patient has to be informed preoperatively about a possibly more radical procedure. In conclusion, we usually refrain from partial resections of the larynx, if subglottic growth of the cancer has been verified.

Moser demonstrated by histological examination of excised specimens that the thyroid cartilage is able to withstand cancer invasion for a long time, even if cancerous infiltration of the internal perichondrium has taken place, and may lead to rarefication of the cartilage. Tumor spread is definitely enhanced in the ossified areas of the cartilage. This may be due to the different conditions of vascularization in both the periosteum and the medullary network. In Moser's serial sections tumor foci could be detected in the medullary spaces, obviously canalized by the granular tissue and vascular routes.

These phenomena are of clinical importance: They underline the necessity of extensive cartilage resections together with partial laryngectomy in the neighbourhood of the tumor, to minimize the risk of local tumor recurrences.

References

Moser F (1966) Glottische Horizontalresektion. Sitzungsberichte d. XXXVII. Jahresversammlung der Deutschen Gesellschaft d. Hals-, Nasen-, Ohrenärzte Saarbrücken, 22. 5.–26. 5.
Moser F (1967) Glottische Horizontalresektion und ihre Indikation. Wiss Zschr Univ Leipzig 16:711
Moser F (1971) Die Erkrankungen an Hals, Nase, Ohr und an den oberen Luft- und Speisewegen, Bd. II. In: Moser (Hrsg) Fischer, Jena
Zöllner F (1941) Die Tumorperichondritis des Kehlkopfes und ihre Beziehung zur Röntgenbestrahlung. Arch Ohr-Nas-Kehlk-Heilk 149:456

Voice and Respiration Before and After Partial Laryngeal Resections

G. KITTEL, Erlangen

Glottic tumours and the different surgical procedures for their treatment always cause alterations of laryngeal phonation and the glottic airflow. For this reason, stroboscopic, voice-analysis and pulmonary function tests should always be carried out before and after a partial laryngeal resection as well as evaluations of the glottic efficiency. In most of the preceding communications the pre- and postoperative vocal and respiratory evaluations were not discussed, and only some authors gave some subjective information which could not satisfy the phoniatrist and phoniatric laryngologist. In a film Labayle demonstrated patients without vocal cords. According to his statement they spoke "relatively well", but from the phoniatric point of view they had severe dysphonia. Vega reported about 86.5% of "good" and 5–10% of "bad" voices after the operation, but according to the objective Erlangen Dysphonia Scale more than 80% of his patients would suffer moderate or severe dysphonia.

These differences in evaluation show that surgeons and phoniatrists speak different languages. A patient after partial resection of the larynx may compare badly with patients with dysphonia of other origin. Nevertheless, a patient with a very poor voice may be able to speak well with a loud voice due to good vocal modulation. The professional needs of the patient should always be considered, because functional restrictions may be very important for the patient although negligible for the surgeon in comparison to tumor removal with an appropriate safety margin.

It was said here "Only a few of our partially resected patients want to become singers!" – but many of our patients wish to remain in the professions they had before. We are always anxious not only to conserve life but also life's quality!

In hospitals which are not yet able to perform objective analyses of voice and breathing capacity, stroboscopic examination at least should be carried out, since it allows evaluation of deep invasion in small tumours and suspicious cases of small squamous cell carcinoma in a simpler and better way than the computerized tomography mentioned by Olofsson. A deeper invasion of the tumour must be assumed in every case of stroboscopic non-vibration of the vocal cord. The evaluation of the depth of invasion of a tumour by palpation only is not exact enough. In complete preoperative immobility of the vocal cord on stroboscopy a simple stripping or a superficial decortication of this vocal cord cannot be recommended, even though the laryngoscopic mobility of this vocal cord may be preserved. It is suggested that the T_1-classification be subdivided into "T_1 with" and "T_1 without" stroboscopic standstill of the vocal cord.

After the operation stroboscopic examination can supply information about the question whether the ability of the vocal cord to vibrate is preserved or not. After the operation we often find an astonishingly well formed compensatory vocal fold often difficult to distinguish from the non-operated vocal cord. In this situation the surgeon often does not understand why the voice is relatively bad. A compensatory vocal fold contributes to better phonation on the first phonatory level by helping to narrow the glottis, but a compensatory vocal cord nearly always remains unable to vibrate. This is the reason why the voice is worse than expected on laryngoscopy. Also the supraglottic sphincter with an enlarged petiolus, the use of the ventricular folds (second phonatory level) and the use of the anteroposterior mechanism of the epiglottic-arytenoid phonation (third phonatory level) augment the phonatory pressure and enable this vocal cord to vibrate better.

A plastic reconstruction of the glottic region (Conley, Draf, Ganz, Kittel, Serafini et al.) can improve the glottic and supraglottic efficiency, though the reconstructed substitute, usually, is unable to vibrate. Even doubling of the fascia (Collo) serves more as a cushion for the remaining healthy vocal cord than as a second vibrator. This is the reason why we have abandoned the endolaryngeal plastic surgical procedures using muscular skin or mucosal flaps. Also the free transplantation of the musculus palmaris brevis as a compensatory vocal cord, which we have performed twice successfully in 1966, is adequate only in very special cases with an extremely large glottis after the operation and in very bad function of the compensatory mechanisms. We agree with Mozolevski, who also has given up the muscular flaps in these cases, because every procedure performed to rebuild a vocal fold can have negative consequences for respiration. In any case, it is very difficult to predict the optimal width of the glottis during the operation. Hence we prefer phoniatric activation of the phonatory compensatory mechanisms to these plastic surgical interventions.

Our experiences also have shown, that a plastic closure of large surgical defects is not necessary, whether the operation is performed with the surgical laser or not.

Surgical techniques which can preserve the superior and recurrent laryngeal nerves and, above all, also the glossopharyngeal nerve, have considerable advantages with regard to the post-surgical phoniatric treatment. Each surgeon should always reconsider not only the organic, but also the functional aims of his operation. After we had realized the important mechanisms of the supraglottic sphincter, we decided not to carry out Moser's partial resection. We do not wish to sacrifice adjacent uninvolved tissue of functional importance which would be the case in removing the false cords for very early cancer of the glottis. Wilke goes too far, in our opinion, in resecting the ventricular folds in T_1 tumours. Whether Guerrier's technique, who even conserves the ventricular folds in cases of recurrences after cordectomies, can be justified, must be proved by further long term follow-up.

In our opinion, a partial laryngeal resection must always be as extensive as necessary, but at the same time as conservative as possible with regard to the functions of the remaining structures. Some of our own cases, in which both vocal cords had to be sacrificed or were lost after injuries, have taught us that the preservation of nerves and supraglottic structures, which do not serve primarily in phonation, may contribute to phonation after intense functional therapy, which must be continued for years in some instances. Oncologic safety and breathing always have the first prevalence, of course, but every surgeon should endeavour to reach the best phonatory result possible.

Functional results after conservation surgery for carcinoma of the larynx must be evaluated with respect to a) tumour size, b) the degree of surgical ablation, and c) the possible activation of the compensatory mechanisms of voice production. They should be documented by tape recording and sonography. Additional stroboscopic, phonetographic, and vitalographic examinations are required. For completeness, objective, computerized measurements of vocal capacities such as the evaluation of the rapid oscillations of the basic frequency and of the vocal amplitude and pitch, or the determination of the glottic efficiency, even of body plethysmography, appear desirable.

D. Horizontal Partial Resection of the Larynx

I. Surgical Techniques and Modifications

Horizontal Partial Laryngectomy. Historical Review and Personal Technique

J. E. ALONSO REGULES, Montevideo

Supraglottic tumours differ both from other laryngeal cancers and from those of the hypopharynx. They arise either in the lower part of the epiglottis (laryngeal surface) or in the ventricular bands, but when they are discovered they usually involve both areas, so that it is often impossible to recognize their starting point. In the past, since the days of Gluck and Soerensen, they were invariably treated by a total laryngectomy.

Why did this trend to mutilating surgery shift to a more conservative tendency? In his book, Soerensen pointed out that epiglottic tumours could be removed through a pharyngotomy without completely removing the larynx. However, he stated that when the ventricular bands had been extensively invaded, conservative surgery was contraindicated, with the sole exception of lateral lesions, which could be treated by hemilaryngectomy.

In the thirties, a number of surgeons tried to operate on isolated cases of vestibule-epiglottis tumours by conservative procedures. Usually, their approach was a transverse or a lateral pharyngotomy, or a laryngofissure. They worked "à la demande", without pre-established schemes, and even if some of their patients were cured, they did not leave guidelines which could be utilized by others. In particular, the laryngofissure approach seems to-day inappropriate to supraglottic tumours. When the glottis is healthy, why should we wound it, carrying out an unnecessary separation of the vocal cords which always affects the voice. Moreover, when the lesion is not completely lateralized, the median incision almost always pierces diseased tissues.

In 1938 Huet described a case of an epiglottic tumour, treated by means of an ingenious technique. Had Huet worked out the procedure without confining it to a single case, supraglottic laryngectomy would now bear his name.

It was Professor Justo M. Alonso from Montevideo, Uruguay, who in 1939 performed the first supraglottic laryngectomy according to the technique which, with some minor modifications, is still in use. In his book "Laryngeal Cancer", published in 1954 by Paz Montalvo in Madrid, he wrote on the first page: "Cancer is a terrible disease, but I do not accept that the surgeon's scalpel may be more destructive than the disease itself. The war against the larynx must stop, since its removal is unnecessary and ineffective in many cases. To take away the disease without excising a healthy glottis, to make an effort to preserve the functions of the organ, to strive not to return a disabled person to the society: that is my motto."

Alonso based the principles of his operation on strong anatomical and embryological arguments as well as on clinical observations. In his times the method of spread of laryngeal tumours already were well known. "Le diagnostic radiologique des tumeurs malignes du pharynx et du larynx" by Baclesse appeared in 1938. Apropos of supraglottic cancer he says: "In short, supraglottic carcinomas often show an exophytic feature and consequently have a good prognosis, in spite of a frequent lymphnodes involvement. They can become considerably large, but even when they fill up the whole vestibule and spread forward on the pre-epiglottic space and backward on the pharyngeal wall, their superficial propagation, i.e. along the mucosa, stops caudad before reaching the vocal cords, as if there were here an obstacle. Also the deep infiltration, which takes place between the mucosal layer and the thyroid cartilage wing is hindered in most cases at the roof of the Morgagni's ventricle by some sort of barrier." Shortly after, Leroux-Robert uttered identical views.

These considerations urge us to meditate. If nature almost invariably stops the supraglottic cancer above the bottom of the ventricle, why not listen to the ever wise voice of nature? Why not excise these tumours incising along that line marked by a wiser hand than ours, rather than sacrifice an organ as noble and useful as the larynx?

Careful examination of several specimens of total laryngectomy, performed in cases of supraglottic cancers, confirmed that Baclesse's and Leroux-Robert's statements were true: tumours arising in the ventricular bands and/or in epiglottis only exceptionally invade the vocal cords.

How can we explain this fact? The blood supply of the upper part of the larynx is provided by the superior laryngeal artery, a branch of the superior thyroid artery, and therefore of the external carotid artery, while the lower part is supplied by the inferior laryngeal artery, derived from the subclavian artery. The plentiful lymphatic vessels of the supraglottic region accompany the superior laryngeal nerves and blood vessels to the upper nodes of the jugular chain. Below the cords, lymph vessels make their way to tracheal and lower jugular nodes. Between the supra- and subglottic regions there is an area, corresponding to the vocal cords, almost devoid of lymphatic vessels.

These differences in blood and lymph supply and in innervation are due to embryological reasons. The epiglottis and the ventricular bands derive from the fourth branchial arch; the fifth arch is represented in the adult only by the Santorini cartilage; the sixth arch forms the arytenoids and the post-arytenoid region. On the contrary, the glottis and subglottis originate from the tracheal tube. Comparative anatomy shows that two different sources for the two parts of the larynx (upper part, branchial; lower part, tracheal) are to be found in many animal classes. In some birds, like the ostrich, the lower part of the larynx is the tracheal glottis.

Supraglottic carcinomas, arising in the branchial portion of the larynx, tend to respect the genetic border of their territory. They may extend to neighbouring areas of the same origin, e.g. the pharynx, but they usually stop at the embryological demarcation, and do not invade the tracheal larynx.

Supraglottic laryngectomy is specifically indicated in lesions which affect the vestibule, the epiglottis, or both. Such lesions can derive from one of the bands and extend forward to the laryngeal surface of the epiglottis or they can start on the posterior surface of the epiglottis and reach either ventricular band or both. When the lesion is discovered, it generally involves both the epiglottis and the vestibule, puzzling us about its actual origin. Such a delay is probably due to the lack of symptoms, since hoarseness is not present until the cords are affected and dysphagia appears only when hypopharynx is involved. Dyspnea may be present, but it is then due to the exophytic character of the growth and not to its site.

Cancers confined to the epiglottis can also be treated by supraglottic laryngectomy. In these instances the removal is excessive, and other techniques, e.g. Huet's, can be considered more suitable.

The most important prerequisite for a correct application of the procedure is a correct identification of the tumour extent. In order to avoid incomplete resections, special care must be paid to what we call the danger points. These are:

1. Toward the front: anterior commissure.
   At this level the tumour may spread downward, not allowing an adequate safety margin to the excision.
2. Toward the back: the anterior aspect of the arytenoids.
3. Outwards: the aryepiglottic folds.
4. Forward and cephalad: the valleculae and base of the tongue and the pre-epiglottic space.

The last direction of spread is rather frequent and symptomless, so that we routinely include this region in the removal. As regards points 2., 3. and 4., they require that the traditional resection be extended, for in these areas no pre-formed barriers exist. Therefore, only a sufficient margin of adjacent healthy tissue may guarantee against local recurrences. Nevertheless, to more extended the removal, the more improbable a satisfactory restoration of laryngeal sphincteric action. The lack of effective protection from food aspiration into the airways is incompatible with life and represents one of the most common reasons for failure of conservative surgery. If this eventuality is feared, we can suture together the vocal cords, either during the operation, or in the postoperative period through endoscopy. This closure of the glottis may be temporary and we performed it in some cases after very wide resections. Some months later, the larynx opens spontaneously, or its lumen is re-established by endoscopy.

The most common general contraindication to traditional supraglottic laryngectomy and even more to the extended procedures is poor respiratory conditions. Patients with chronic bronchitis or emphysema, with poor cough and a low vital capacity are usually bad candidates for this kind of surgery. Aspiration of saliva and foods, which cannot be avoided in the immediate postoperative period, may cause severe and even fatal bronchopulmonary infections.

The operation should not be performed in old patients, owing to difficulties in compensation of the swallowing mechanism. Limitations however arise more frequently from bad respiratory conditions related to age, than from age itself.

Radiotherapy does not restrict the indications if it is used before surgery in a well planned programme of combined treatment. However, some postoperative complications, such as necrosis of the tissues, chondritis or chronic edema with permanent laryngeal stenosis are to be expected.

Finally, there are limitations due to the surgeon's skill. If he is not perfectly acquainted with the principles and technique of the operation, irreparable mistakes can be made. Functional surgery of laryngeal cancer is exciting, but we must pay all tention to the risk of emphasizing its advantages without considering its dangers and harms.

Outline of the Technique

We prefer a vertical skin incision parallel to the midline and a few centimeters from it. The incision is drawn on the healthy, or less-involved side, and runs from the hyoid bone to the inferior border of the thyroid cartilage. Two horizontal incisions start from its upper and lower ends, reaching the sternomastoid muscle. When a neck dissection is indicated, these two lines are prolonged laterally.

After elevation of the skin flap, which must include the platysma muscle and the external cervical aponeurosis, the anterior border of the sternomastoid muscle is retracted backward and the carotid space is inspected. Our policy towards neck lymphnodes, which may range from abstention to localized dissection or the en-bloc removal is always based on direct surgical exploration.

The half of the hyoid bone on the most affected side, i.e. on the side we are operating, and the upper part of the ipsilateral strap muscles are removed. The superior thyroid horn is divided at its base and excised. The superior laryngeal vessels are identified and divided between two ligatures.

Pharyngeal entrance is gained along its lateral wall, with a vertical cut performed at the site of the upper thyroid cornu. The index finger is introduced into the lumen to palpate the glosso-epiglottic groove. If it is healthy, as in standard cases, the tissues above the finger are severed with scissors, stopping soon after the midline has been crossed.

The epiglottis is retracted by means of a thread inserted in its base and the laryngeal cavity is inspected, both by sight and by finger. If it is confirmed that the glottis is not involved, the pyriform sinus mucosa is released both on the external and on the internal side of the pharyngolaryngeal gutter. The superior half of ipsilateral thyroid ala is elevated from the underlying tissues and cut horizontally. Along the midline, a thread is passed through the cartilage cut portion, as it will be removed later, together with the specimen.

The excision commences by incising the ipsilateral aryepiglottic fold. The cut runs nearly vertical, just in front of the arytenoid, until it reaches the posterior end of the ventricle. From here it runs along the ventricle and meets the midline. On the contralateral thyroid wing an incision is drawn, starting from the midline, i.e. from the endpoint of the previous cartilage cut, and ascending obliquely to the upper margin. This allows the contralateral ventricle to be exposed and incised up to the aryepiglottic fold. The specimen is then removed.

The redundant pyriform sinus mucosa is approximated to the vocal cords. Then two or three strong threads are passed round the hyoid bone remnant and below the inferior edge of thyroid cartilage. Once they have been tied, the larynx stump rises and the gap left by the excision is almost completely closed. Further sutures are placed in the pharyngeal mucosa and finally the strap muscles are replaced.

Horizontal Supraglottic Laryngectomy: Surgical Technique

C. CALEARO, G. P. TEATINI, and A. STAFFIERI, Ferrara

Horizontal supraglottic laryngectomy is characterized by the removal of the entire laryngeal vestibule. The section plane passes horizontally along the floor of the laryngeal ventricle of Morgagni (Fig. 1).

The excision must be carried out in a single block with the pre-epiglottic space. The hyoid bone can be preserved (Fig. 2). Thus the laryngeal stump includes the glottic plane, the arytenoids and the subglottic portion.

Surgery can be divided into the following stages:
1. exposure and preparation of the larynx;
2. excision;
3. reconstruction.

1. After having carried out a tracheotomy, an apron skin flap is drawn. The limits of the surgical field are as follows: the tracheotomy below, a line passing 1–2 cm over the hyoid bone above, and laterally the medial margins of the sternomastoid muscles.

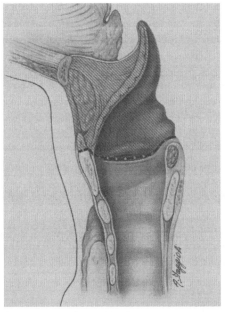 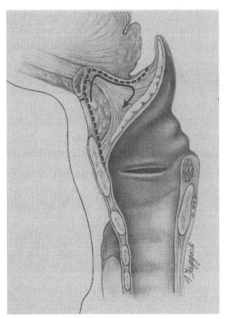

Fig. 1   Fig. 2

Fig. 1. The dashed line crossing the ventricle indicates inferior section plane. Hatched area corresponds to the portion of larynx to be removed

Fig. 2. Pre-epiglottic space (*arrow*) must be included in resection. Thus dashed line indicates the anterior and superior limits of removal

The strap muscles are isolated, sectioned at their hyoid bone insertions and reflected downward.

On the side chosen for the pharyngotomy, the superior laryngeal vessels are identified, ligated and cut. It is not necessary to try to save the superior laryngeal nerve since no appreciable difference in deglutition recovery has been found between patients with either intact or sectioned nerves.

2. The next stage starts with the dissection of the pre-epiglottic space.

From an oncological point of view, conservation of the hyoid bone is acceptable, provided that it is stripped of its periostium, which is incised along the entire length of the hyoid bone and elevated.

Dissection continues caudad along the hyoid-epiglottic membrane until the mucosa of the valleculae appears in transparency (care must be taken on that side where the superior laryngeal vessels are preserved).

Starting from the thyroid notch and proceeding laterally, the cranial edge of the thyroid cartilage is skeletonized and the superior cornu is amputated at its base. Along the lateral edge, the fibres of the inferior pharynx constrictor muscle are cut, and the pyriform sinus mucosa can be easily elevated from the inner aspect of the thyroid wing.

The perichondrium is then incised along the thyroid cartilage cranial edge and elevated both from the outer and from the inner aspect.

This stripping should extend up to a horizontal line passing a few millimeters below the thyroid notch.

The thyroid cartilage can be cut with a burr or with Moure scissors. The section line should coincide with the lower level of the laryngeal vestibule just above the glottis, that is from a point approximately one centimeter below the base of the previously amputated horn to the thyroid notch. The cut is almost symmetrical on both alae (Fig. 3).

After the removal of the cartilage fragments, the pharyngotomy is carried out on the lateral wall. The incision begins in correspondance to the cartilage section surface, rises cephaled towards the hyoid bone, then it bends at a right angle and crosses the valleculae. The epiglottis is grasped with a tenaculum and the vestibulum is exposed by rotating the larynx.

The vestibular resection is initiated on the ary-epiglottic fold. The incision line anteriorly grazes the arytenoid and enters the ventricle at its posterior angle (see Fig. 1). From this point the exeresis corresponds to the ventricle floor, tangentially to the true cord which lies below.

On the contralateral side, a similar incision meets the first at the anterior commissure level. Then the specimen can easily be freed from the pharynx by sectioning the pyriform sinus mucosa on the side opposite to the pharyngotomy.

If the supraglottic excision is properly executed the loss of substance on the side of the pharyngotomy is nearly the same as contralaterally.

3. The reconstruction of the air channel continuity must be particularly accurate. It consists of the following steps:

– reduction of the pharynx defect;
– pexy between the thyroid cartilage and the hyoid bone;
– reinforcement of the pexy by means of the perichondrium and the strap muscles.

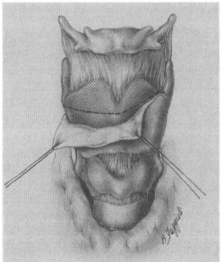 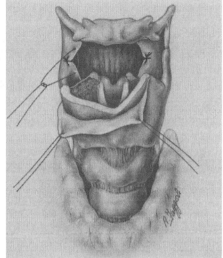

Fig. 3   Fig. 4

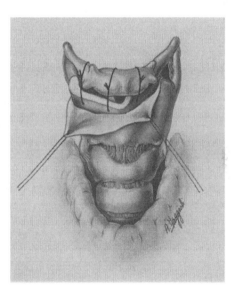

Fig. 5

Fig. 3. Thyroid perichondrium has been elevated starting from the cartilage upper margin and is stretched by means of threads. Dashed line shows incision on cartilage denuded surface. Hatched area indicates cartilage fragment to be removed

Fig. 4. After removal of specimen the gap between hyoid bone (*above*) and laryngeal stump (where vocal cords and arytenoids are clearly discernible) is reduced by means of some sutures in pharyngeal mucosa

Fig. 5. The pexy which approximates hyoid bone to thyroid cartilage is carried out by means of threads encompassing bone and going across holes drilled in cartilage

First of all, the pyriform sinus mucosa is approximated by means of only one suture to the remnants of the arytenoid mucosa, in order to cover the cartilage aspect.

The pharynx gap is reduced, placing sutures in the upper corners, i.e. between the vallecula and the lateral pharyngeal wall (Fig. 4). Two or three stitches are generally sufficient.

The remaining defect is closed through the pexy between hyoid bone and thyroid cartilage. Several thick chromic catgut threads are passed through holes drilled in the thyroid cartilage and clasp the hyoid bone, thus recreating the continuity of the air tube.

The ventral axis of the new channel is slightly anterior to the anatomic conditions preceeding surgery.

In order to facilitate the pexy, the patient's head should be bent forward.

The external perichondrium of the thyroid cartilage is now reflected up and sutured to the suprahyoid muscles to reinforce the pexy and to close any small lateral pharyngostomas (Fig. 5).

Finally the strap muscles are returned to their natural positions and sutured to the muscles above the hyoid bone.

My Personal Surgical Technique of Supraglottic Horizontal Laryngectomy

I. SERAFINI, Vittorio Veneto

In my opinion the bilateral cervical approach, inaugurated by André, is the method of choice for this procedure. It provides adequate exposure of the larynx and of both laterocervical regions by a single skin incision. It also allows a tracheostomy below the thyroid gland (Fig. 1).

In all cases of carcinoma of the epilarynx, irrespective of their extension and localization, a complete excision of the supraglottic compartments of the larynx is carried out. This procedure includes removal of the hyoid bone and a bilateral neck dissection, which might be functional on one side, at least, if performed simultaneously on both sides (Fig. 2).

If a lesion is situated on the lingual surface of the epiglottis, in the vallecula or in the paralaryngeal portions of the base of the tongue, the resection is continued into the base of the tongue. Care has to be taken, however, not to trespass the foramen caecum and the terminal sulcus (Fig. 3).

When tumours are localized to one aryepiglottic fold or the upper portion of the medial partition of the piriform sinus the resection must include an appropriate block of the hypopharynx. In this case the ipsilateral vocal cord and its arytenoid cartilage must usually be sacrificed (Fig. 4).

If supraglottic carcinomas involve the anterior mucosa of one arytenoid this cartilage will be excised, with possible preservation of its base with the apophysis of the vocal process, if possible (Fig. 5).

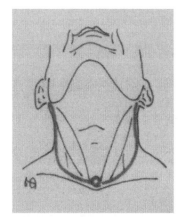

Fig. 1

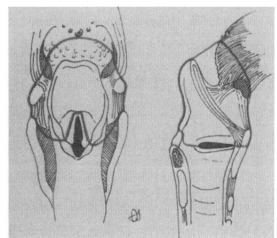

Fig. 2

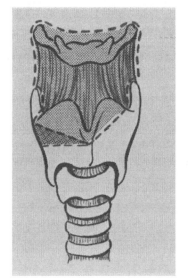

Fig. 3

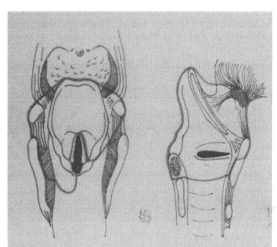

Fig. 4

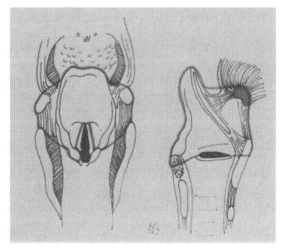

Fig. 5

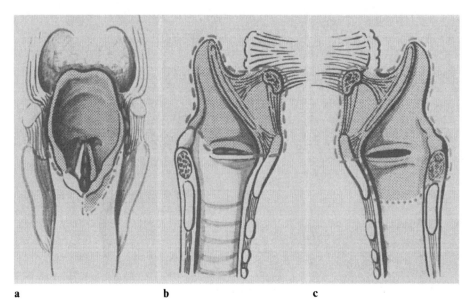

a b c
Fig. 6

A three quarters laryngectomy (Fig. 6) with removal of one arytenoid, one vocal cord and parts of the subglottic mucosa, is available for supraglottic lesions extending superficially into one vocal cord which is still mobile.

We always reconstruct the glottis, utilizing both the external perichondrium of the thyroid cartilage, which is folded medially, and the mucosa of the piriform sinus, folded dorsally. In 3/4 laryngectomy the wide excision of the thyroid cartilage always releases enough perichondrium to provide material for the reconstruction of a new vocal cord (Fig. 7).

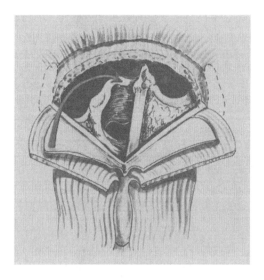

Fig. 7

Continuity between the hypopharynx and the inferior laryngeal stump is accomplished by medial anchoring using a steel wire suture (clasping together the thyroid cartilage via the crico-thyroidal membrane and the tongue base in a centimeter of its diameter). Two additional lateral sutures, using chromic gut, help to reconstitute the pharyngo-laryngeal tube by connecting the bases of the great thyroid horns with the mucosa of the tonsillo-lingual fold. Further sutures of fine cat gut fix the mucosa of the base of the tongue to the external perichondrium along the resection line of the thyroid cartilage.

Finally, the supra- and subthyroid strap muscles are reunited. A tracheostomy tube is inserted into the subthyreoid tracheostomy and retained for 2 to 3 days. Insertion of transcutaneous vacuum drains, and skin closure in two layers end the procedure.

Conservation Surgery for Supraglottic Carcinoma

M. F. Vega, B. Scola, and M. Catalá, Madrid

One long-term goal of those treating laryngeal cancer has been to reduce the severe disability of total loss of the voice. This desire has lead to the development of various procedures for partial laryngectomies. Such procedures are based on the knowledge of the natural history of the tumor and its spread, which will be conditioned by the primary site of the tumor and by the resistance to its progression. This first consideration defines the limits and indications for partial horizontal surgery of the larynx.

It is impossible to establish a rigid scheme, which will be valid for all situations, but the surgeon should know how to adapt the scheme to each case, using the proper technique required for each case.

The author's experience is based upon the data of 240 patients with supraglottic carcinoma who have had conservation surgery at the Provincial Institute of Oncology in Madrid.

In this chapter, we present our views about the indications, contraindications, choices of techniques and results obtained, as well as the complications, recurrences and the postoperative care.

Surgical Procedures of Partial Horizontal Laryngectomy

Incision

During the last twenty years the incisions have been adapted to the different approaches, as well as to the needs of the neck dissection. Thus, we used Maspétiol's horizontal incision for the Leroux-Robert type of laryngectomy, a T shape when we needed a Tapia type approach, the Alonso incision when doing a lateral approach, the Conley and Hayes Martin exposure if we performed a neck dissection. However, for the last ten years, in almost every case, we have used a U shaped incision extended on one side by a lateral supraclavicular branch.

In the first table the frequency of the different approaches is listed.

Table 1

Incision	Cases
S.H.L. Alonso's midline approach	146
S.H.L. Alonso's lateral approach	32
S.H.L. Leroux-Robert's approach	46
S.H.L. Tapia's approach	16
Total	240

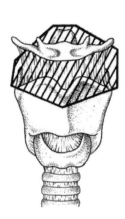 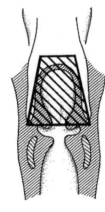

Fig. 1

Our opinion concerning the adequacy of the different ways of approach is as follows:

1. Alonso's Midline Approach. Nowadays we use this incision routinely except in exceptional cases which we will discuss, when we come to discuss the other incisions (Fig. 1).

2. Alonso's Lateral Approach. We use this type of approach in lesions limited to the aryepiglottic fold and to the external angle of the "aditus" (Fig. 2).

3. "A Minimum" Approach After Leroux-Robert. Is used rarely because the small tumors of the suprahyoid-epiglottis which could be treated by this technique, are frequently multifocal and should be treated by a wider Supraglottic H.L. (Fig. 3).

4. Approach by Tapia's Laryngofissure. Is also seldom used for lesions of the ventricular band of doubtful extension to the vocal cord, which need a laryngofissure examination, or an intraoperative biopsy, taking advantage of this entry to resect the laryngeal vestibule and the superior part of both thyroid wings (Fig. 4).

Surgical Techniques and Modifications

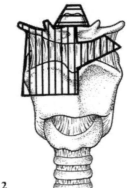
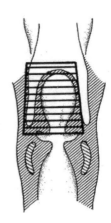

Fig. 2

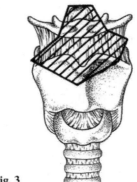
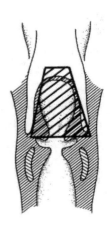

Fig. 3

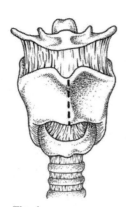
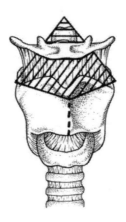
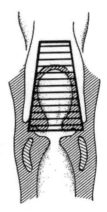

Fig. 4

Opening of the Pharyngo-Laryngeal Cavity

1. Midline Subhyoid Pharyngotomy. Is used for epiglottic tumors which do not affect the "aditus" and the vallecula.

2. Transthyroid in the Alonso "O" Point. Recommended for lesions of the aditus laryngis inlet, but contraindicated when the base of the epiglottis and the ventricular band are involved because of the risk of meeting the tumor if the tumor spreads along the anterior commissure or along the paraglottic space.

3. Pharyngotomy Contralateral to the Lesion. We use it routinely as it permits a perfect examination of the laryngeal vestibule and an excision with a good margin, even if the tumor extends downwards, upwards or laterally.

Hyoid Bone

Except in cases with invasion of the vallecula whose partial or total excision is necessary, the preservation of the hyoid bone permits a better adaptation of the remaining larynx to the base of the tongue. In certain cases of a wider excision of the thyroid alae, division of the hyoid bone aids in closure of the surgical defect, permitting a greater displacement of the hyoid bone.

Extended Horizontal Supraglottic Laryngectomies

The following table shows the type and number of partial horizontal laryngectomies with extended resections we have performed:

Table 2

Extended supraglottic horizontal laryngectomy	Cases
S.H.L. extended to the base of the tongue	24
S.H.L. extended to a piriform sinus and hypopharynx	8
S.H.L. extended to one arytenoid	34
S.H.L. extended to a vocal cord	17
Subtotal horizonto-vertical laryngectomy	8
Total	91

From the oncological and functional results observed in our series, our opinion on the Extended Supraglottic Laryngectomies is a follows:

1. H.S.L. Extended to the Base of the Tongue. Involvement of the vallecula compels us to extend the excision over the hyoid bone with an extended partial resection of the base of the tongue, when the lesion does not exceed a size of 1 cm (Fig. 5). If the involved part exceeds this limit partial surgery is contraindicated.

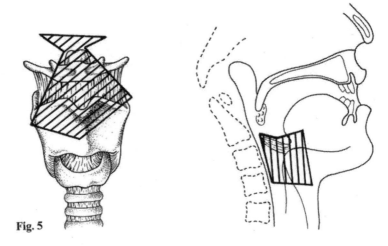

Fig. 5

2. *H.S.L. Extended to a Piriform Sinus and Lateral Wall of the Hypopharynx.* The lateral approach permits excision of tumors within the area of the three folds and with extension to the upper part of the lateral wall of the hypopharynx, performing a partial hemilaryngo-pharyngectomy. In involvement of the lower part, and of the piriform sinus, in our opinion all kinds of partial surgery are contraindicated (Fig. 6).

3. *H.S.L. Extended to an Arytenoid.* When the arytenoids are involved, but their mobility is preserved, the patient is perfectly suitable for H.S.L., and this does, in our opinion, not mean a worse prognosis.

4. *H.S.L. Extended to a Vocal Cord.* In invasion of the glottis it is necessary to distinguish the superficial forms preserving mobility which permit the performance of

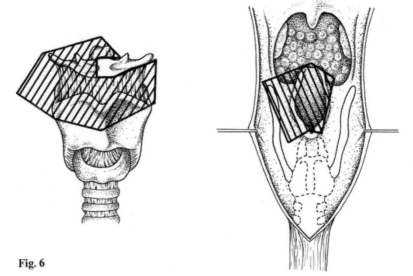

Fig. 6

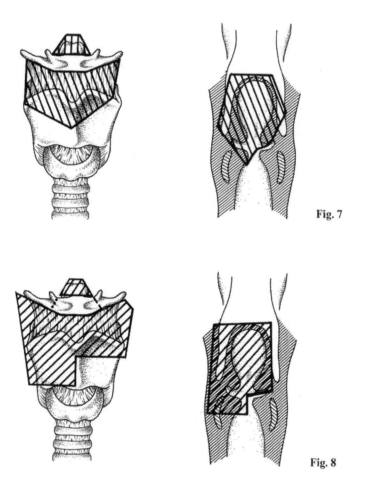

Fig. 7

Fig. 8

a Three Quarter Laryngectomy, preserving the inferior third of the thyroid wing from the infiltrating forms, in which the paraglottic space is involved and mobility impaired requires excision of all thyroid ala (Horizonto-vertical Laryngectomy). In these cases we perform reconstruction with the constrictor muscles and reinforce it with the prelaryngeal muscles (Figs. 7 and 8). However, it is necessary to point out that these extremes of extended partial laryngectomies shouldn't be combined with each other.

Table 3

N-stage	Policy
I) N_0, N_{1a}, N_{1b}	Homolateral neck dissection
II) N_{2a}, N_{2b}	Bilateral neck dissection
III) N_3	Radical neck dissection

Neck Dissection

Our attitude to the treatment of the neck nodes has changed down the years, and so in earlier years we only performed laryngeal surgery associated at a later stage with telecobalt therapy over the ganglionar areas. But for the last 12 years our system has been as indicated by Table 3.

In all cases in which the histopathological study of the specimen indicates tumor involvement, we carry out complementary treatment by telecobalt therapy (60 Gy in 6 weeks).

Horizontal Glottic Laryngectomy (Horizontal Glottectomy): Surgical Technique

C. Calearo and G. P. Teatini, Ferrara

During a horizontal glottectomy both vocal cords are removed together with the corresponding portion of the thyroid cartilage. When indicated, surgery can be extended to either or both of the false cords as well as to one arytenoid. Once the removal has been completed the air channel continuity is repaired by approximating the cricoid to the thyroid cartilage stump, in other words by carrying out a thyroid-cricoid-pexy.

Surgery can be divided into the following stages:
1. exposure of the larynx;
2. removal of the glottic plane;
3. reconstruction.

1. After having first carried out a tracheotomy, an apron skin flap is made. The vertical branches of the incision run along the anterior margins of the sternomastoid muscles.

The strap muscles are isolated. Those closest to the surface, i.e. the sternohyoid and omohyoid muscles, are cut a short distance from their attachments to the hyoid bone and reflected downward. The second layer muscles, i.e. the thyroid-hyoid muscles, are incised at their thyroid cartilage junctions and reflected upward.

The upper horns of the thyroid cartilage are isolated at their bases and amputated, permitting good mobilization of the larynx. After rotation of the larynx, a few centimeters of the thyroid cartilage lateral margin are isolated on each side by severing the lower pharynx constrictor fibres. The pyriform sinus mucosa is then stripped from the inner surface of both thyroid cartilage wings.

The cricothyroid articulations are sectioned, thus isolating the thyroid cartilage lower horns.

The perichondrium is cut along the lower edge of the thyroid cartilage and stripped upwards. In this way the lower two thirds of the cartilage are denuded (Fig. 1).

The cricothyroid membrane is incised along the lower edge of the thyroid cartilage which is lifted, making it possible to expose the caudal aspect of the vocal cords.

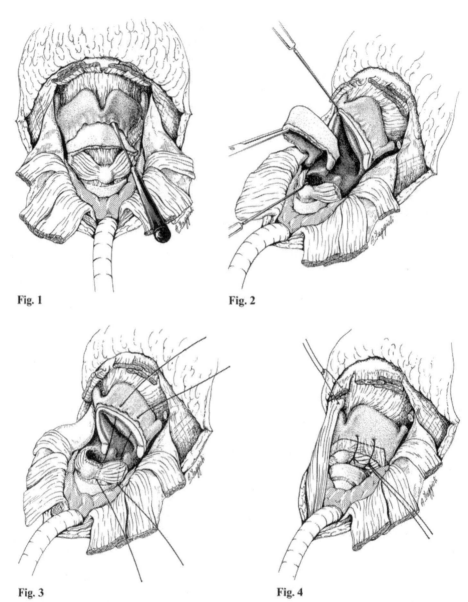

Fig. 1. Strap muscles have been sectioned at their attachments to hyoid bone and reflected downward. Perichondrium is incised along thyroid cartilage lower edge and elevated

Fig. 2. Larynx is trisected by two incisions. The lower crosses cricothyroid membrane and runs along thyroid cartilage inferior border. The higher starts on mid-line, 5 mm below thyroid notch. Hence it traverses horizontally both wings, ending at their lateral margins. Middle portion contains the glottis and can be removed after having severed vocal cords by means of two vertical incisions grazing vocal processes

Fig. 3. Threads are passed through holes drilled in thyroid cartilage stump (cephalad). Caudad, they encompass cricoid ring, without projecting into the lumen

Fig. 4. The pexy between cricoid cartilage and thyroid remnant is accomplished. Strap muscles are then replaced in their original positions

2. The thyroid cartilage incision line must intersect the mid-line 5 mm below the thyroid notch, i.e. at a point which lies above the anterior commissure. Hence the line runs horizontally over the thyroid wings. Near the lateral margin, it folds obliquely in a caudal direction, forming a new inferior horn.

The cartilage is cut with a wheel burr. Then the mucosa is sectioned by a knife and the incision is widened by means of hooks.

At this point it is possible to check the upper aspect of the vocal cords and – in the thyroid cartilage stump over the incision line – the lower surface of the false cords.

At the level of the vocal processes, the vocal cords are sectioned by means of two vertical incisions and the specimen is removed (Fig. 2).

3. One or two holes are made in the remainder of each thyroid wing with a burr. Through these holes threads are passed which caudally clasp the cricoid ring and yet remain below the mucosa (Fig. 3).

Before knotting the threads, the cricoid must be brought close to the thyroid cartilage stump using small hooks. In order to facilitate this maneuver the patient's head must be bent forward. Once the threads are knotted the thyroid-cricoid-pexy is complete.

The thyroid perichondrium is lowered into place and sutured to the cricoid (Fig. 4). The muscle plane is then reconstructed.

Modifications of Supraglottic Resection of the Larynx

J. CZIGNER, Budapest

The principle of conservation surgery for supraglottic carcinoma of the larynx is widely accepted. However, we are not yet through the period of techniqual improvement as recently was suggested by Ogura (1979). Our personal modifications are the following.

Simplified Supraglottic Horizontal Laryngectomy

Indication

T_{1a} and T_{1b} supraglottic carcinomas, which are confined to the supraglottic compartment, are removable by this technique when there are no palpable cervical lymph nodes.

107 simplified supraglottic horizontal laryngectomies have been performed by the following technique which has been modified in several details from the well described techniques of Alonso (1947), Ogura (1958), Bocca et al. (1968).

Technique

A separate tracheotomy is performed via a short vertical skin incision, and an infrahyoid transverse neck incision is used for horizontal resection of the larynx. The

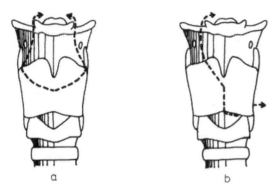

Fig. 1. a Schematic drawings of a simplified supraglottic horizontal laryngectomy (S.S.H.L.), and in **b** of an extended supraglottic subtotal laryngectomy including one vocal cord and arytenoid (E.S.S.L.)

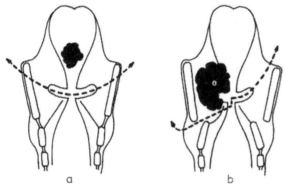

Fig. 2a, b. Schematic drawings of a S.S.H.L. (**a**) and a E.S.S.L. demonstrating the lower resection lines (**b**)

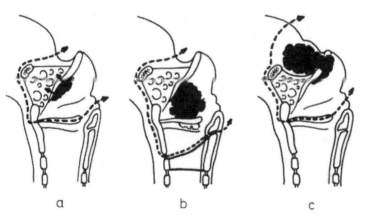

Fig. 3a–c. Schematic drawings of the sagittal view of a S.S.H.L. (**a**), an E.S.S.L. (**b**), and a supraglottic horizontal laryngectomy extended to the base of the tongue (**c**)

suprahyoid and infrahyoid muscles are dissected off the hyoid bone between the two lesser cornua. Both greater cornua are then resected. The preserved infrahyoid muscle flaps are reflected from the thyrohyoid membrane and the thyroid cartilage on both sides to the superior horns and the inferior border of the cartilage. The upper third of the thyroid cartilage is cut by a saw in a wide and flat "V" shaped cut (Fig. 1a). The superior laryngeal nerve is preserved on the less involved side or, if possible, on both sides.

A suprahyoid pharyngotomy is used which is adequate for the most satisfactory visual control of the supraglottic lesion prior to excision. The resection proceeds with an electrocautery cut from the arytenoids above the vocal cords. The cuts are continued on both sides along the floor of the ventricle and just above the anterior commissure (Fig. 2a). By these cuts, the ary-epiglottic folds, false cords and the epiglottis with the entire pre-epiglottic space, the adjacent V-shaped part of the thyroid cartilage, the hyoid bone (without its two greater cornua) are removed in one block (Fig. 3a).

A helpful technique was designed by Banfai (1962) for closure in which the base of tongue is transversely dissected, producing two layers to cover the transsected

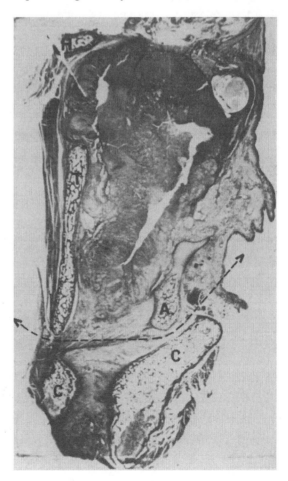

Fig. 4. Sagittal para-median section of a large supraglottic carcinoma with right glottic extension submitted to primary surgery. *A*, arytenoid cartilage; *C*, cricoid cartilage; *H*, hyoid bone; *T*, thyroid cartilage. Dotted line indicates the resection line

surface of the thyroid cartilage. The reconstruction should be performed carefully: a) by appropriate suturing of the new laryngeal vestibule; b) by fixation of the laryngeal remnant to the base of tongue; and c) by the careful suturing of the pharyngeal defect on both sides. The infrahyoid muscles are sutured to the suprahyoid tongue musculature, and the skin incision is then closed.

The voice preservation is excellent and the deglutition has been restored in most patients relatively rapidly. Of the 107 patients who had been operated on by this technique (without neck dissection) 19 underwent secondary radical neck dissection later because of subsequent development of cervical lymph node metastasis. Survival rate at 3 years was 74% and at 5 years it was 72%.

Extended Supraglottic Subtotal Laryngectomy

There is no standard surgical subtotal technique; however, there are some suitable techniques (Miodonsky 1962; Ogura and Dedo 1965; Iwai et al. 1970; Czigner 1972) which can be applied to a selected group of T_2 supraglottic tumors. These were used in 20.4% of our supraglottic conservation surgery procedures.

Indication

Supraglottic tumors which penetrate through the quadrangular membrane on one side and invade downwards between the ventricle and thyroid ala below the glottic

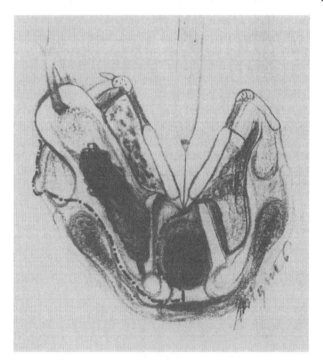

Fig. 5. Schematic drawing of E.S.S.L. to demonstrate the superior aspect of resection

level (Fig. 4). This compartmentalization by the thyro-arytenoid muscles and their fascia allows an extended supraglottic laryngectomy which is designed for resection of the entire supraglottis and one true vocal cord with the arytenoid and ipsilateral thyroid ala below the thyro-arytenoid muscles and through the cricoarytenoid joint (Figs. 2b, 3b and 4).

Technique

Tracheostomy and soft tissue incisions are made as in the method previously described. The hyoid bone is transsected at the lesser cornu of the uninvolved side. The infrahyoid muscles are preserved as a "muscle flap" on both sides. The thyroid cartilage is cut obliquely in the upper third and inferiorly in the middle (Fig. 1b). A suprahyoid pharyngotomy follows.

The cautery is used to cut through the normal aryepiglottic fold, false cord and ventricle, and through the anterior commissure to the inferior border of the thyroid cartilage (Fig. 5). The incision is continued posteriorly on the involved side to the interarytenoid space.

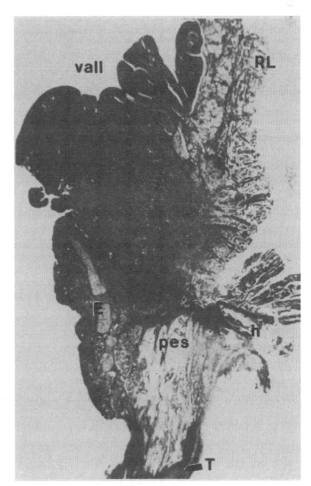

Fig. 6. Epiglottic suprahyoid tumor with large submucosal invasion to the vallecula (*vall*) and limited involvement of radix linguae (*RL*). Sagittal section of the specimen of a supraglottic horizontal laryngectomy extended to the base of tongue. *E*, epiglottic cartilage; *T*, superior part of thyroid cartilage; *h*, hyoid bone; *pes*, pre-epiglottic space

It should be emphasized that to reconstruct a functioning larynx, the minimum unit of the larynx should include the cricoid cartilage with one functioning arytenoid cartilage and one vocal cord. The excised vocal cord is reconstructed utilizing the adjacent mucous membrane. The laryngeal remnant is elevated and fixed to the base of tongue. The wound closure is then continued as in the previously described method.

46 patients were operated on by this method. The survival rate was 78% for 3 years and 77% for 5 years.

Supraglottic Horizontal Laryngectomy Extended to the Base of the Tongue

Conservation surgery can be employed in selected instances of supraglottic carcinomas with limited involvement of the vallecula or base of tongue (Figs. 3c and 6). The prognosis is not as hopeless as the T_4 classification would indicate. The extended technique of the supraglottic laryngectomy starts with a lateral transhyoid pharyngotomy, and it requires a careful dissection with preservation of the lingual artery and hypoglossal nerve. Otherwise difficulties in rehabilitation of deglutition have to be expected. 24 such operations were performed as 10% of our supraglottic conservation surgery procedures. The 3-year survival rate was 45%, and it was 36% after five years.

References

Alonso JM (1947) Conservative surgery of cancer of the larynx. Trans Am Acad Ophthalmol Otolaryngol 51:633–642
Banfai I (1963) Anatomische Rekonstruktion des Kehlkopfs nach horizontaler Resektion. Z Laryngol Rhinol 42:32–38
Bocca E, Pignataro O, Mosciaro O (1968) Supraglottic surgery of the larynx. Ann Otol Rhinol Laryngol 77:1005–1026
Czigner J (1972) Vertical subtotal laryngectomy. Laryngoscope 82:101–107
Iwai H, Tamura M, Yoshioka A, Okumara H, Yanagihara N (1970) Subtotal Laryngectomy. Arch Ohr-Nas-Kehlk-Heilk 197:85–96
Miodonski J (1962) Enlarged hemilaryngectomy. J Laryngol Otol 76:266–273
Ogura JH (1958) Supraglottic subtotal laryngectomy and radical neck dissection for carcinoma of the epiglottis. Laryngoscope 68:983–1003
Ogura JH, Dedo HH (1965) Glottic Reconstruction Following Subtotal Glottic-Supraglottic Laryngectomy. Laryngoscope 75:865–878
Ogura JH (1979) Hyoid muscle flap reconstruction in subtotal supraglottic laryngectomy etc. Laryngoscope 89:1522–1524

Vascular Pedicle Flap of the Thyroid Gland in Horizontal Supraglottic Laryngectomy

E. MOZOLEWSKI, P. MAJ, P. WDOWIAK, K. JACH, C. TARNOWSKA, and M. WASILEWSKA, Szczecin

Supraglottic laryngectomies formed 68% of 322 partial laryngectomies performed between 1971–1981 or 52% of all our operated cases of laryngeal carcinoma. No X-ray therapy was applied. They include 26% of extended partial resections limited to the larynx itself and 10% with extension into the tongue. Surgical problems with the operation were mentioned in our report on the three quarters laryngectomy. In the remaining cases of partial extended laryngectomies limited to the larynx, functional consequences of excision of the arytenoid cartilage were pointed out. The technique of reconstruction of the arytenoid cartilage eminence by use of a vascular pedicle thyroid flap was presented above. In our supraglottic carcinoma cases with tongue base involvement the results were poor, due mainly to local recurrences. There were 8% deaths due to tumor. One of the reasons seemed to be a too narrow safety margin around the tumor, due to our fear of the well known functional consequences. The possibility of tongue base reconstruction with use of vascular pedicled thyroid or submandibular gland flap was presented. Functional result was uniformly good in all three cases where this technique was applied.

One case with an observation period of one and a half year (vallecular tumor T_2) is alive without recurrence. Other cases had relatively short follow-up intervals of 6 months and 6 weeks.

The crude three years survival rate of patients with a typical horizontal laryngectomy was 77% (54 of 70 cases), in 3/4 laryngectomy 68% (41 of 61 cases), and in horizontal partial laryngectomy with tongue resection it was only 8% (2 of 25 cases).

Conclusions

1. In supraglottic carcinoma a unilateral extension of the excision in the larynx, resecting one arytenoid cartilage or one arytenoid together with one vocal cord, has relatively little oncological risk in comparison to the typical horizontal laryngectomy.

2. The excision of one arytenoid cartilage may be successfully reconstructed by a vascular pedicled flap of the thyroid gland.

3. The oncological results in involvement of the base of the tongue were extremely poor. One of the reasons seems to be the narrow safety margin, due to the surgeon's fear of the well known functional consequences such as aspiration.

4. The application of a vascular pedicled flap of the thyroid gland or submandibular salivary gland allows adequate repair even in large defects of the tongue base, thus encouraging the surgeon to broaden the margin.

Three Quarters Laryngectomy

G. P. Teatini, Ferrara

Principle of the Operation

As its name indicates, the three quarters laryngectomy associates the removal of the supraglottic portion of the larynx (horizontal resection) with the excision of one arytenoid plus the corresponding vocal cord (vertical resection). Before closing the gap by means of a pexy between the hyoid bone and the thyroid cartilage remnants, a neocord must be shaped, in order to allow the larynx to recover its phonatory and sphincteric function.

Indications

Whenever the typical excision of a supraglottic laryngectomy has to be enlarged to include an arytenoid and a vocal cord: e.g., lateral vestibular tumours which penetrate into the ventricle and come into contact with the vocal cord.

Preserved mobility of both vocal cords is mandatory.

Surgical Technique

Exposure of the larynx and dissection of the pre-epiglottic space: See chapter on horizontal supraglottic laryngectomy. Removal of the thyroid cartilage. The perichondrium is incised along the cranial margin of the thyroid cartilage, elevated and reflected downwards. About two thirds of the thyroid wings should be denuded.

The thyroid cartilage is cut by means of a Stryker saw or a wheel burr. The first incision starts from the thyroid notch and runs along the vertical midline for 1.2–1.5 cm. Thus its end point lies *below* the glottic plane.

The second incision is drawn on the side where the vocal cord must be removed. Beginning from the lowest point of the vertical incision one moves quasi-horizontally across the ala as far as the previously isolated lateral margin.

Although the third incision is also perpendicular to the vertical one, it starts just 0.5 cm from the thyroid notch, i.e. from a point situated *above* the glottic plane (Fig. 1).

The two cartilage fragments are elevated and removed.

Lateral Pharyngotomy

Entrance to the pharynx is gained through the lateral pharyngeal wall, a few millimeters before (medially to) the thyroid upper horn, which has been left in place after its section. As soon as the level of the hyoid bone is reached, the incision bends at a right angle and stops about 1 cm beyond the midline (Fig. 2).

The epiglottis is grasped and rotated towards the opposite side, the arytenoids are gently retracted outwards and the larynx inside is exposed.

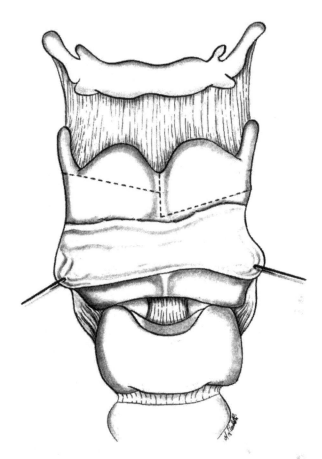

Fig. 1. Cartilage incisions. The thyroid perichondrium has been incised along the cartilage cranial margin, elevated and retracted caudad by means of two hooks. Dashed lines show cartilage incisions. The vertical cut starts from thyroid notch and runs along the midline for 1.5 cm, i.e. its endpoint lies *below* the glottic plane. Hence moves the horizontal incision on the side where the vocal cord must be removed (in the scheme, on the left), while on the side where the vocal cord must be spared (in the scheme, on the right) the horizontal incision starts from the vertical one just 0.5 cm from thyroid notch, i.e. *above* the glottis

Tumour Removal

The excision begins by sectioning the aryepiglottic fold just in front of the arytenoid to be preserved. One proceeds obliquely caudad, always close to the arytenoid anterior edge, until the posterior horn of the ventricle is reached. Hence, the incision horizontally crosses the whole ventricle up to the anterior commissure (Fig. 3a).

On the opposite side, the posterior commissure between the two arytenoids is severed first. Then the cricoarytenoid joint is transsected and the cut continues along the lateral laryngeal wall below the vocal cord. As the ventral midline is reached, the incision vertically crosses the anterior commissure and meets the contralateral cut (Fig. 3b).

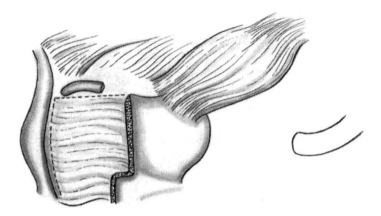

Fig. 2. Pharyngotomy incisions. Dashed line shows the pharyngotomy incision. The cut starts from the upper border of thyroid cartilage stump, just medially to the upper horn which has been left in place after its section. Cephalad, as the level of the hyoid bone is reached, the incision bends at a right angle and stops soon beyond the midline

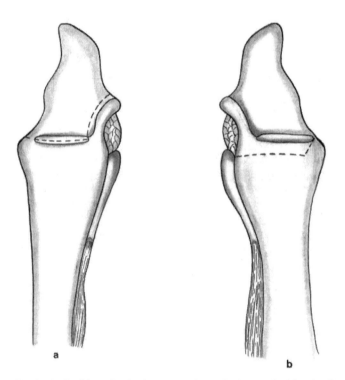

Fig. 3a, b. Incisions in the larynx cavity. **a** In larynx inside, the first incision starts from the aryepiglottic fold on the side where the vocal cord must be preserved. The section grazes the arytenoid anterior aspect, then crosses the ventricle and reaches the anterior commissure. **b** On the opposite side, i.e. where the vocal cord must be removed, after having divided the posterior commissure between the two arytenoids, the cricoarytenoid joint is transsected. Then the incision continues horizontally below the vocal cord until the midline. Here it crosses vertically the anterior commissure and meets the contralateral cut

Finally, the specimen is separated from the opposite side pyriform sinus and removed.

Formation of the Neo Cord

The thyroid perichondrium is raised and severed along the midline. From the side where the vocal cord has been removed, it is reflected dorsally and fixed by sutures and/or glueing to the cricoid upper aspect (Fig. 4a).

A second flap, built from the strap muscles and inferiorly pedicled, is also reflected dorsally and sutured to the cricoid over the perichondrium (Fig. 4b). The third, cranial layer of the neocord is made up of the redundant pyriform mucosa, which is pulled to completely cover the muscle flap.

Along the free edge of the neocord the mucosa is accurately approximated to the perichondrium by means of several very fine Dexon sutures, reinforced by fibrin glue.

Caution. To attain a good restoration of phonatory and sphincteric functioning the neocord should
a) not be too bulky (take care during preparation of the muscular flap);
b) extend as far as the median line, mainly forward (in due time, the uninvolved vocal cord may compensate for posterior minor displacements from the median line through hyperadduction);
c) be located exactly on the same horizontal plane as the unaffected cord (to reach this goal, it is sometimes necessary to lower the section of the thyroid cartilage by some millimeters).

Repair

The repair steps are quite the same as in supraglottic laryngectomy:
- one or two stitches approximate the mucosal wound on the arytenoid;
- the pharyngeal gap is narrowed by means of sutures;
- the gap is then bridged through a pexy between the hyoid bone and the thyroid cartilage stump (to this purpose, holes have been previously drilled in the cartilage);
- finally, the strap muscles are replaced and the wound is closed.

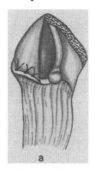 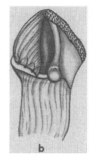

Fig. 4a, b. Formation of the neocord. **a** To build the neocord, a perichondrium flap is reflected dorsally and fixed to the cricoid upper aspect. **b** A second flap, built from the strap muscles, is likewise fixed to the cricoid. It will be covered by a third layer, made up of the redundant mucosa of ipsilateral pyriform sinus

II. Posttherapeutic Histology and Microstaging in Horizontal Partial Laryngectomy

Horizontal Partial Resections of the Larynx. Posttherapeutic Histology and Microstaging[1]

J. A. KIRCHNER, New Haven (Connecticut)

Horizontal supraglottic laryngectomy depends upon the concept of a barrier between the glottic and supraglottic parts of the larynx. Although a definite anatomical structure is not identifiable, cancer often remains confined to the epiglottis and ventricular bends, leaving the ventricle free of tumor (Baclesse 1949; Bocca et al. 1968; Leroux-Robert 1937). The sharp division between the glottic and supraglottic areas has been further demonstrated by injections of fluid and dyes into various parts of the larynx (Hajek 1891; Pressman et al. 1960).

Sixty-one supraglottic tumors removed by partial or total laryngectomy have been studied by serial section. These studies support the validity of horizontal supraglottic partial laryngectomy for the following reasons:

1. In every tumor which has remained confined to the ventricular band and/or epiglottis, regardless of size, the thyroid ala has been found to be intact. It is only in the "transglottic" lesion, i.e., one that has extended downward across the anterior commissure or ventricle, that invasion of the thyroid cartilage has been observed. Where any doubt exists as to the lower margin of the tumor, this extension can usually be recognized by lateral laryngography before operation, and definitely identified as the larynx is being opened after lateral pharyngotomy. Downward extension of tumor below the anterior commissure requires total laryngectomy (Kirchner and Som 1971).

2. Gross examination of the inferior extent of the lesion after pharyngotomy is sufficient to define its limits of infiltration. In not a single instance was the line of resection violated inferiorly by cancer when horizontal partial laryngectomy was performed after adequate exposure. This has been confirmed by our histological studies, and supported further by the observation that when cancer recurs locally after horizontal supraglottic resection (Fig. 1), it is in the base of the tongue, and not in the true cords (Som 1970).

3. The pre-epiglottic space, into which infra-hyoid cancer tends to spread, can be removed just as completely with horizontal supraglottic as with total laryngectomy (Figs. 2–3). In fact, the hyoid bone can be safely preserved during horizontal supraglottic resection, unless the tumor mass is palpable in the base of the tongue or

---

1 Supported by U.S.P.H.S. Grant CA 22101-06 National Cancer Institute, DHHS

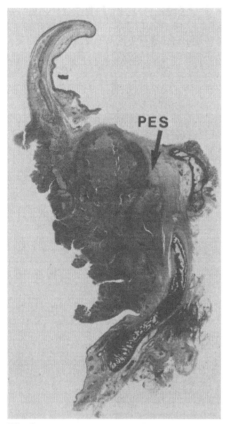
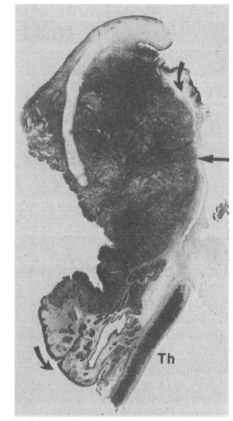

Fig. 1

Fig. 3

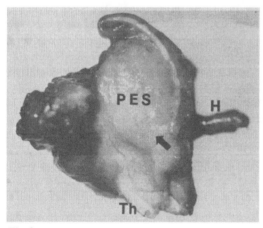

Fig. 2

Fig. 1. Sagittal section of laryngectomy specimen removed for supraglottic cancer. The pre-epiglottic space (*PES*) has been invaded, and the tumor exhibits the characteristic spread upward and forward into the base of the tongue

Fig. 2. Epiglottic cancer removed by horizontal partial resection, cut sagitally near midline for demonstration. Cancer invades the pre-epiglottic space (*PES*) from its origin in the base of the epiglottis

Fig. 3. Sagittal section of specimen shown in Fig. 2, illustrating three favorable features of many supraglottic growths: a) Adequate inferior margin (*lower arrow*), b) "Pushing" edge (*middle arrow*), c) Free space behind hyoid bone (*top arrow*)

the thyro-hyoid membrane at the time of operation. Preservation of the hyoid bone facilitates postoperative deglutition (Kirchner 1979).

Invasion of the pre-epiglottic space as shown in Fig. 2 is a major cause of failure to cure supraglottic cancer by radiotherapy (Fletcher et al. 1975). Such invasion can sometimes be identified by computerized axial scanning, but this requires very careful study with the latest scanning equipment. On the other hand, invasion of the pre-epiglottic space can be anticipated when the lesion is located in the infra-hyoid portion of the anterior larynx, when it is ulcerative rather than exophytic, and when fullness or induration in this area can be appreciated on inspection or by palpation with the tip of the laryngoscope.

For all of the above reasons, and because of superior results obtained by surgery with or without radiotherapy (Fletcher et al. 1970), horizontal supraglottic partial laryngectomy is our treatment of choice for advanced supraglottic cancer. Local recurrence after horizontal supraglottic partial laryngectomy is relatively rare, whereas cervical node metastasis is the greatest single cause of failure.

References

Baclesse F (1949) Carcinoma of the larynx. Br J Radiol [Suppl] 3: 1–62
Bocca E, Pignataro O, Mosciaro O (1968) Supraglottic surgery of the larynx. Ann Otol 77: 1005–1026
Fletcher GH, Jesse RH, Lindberg RD, Koons CR (1970) The place of radiotherapy in the management of the squamous cell carcinoma of the supraglottic larynx. Am J Roentgenol 108: 19–26
Fletcher GH, Lindberg RD, Hamberger A, Horiot JC (1975) Reasons for irradiation failure in squamous cell carcinoma of the larynx. Laryngoscope 85: 987–1003
Hajek M (1891) Anatomische Untersuchungen über das Larynxödem. Arch Klin Chir 42: 46–93
Kirchner JA (1979) Closure after supraglottic laryngectomy. Laryngoscope 89: 1343–1344
Kirchner JA, Som ML (1971) Clinical and histological observations on supraglottic cancer. Ann Otol Rhinol Laryngol 80: 638
Leroux-Robert JL (1937) Formes anatomocliniques et indications therapeutic des epitheliomas intra-larynges. Ann Otolaryngol Chir Cervicofac 1003–1044
Pressman JT, Simon MB, Monell C (1960) Anatomical studies related to the dissemination of cancer of the larynx. Trans Am Acad Ophthalmol Otolaryngol 64: 628–638
Som ML (1970) Conservative surgery for carcinoma of the supraglottis. J Laryngol Otol 84: 644–678

Supraglottic Carcinoma – Posttherapeutic Histology

J. OLOFSSON, Linköping

The growth and spread of supraglottic carcinoma is well studied by the use of whole organ (specimen) serial sections (Kirchner and Som 1971; Olofsson and van Nostrand 1973; McDonald et al. 1976). The supraglottic region is bounded inferiorly by

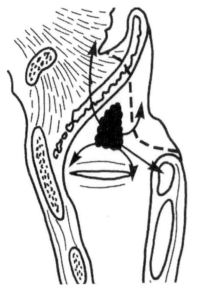 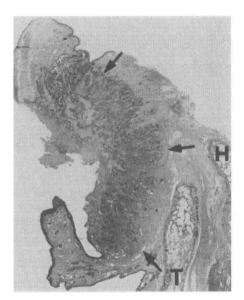

Fig. 1 **Fig. 2**

Fig. 1. Supraglottic carcinoma – modes of extension

Fig. 2. Sagittal section. Ulcerated supraglottic carcinoma growing with "pushing" margins. The epiglottic cartilage is destroyed and the tumour invades the preepiglottic space and extends to the base of the tongue but respects the anterior commissure and does not invade the thyroid cartilage (*T*). This patient received preoperative radiotherapy followed by a total laryngectomy and right neck dissection. An extended supraglottic laryngectomy including a part of the base of the tongue could have been performed in this case. *H* Hyoid bone

the vocal cords and superiorly by the free margins of the epiglottis, aryepiglottic folds and arytenoids. The posttherapeutic histology depends on the previous therapy i.e. primary surgery, preoperative radiotherapy or primary radiotherapy with surgery for recurrent disease. Certain characteristics are, however, typical for the growth and spread of supraglottic carcinoma (Figs. 1 and 2).

McGavran et al. (1961) noticed that supraglottic carcinomas often had a "pushing margin". They often involve both sides of the supraglottic larynx. Bocca et al. (1968) pointed out that "the larynx consists of two distinct parts, an upper and a lower part, whose line of demarcation runs at the level of the vocal cord". The different embryologic derivations and the different lymphatic supplies were also stressed. This strict limitation of supraglottic carcinomas does not prove true in all cases but the differences in reported series may to a certain extent depend on the selection of the material examined (Szlezak 1966; Olofsson and van Nostrand 1973).

Kirchner and Som (1971) differentiated between exophytic lesions that tend not to extend to the glottic region and not to invade the thyroid cartilage, and ulcerative lesions that may extend down crossing the anterior commissure, and when doing so exhibit a great risk to invade the thyroid cartilage. However, invasion of the cartilage does not seem to occur unless the tumour macroscopically extends below the anterior commissure, an observation of great clinical importance in selecting patients suitable for a horizontal supraglottic laryngectomy.

Invasion of the preepiglottic space (PES) is a common finding (Fig. 2), when studying supraglottic carcinomas. The epiglottic cartilage is fenestrated and carcinomas involving the laryngeal surface of the epiglottis may easily penetrate into the PES either through these fenestrations or by destruction of the cartilage. The lateral parts of the PES is in direct continuity with the paraglottic space (Tucker and Smith 1962) and this is another pathway for tumours to reach the PES but is less commonly used.

In a series of 110 carcinomas, all studied by whole organ serial sections, 18 involved the PES. All but one involved the laryngeal surface of the epiglottis (Olofsson and van Nostrand 1973). However, McDonald et al. (1976) did not find any specific patterns in the mucosal involvement or in the configuration of the tumour, when invasion of the PES was seen. Invasion of the PES occurs in about 40% of all supraglottic carcinomas and in about 70% of all epiglottic primaries (Ogura 1955; Szlezak 1966; Kirchner 1969; Olofsson and van Nostrand 1973; McDonald et al. 1976).

The tumours may extend further up to the vallecula and to the base of the tongue, which limits the possibilities for conservation surgery mainly by increasing the swallowing problems postoperatively if too much of the tongue is resected (Fig. 2).

Posterior extension to the arytenoid region is also a limiting factor for partial surgery. Kirchner and Som (1971) found invasion of the arytenoid cartilage only in those cases with gross involvement of the mucosa overlying the arytenoid.

The pyriform sinus may be involved by marginal tumours overriding the aryepiglottic fold and sometimes making the classification difficult. The tumour may also reach the pyriform sinus by deep invasion.

The supraglottic carcinomas present with diffuse symptoms and are often in an advanced stage before diagnosed, which in combination with a rich lymphatic supply explains the high incidence of lymph node metastases, 32% as reported by Som (1970) and 73% as reported by Baclesse (1949). Systematized studies in surgical pathology are necessary to achieve the knowledge to be able to safely select patients suitable for conservation surgery and to modify and improve our surgical techniques. We must make full use of our clinical and radiographic examination methods including laryngography and computed tomography to give more patients the chance to retain their voice and airway but still to have radical cancer surgery performed.

References

Baclesse F (1949) Carcinoma of the larynx. Radiotherapy of laryngeal cancer. Clinical, radiological and therapeutic study. Follow-up of 341 cases treated at the Foundation Curie, from 1919 to 1940. Br J Radiol [Suppl] 3: 1–62

Bocca E, Pignataro O, Mosciaro O (1968) Supraglottic surgery of the larynx. Ann Otol Rhinol Laryngol 77: 1005–1026

Kirchner JA (1969) One hundred laryngeal cancers studied by serial section. Ann Otol Rhinol Laryngol 78: 689–709

Kirchner JA, Som ML (1971) Clinical and histological observations on supraglottic cancer. Ann Otol Rhinol Laryngol 80: 638–645

McDonald TJ, DeSanto LW, Weiland LH (1976) Supraglottic larynx and its pathology as studied by whole laryngeal sections. Laryngoscope 86:635–648
McGavran MH, Bauer WC, Ogura JH (1961) The incidence of cervical lymph node metastases from epidermoid carcinoma of the larynx and their relationship to certain characteristics of the primary tumor. A study based on the clinical and pathological findings for 96 patients treated by primary en bloc laryngectomy and radical neck dissection. Cancer 14:55–66
Ogura JH (1955) Surgical pathology of cancer of the larynx. Laryngoscope 65:867–926
Olofsson J, van Nostrand AWP (1973) Growth and spread of laryngeal and hypopharyngeal carcinoma with reflections on the effect of preoperative irradiation. 139 cases studied by whole organ serial sectioning. Acta Otolaryngol [Suppl] (Stockh) 308:1–84
Som ML (1970) Conservation surgery for carcinoma of the supraglottis. J Laryngol Otol 84:655–678
Szlęzak L (1966) Histological serial block examination of 57 cases of laryngeal cancer. Morphological and clinical correlations. Oncologia 20:178–194
Tucker GF, Smith HR (1962) A histological demonstration of the development of laryngeal connective tissue compartments. Trans Am Acad Ophthalmol Otolaryngol 66:308–318

Histological Examination of the Excised Specimen After Supraglottic Laryngectomy

I. SERAFINI, Vittorio Veneto

After any kind of laryngectomy or neck dissection all tissues were submitted to serial section and histological examination by our pathologist. Prof. Carlon after removal of its skeleton and of the hyoid bone the larynx was cut into 37 slices (Fig. 1): one medioanterior plane (slide 0) included the epiglottis, the anterior commissure, and the subglottic mucosa. A greater part of the vestibule was cut in the transverse direction (slices 1–9 and 11–19). The inferior part of the ventricular fold, the ventricle itself, and the subglottic area were sectioned in the longitudinal plane (slices 21–27 and 31–37).

The histological slides were exposed to photographic magnification and projected on white paper. By this method the following compartments of the larynx could be graphically reconstructed: The tumour was dyed in grey, the normal tissues remained white, while the cartilage (if present) appeared in black. Figure 2 gives an example of the graphical reconstruction of a carcinoma of the laryngeal vestibule, localized to the laryngeal surface of the epiglottis.

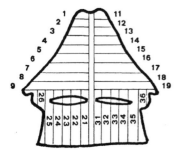

Fig. 1

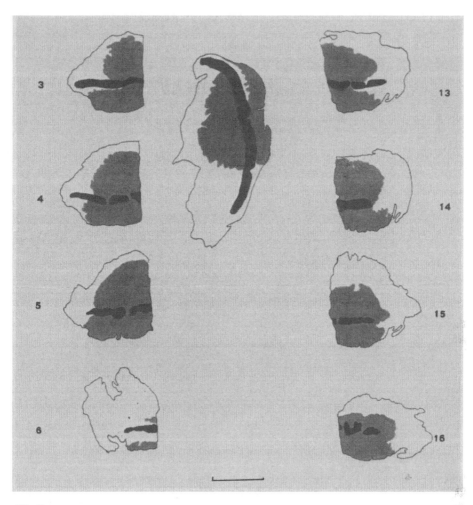

Fig. 2

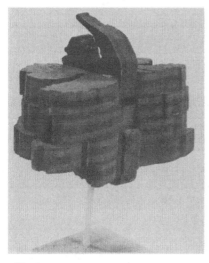

Fig. 3

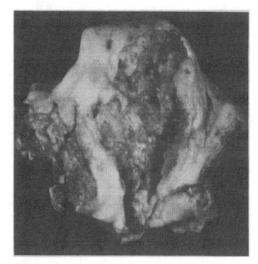

Fig. 4

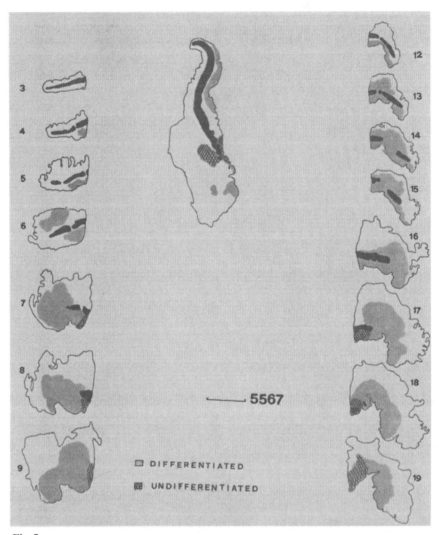

Fig. 5

This method allows a three-dimensional reconstruction of magnified tumour models, grossly featuring form, size and volume of the tumour. Figure 3 illustrates one case by a wooden model, equivalent to the preceding lesion of Fig. 2.

Systematical studies like these allow scrutiny of the superficial spread of a tumour, and also documentation of its macroscopic and microscopic details of infiltration into the preepiglottic space, the ventricular folds, the piriform sinus and the periarytenoidal space. They also convey an intimate knowledge of the micrograding and microstaging of the particular lesion including all local tissue reactions of the host.

Our histological investigations have frequently shown both cytological and structural variations between different parts of one tumour. One example is given

Posttherapeutic Histology and Microstaging in Horizontal Partial Laryngectomy

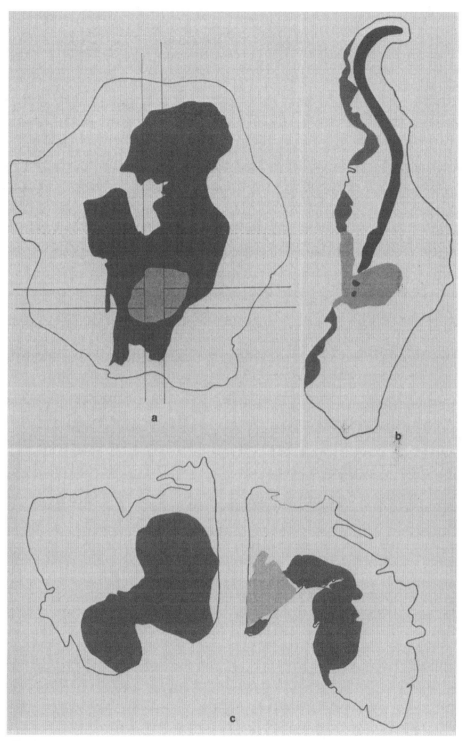

Fig. 6

by Fig. 4 demonstrating partly epidermoid configuration of the tumour cells, and partly zones of undifferentiated cells. The graphic reconstruction (Fig. 6a) gives an idea of the geometric distribution of both of these tumour components.

In the median plane (Fig. 6b) the extension of the undifferentiated (clear) and of the differentiated dark areas may well be studied together with the involvement of the epiglottic cartilage.

Similar information is provided by reconstruction in the transverse planes (Fig. 6c). This picture illustrates the squamous cell carcinoma of medium differentiation, consisting of polygonal, partly keratinizing cells, while the undifferentiated focus contains smaller, polygonal cells with clear cytoplasm without any signs of maturation.

In the cervical lymph nodes affected by metastases, chains of undifferentiated cells are visible, mainly situated in the lymphatic sinuses. This case will emphasize the necessity of serial sections, because a single biopsy cannot be representative of the whole tumour.

III. Oncological and Functional Results of Horizontal Partial Resections as the Basis of Surgical Indications

Horizontal Supraglottic Laryngectomy: Results

A. STAFFIERI, Ferrara

A follow-up study of cases of horizontal supraglottic laryngectomy (HSL) at the E.N.T. Clinic of the University of Ferrara was carried out. In order to permit a minimum observation time of three years for all patients this study includes only those patients who underwent horizontal supraglottic laryngectomy during the period from 1965 through 1978. In Table 1 these cases are listed according to the modalities of therapy.

The data reported in the first row of Table 1 concern a homogeneous sample of patients who had undergone horizontal supraglottic laryngectomy with no associated radiation therapy nor with any extension of the surgery beyond its classical limits. Of this group (Table 2) composed of 143 cases, only 5% (7 patients) underwent no neck dissection because of high operative risk. Since the great majority of these cases were supraglottic laryngectomies with bilateral functional neck dissections, the results of both the horizontal supraglottic laryngectomy and the neck dissections can be considered together. The operative mortality in this group was 2%.

Table 1. Horizontal supraglottic laryngectomy (HSL). Number of interventions between 1965 and 1978. Combination with radiotherapy (RX) and neck dissection

a) HSL	n = 143
b) Enlarged HSL	n = 20
c) HSL + RX postop	n = 42
d) Enlarged HSL + RX preop	n = 21
e) Enlarged HSL + RX postop	n = 9
Total	n = 235

Age: mean 54 years
 min. 28 years
 max. 74 years

Neck dissection: not dissected 16 cases (6.8%)
 functional 208 cases (88.5%)
 classic 11 cases (4.7%)

Post-operative deaths: 4 cases (1.7%)

Table 2. Modes of functional neck dissection in 143 cases of horizontal supraglottic laryngectomy

Bilateral neck dissection	136 cases (95%)
No neck dissection	7 cases (5%)
Operative mortality	3 cases (2%)

Table 3. Stages of lymph node metastasis (N-stage) in 143 cases of horizontal supraglottic laryngectomy for T_1- and T_2-tumours of the larynx

	N_0 −	N_0 +	N_{1-2} −	N_{1-2} +	N_3+	not diss. N_0	
T_1	32	6	7	−	2	2	49
T_2	54	6	21	6	2	5	94
	86	12	28	6	4	7	143

Table 4. Survival rates (in percent) of 143 cases of supraglottic cancer, treated by horizontal supraglottic laryngectomy, with regard to the T- and N-stage

		N_0 −	N_0 +	N_{1-2} −	N_{1-2} +	N_3+	not diss. N_0
T_1	3 years	93.9	83.3	71.4	−	0	50.0
	5 years	85.7	66.7	71.4	−	0	50.0
T_2	3 years	90.6	33.3	73.7	50.0	50.0	60.0
	5 years	87.2	25.0	61.1	40.0	50.0	50.0

Table 3 gives the preoperative tumor stage in relation to three factors: a) clinical condition of the lymph nodes; b) postoperative histology; and, finally, c) comparison to patients who did not undergo neck dissection. The majority of the cases had the clinical stage N_0-. However, a considerable number of false negative cases turned out to be positive in lymph node histology. There were 4 cases of N_3, all of which underwent classic neck dissection.

Table 4 shows the survival rates of the patient categories listed in table 3. The survival rates for T_1 and T_2N_0- were essentially identical. The T_2 survival rate dropped only in cases of histologically positive lymph nodes, fixed lymph node metastases, and in those cases which did not undergo neck dissection.

The survival table (Table 5) shows that after 5 years the overall survival rate of the 143 cases examined was 79.4%.

Table 6 examines the site of 11 local recurrences (7.7%). Six cases recurred at the base of the tongue above the laryngeal stump, 1 case to the anterior commissure and 4 to the vocal cords. Of these 11 patients (Table 7), who were submitted to various

Table 5. Over-all survival table after horizontal supraglottic laryngectomy (n = 143)

Key
Alive   = alive at start of interval
Died   = died during the interval
Lost   = lost to follow-up
At risk = exposed to risk
% D.   = proportion dying
% A.   = proportion surviving
Cum.   = cumulative survival

Years	Alive	Lost	At risk	Died	% D.	% A.	Cum.
1	143	–	143	13	0.0909	0.9091	909
2	130	2	121	5	0.0413	0.9587	871
3	115	2	100	3	0.0300	0.9700	845
4	96	–	88	4	0.0454	0.9546	806
5	84	2	72	1	0.0138	0.9862	794
6	70	–	69	–	0.0000	1.0000	794
7	69	21	54.5	–	0.0000	1.0000	794
8	44	5	39.5	–	0.0000	1.0000	794
9	37	6	27	–	0.0000	1.0000	794
10	24	1	10.5	–	0.0000	1.0000	794
11	10	1	6.5	–	0.0000	1.0000	794
12	6	1	4.5	–	0.0000	1.0000	794
13	4	1	0.5	–	0.0000	1.0000	794

Table 6. Frequency and localization of local recurrences after horizontal supraglottic laryngectomy (n = 143)

Superior	6 cases
Inferior:	
Anterior	1 case
Lateral	4 cases

treatments, 46% (5 patients) survived. It is worth noting that two of the surviving patients were given a combination of surgical and radiation therapy. For those patients who did not survive, death occurred after an average of 13 months after the recurrence appeared.

Lymph node recurrence was present in 6 cases (Table 8): only 2 patients (33.3%) are still alive. One of these was preoperative stage N_0- and the other one N_{0^+}. The

Table 7. 5 years survival of patients with local recurrence after horizontal supraglottic laryngectomy (n = 143)

Treatment	Patients	Died	Alive
TL + RX	2	–	2
RX	5	2	3
TL	1	1	–
Palliation	3	3	–
	11	6 (54%)	5 (46%)
		⋮ mean 13 months	

Table 8. 5 years survival of patients with recurrences of lymph node metastases after horizontal supraglottic laryngectomy (n = 143)

	Patients	Died	Alive
N_{0-}	2	1	1*
N_{0+}	3	2	1
N_{3+}	1	1	–
	6	4 (66.6%)	2 (33.3%)
		⋮ mean 20 months	

Treatment: RX therapy, excepted surgery + RX (*)

Table 9. Complications after horizontal supraglottic laryngectomy (n = 143)

Fixed cord	11%
Mucosal flap	7%
Early oedema	5%
Vestib. stenosis	5%
Late tracheotomy	5%
Late fistulas	1%

former was treated by surgery in combination with postoperative radiation therapy, the latter with radiation therapy alone.

Local complications are considered in Table 9. On the average the feeding tube was removed on the 17th day, the earliest being the 6th and the maximum the 56th day. However, no patient was released before the tube had been removed. The tracheostoma was closed and the cannula removed after the patient had started to eat. The average of 57 days which is shown in the table is somewhat distorted by the fact that 8 patients (13%) were discharged with the cannula still in place, to be removed at a later date. Three of these patients (2% of the total) were never decannulated.

Results of Supraglottic Horizontal Laryngectomy

I. SERAFINI, Vittorio Veneto

The clinical material of the author consisted of 487 patients with carcinoma of the larynx:
180 (=37%) underwent horizontal partial laryngectomy,
105 (=21%) underwent vertical partial laryngectomy,
144 (=30%) had a total laryngectomy, while
49 (=10%) had other kinds of reconstructive surgery, and
9 cases (=2%) were treated by radiotherapy alone.

Horizontal partial resection of the larynx by Alonso's method comprised more than one third of all surgical interventions for carcinoma of the larynx.

In 97 cases the classical supraglottic resection was carried out. It was extended to excision of the base of the tongue, one arytenoid cartilage, or one piriform sinus in 36 cases. A three quarters resection of the larynx was carried out in 47 cases. Functional neck dissection was performed bilaterally in 100 cases, unilaterally in 48, and no neck dissection was indicated in 32 cases.

Regarding the TNM-classification, our material (Table 1) appeared heterogeneous in so far as T_1 and T_2 cases (with classical Alonso procedure), T_3 tumours (submitted to 3/4 resection) and T_4 tumours (with extended horizontal laryngectomy) were also represented.

With respect to the histological grading most frequently (37%) well differentiated squamous cell carcinomas were observed, followed by low grade differentiation in 30% and by medium grade malignancies in 27%. There were only 4% carcinomata in situ and 2% undifferentiated carcinomas.

The most frequent postoperative complications were
unilateral paresis of the N. hypoglossus   7%
hemorrhage from the tracheostomy   5%
bronchopneumonia due to aspiration   4%
obstructive edema and absolute dysphagia   3%
postoperative mortality   2%

In 174 cases (=97%) the feeding tube could be removed after 21 days on average, ranging from 14 to 30 days. In 169 cases (=94%) the definite closure of the tracheo-

Table 1. T- and N-stages of 180 cases of supraglottic horizontal laryngectomy operated from 1974 to 1981

$T_{is} N_0$	2	$T_2 N_1$	17
$T_{1a} N_0$	13	$T_2 N_2$	3
$T_{1a} N_1$	5	$T_3 N_0$	12
$T_{1a} N_2$	1	$T_3 N_1$	5
$T_{1b} N_0$	36	$T_3 N_2$	2
$T_{1b} N_1$	20	$T_4 N_0$	9
$T_{1b} N_2$	6	$T_4 N_1$	17
$T_2 N_0$	26	$T_4 N_2$	5
		$T_4 N_3$	1

stoma could be performed after 29 days on average (4–60 days), and all patients started phonation after a few postoperative days.

Table 2 shows all our oncological results: Local recurrence was detected in 16 patients (=9%), regional lymph node metastases occurred in 23 patients (=13%), distant metastases were diagnosed in 11 cases (=6%). It has to be emphasized, however, that in the group without prophylactic neck dissection subsequent lymph node metastases were observed in 18%, while recurrence of regional lymph nodes occurred in only 10% of the cases with prophylactic neck dissection. There was a slight increase of local recurrences (+1%) in those 135 cases operated before more than three years. The same was true (+2%) of lymph node recurrence.

The site of local recurrences is illustrated by Table 3: the base of the tongue in 4%, the glottis in 3%, the piriform sinus in 1%, and the arytenoid or the tonsils in 0.5% each.

Distant metastasis was most frequent in the lungs (4%), while other sites (pancreas, skin, intestinum) totalled less than 0.5%. They may be due to another primary tumour (Table 4).

40 patients (22%) required further surgery: total laryngectomy for absolute dysphagia became necessary in 6 cases (3%), total laryngectomy for local recurrence

Table 2. Oncological results of supraglottic horizontal laryngectomy (180 cases between 1974 and 1981)

Overall	
Local recurrence	16 (9%)
Lymph node metastasis	23 (13%)
Distant metastasis	11 (6%)
Cases with over 3 years survival (n = 135)	
Local recurrence	14 (10%)
Lymph node metastasis	20 (15%)
Distant metastasis	8 (6%)

Table 3. Analysis of local recurrences after supraglottic horizontal laryngectomy (n = 180)

Base of the tongue	7 (4%)
Glottis	5 (3%)
Piriform Sinus	2 (1%)
Arytenoid	1 (0.5%)
Tonsil	1 (0.5%)

Table 4. Localization of distant metastases after supraglottic horizontal laryngectomy (n = 180)

Lung	8 (4%)
Pancreas	1 (0.5%)
Intestine	1 (0.5%)
Skin	1 (0.5%)

Table 5. Analysis of the causes of death after supraglottic horizontal neck dissection

Overall (n = 180, between 1974 and 1981)	
Distant metastases	11 (6%)
Lymph node metastases	8 (5%)
Local recurrence	4 (2%)
Postoperative complications	4 (2%)
Reasons not due to tumour	4 (2%)
135 Cases with more than 3-years survival (n = 135)	
Distant metastases	8 (6%)
Lymph node metastases	7 (5%)
Local recurrence	3 (2%)
Postoperative complications	4 (3%)
Reasons not due to tumour	3 (2%)

Table 6. Synopsis of oncological and functional results after supraglottic horizontal laryngectomy (180 cases operated between 1974 and 1981)

Alive	149 (83%)
More than 3-years survival	110 (81%)
Larynx preserved	133 (74%)
Salvage laryngectomy	16 (9%)

was required in 14 patients (8%), and we had a mortality rate of 4 (=2.9%). A second procedure for recurrent regional lymph node metastases after functional neck dissection became necessary in 20 patients (=11%) of whom 8 died later (=40%).

According to these data there was a total mortality rate of 31 out of 180 cases (=17%). Among the causes of death distant metastases were the most important (6%), followed by regional lymphatic spread (5%). Local recurrences, postoperative complications (in two cases a massive hemorrhage from the tracheostomy), one cardial infarction, one acute lung edema, and other unrelated problems, totalled two percent each (Table 5). In the group operated more than three years ago the mortality rate increased from 17 to 19%.

In conclusion: out of a group of 180 patients operated between 1974 and 1981 for laryngeal supraglottic carcinoma by a horizontal partial laryngectomy 149 (=83%) are still alive. 110 (=81%) patients had a crude survival time of more than three years, in 133 cases (=74%) of this population the larynx could be preserved. 16 patients (=9%) were submitted to subsequent salvage total laryngectomy (Table 6).

Oncological and Functional Results of Horizontal Partial Laryngectomy

M. F. Vega, Madrid

240 patients with supraglottic carcinoma were treated by horizontal partial laryngectomy (H.P.L.). Additional prophylactic radiotherapy with telecobalt was applied to the cervical nodes. During the last twelve years a homolateral functional neck dissection was complemented by telecobalt therapy if the neck specimen indicated lymph node involvement. In this retrospective study all patients who had died either of a second disease or were lost to follow up were considered as dead at the date of their last examination.

There were 12 deaths caused by postoperative complications, and 3 deaths caused by secondary diseases.

4 patients were lost to follow up before the first postoperative year,
11 patients were lost to follow up between the 1st to 3rd postoperative year,
12 patients were lost to follow up between the 3rd and 5th postoperative year.

Table 1 gives the survival rates of all patients with H.P.L., and Table 2 the survival rates correlated to the post-surgical state of the tumor.

The prognosis depends on the extension of the laryngeal lesion into the hypopharynx, while H.P.L. offers a fair chance of survival even for the advanced tumor confined to the endolarynx (Table 3).

The presence of metastatic nodes is the principal prognostic index as can be observed in Table 4, which shows the survival rate correlated to the postsurgical stage of regional lymph node metastases. As mentioned before, the therapeutic regimen was changed from an expectant attitude with prophylactic regional radiotherapy to

Table 1. Survival rate after horizontal partial laryngectomy

Alive after one year	207/240 (=86.25%)
Alive after three years	147/215 (=68.37%)
Alive after five years	100/185 (=54.00%)

Table 2. Global survival rates after H.P.L. according to the post-surgical tumor stage

	1 year	3 years	5 years
Stage I	118/119 (93.0%)	89/114 (78.0%)	64/99 (65.0%)
Stage II	35/40 (87.5%)	26/34 (76.5%)	18/29 (62.0%)
Stage III	19/20 (95.0%)	13/19 (68.0%)	7/15 (47.0%)
Stage IV	25/34 (65.0%)	19/48 (35.5%)	11/42 (25.0%)

Results of Horizontal Partial Resections as the Basis of Surgical Indications 227

Table 3. Survival rates after H.P.L. according to the T-stage

	1 year	3 years	5 years
T_1N_0	119/128 (93.0%)	89/114 (78.0%)	64/99 (65.0%)
T_2N_0	35/40 (87.5%)	26/34 (76.5%)	18/29 (62.0%)
T_3N_0	5/5 (100%)	4/4 (100%)	3/5 (100%)
T_4N_0	14/22 (64.0%)	10/22 (45.5%)	5/18 (25.0%)

Table 4. Survival rates after horizontal partial laryngectomy according to the postsurgical N

	1 year	3 years	5 years
N_0	173/195 (89.0%)	129/174 (74.0%)	90/149 (60.5%)
N_+	34/45 (75.5%)	18/41 (44.0%)	10/36 (28.0%)

Table 5. Survival rates of N_0-stages after H.P.L. according to prophylactic treatment of the lymphatics

	1 year	3 years	5 years
H.P.L.$\pm$Co^{60}	74/87 (85.0%)	51/81 (63.0%)	40/76 (52.5%)
H.P.L.+Neck diss.	106/115 (92.0%)	84/100 (84.0%)	51/76 (67.0%)

prophylactic homo- or bilateral functional neck dissection with additional telecobalt therapy in the event of postsurgical verification of lymph node involvement.

Table 4 correlates the survival rates with the existence of lymph node metastases at the time of surgery. Table 5 shows the effect of prophylactic treatment of the regional lymph nodes in N_0-stages. It became evident that prophylactic functional neck dissection increased the survival rate by about 15%.

Functional Results of Partial Horizontal Laryngectomies

We have classified the functional results as follows:
a) Good: Good voice, no problems in swallowing, patient decannulated.
b) Fair: Voice slightly hoarse, some problems in swallowing liquids, patient with a plugged cannula.
c) Poor: Voice very hoarse, serious problems in swallowing liquids, patient with an open cannula.

Phonation: The phonation is usually normal 30 to 45 days after the operation. It is necessary to make the patient speak on the 4th or the 5th day after the operation to prevent arytenoid paralysis and fibrosis of the remaining larynx. However, in a 13% of the cases the patient never recover a normal voice:

Good	86.50%
Fair	8.10%
Bad	5.40%

Deglutition: If we ask a patient after a supraglottic laryngectomy, how he eats, he will usually answer that he eats very well, but if we investigate a little further we will find that he has some problems in swallowing liquids.

In our series those were the deglutition results:

Good	82.15%
Fair	11.35%
Bad	6.50%

Respiratory Status: In the majority of the cases the cannula can be removed between 15 and 45 days. However, sometimes, especially in cases of postoperative radiotherapy, if the remaining larynx has not been protected, laryngeal stenosis occurs which means that the patient has to wear a tracheostomy tube for life, or at least for a long period, which has occurred in 15% of our patients:

Good	90%
Fair	8%
Bad	2%

Horizontal Glottectomy: Results

A. STAFFIERI, Ferrara

The present study, carried out in May 1982, deals with the results of horizontal glottectomies performed at the E.N.T. Clinic of the University of Ferrara from February 1973 to December 1978. The dead line of December 1978 was established in order to have a minimum follow-up of 3 years for all patients. A total of 22 horizontal glottectomies were performed during that period. All patients were males, and their ages ranged from 43 to 70.

The tumor sites were as follows:
2 bilateral cancers of the vocal cords;
5 diffuse hyperkeratoses associated with carcinoma in situ;
4 verrucous cancers of the glottis;
11 cancers of one vocal cord invading the controlateral vocal cord via the anterior commissure.

Two patients expired shortly (on the 7th and 14th day) after the surgical procedure due to cardiovascular complications. Another patient expired after 2 years due to a pre-existing cirrhosis of the liver.

Table 1. Stages of functional recovery after horizontal glottectomy (n=22)

Decannulation		Deglutition (removal of nasogastric tube)	
Mean	9th day	Mean	7th day
Minimum	6th day	Minimum	6th day
Maximum	20th day	Maximum	13th day

Table 2. Incidence of local recurrence after horizontal glottectomy (n=22)

2 verrucous cancers .... TL .... over 5 years survival
1 carcinoma .... TL .... over 5 years survival
1 carcinoma .... RX therapy .... over 5 years survival
1 carcinoma .... RX therapy .... lost at 3rd year

Table 3. 3- to 5-years survival rates after horizontal glottectomy (n=22)

	at risk	dead	survival rate	
"fair"	22	3	86.4%	3rd year
	21	4	80.9%	4th year
	17	4	76.5%	5th year
"unfair"	22	6	72.7%	3rd year
	21	7	66.6%	4th year
	17	8	52.9%	5th year

4 patients were lost: 1 at the first year,
2 at the second year,
1 at the third year.

Table 1 indicates the stages of functional recovery: removal of the tracheotomy tube, closing of the stoma and initiation of natural swallowing. Only one patient had problems with tube removal since he had a voluminous mucosal flap which had to be surgically removed before discharge.

There were 5 local recurrences (Table 2) all of which recovered and, with the exception of one with whom contact was lost after 3 years, all are still alive 5 years after the first surgical procedure.

Only one patient, a year after surgery, manifested a N_3 lymph node. Although he underwent a classic neck dissection he expired a year later of generalized metastases.

Table 3 examines the 3-, 4- and 5-years survival rates. Since the total sample was extremely small it was impossible to draw up a statistical calculation. Thus "fair" and "unfair" percentages were derived including those patients lost to follow-up as alive and expired respectively.

Based on the above, overall survival is comprised between 72.7% and 86.4% for 3 years and between 52.9% and 76.5% for 5 years.

Phonatory Function of the Larynx Following Partial Laryngectomy

S. Vecerina and Z. Krajina, Zagreb

With regard to the importance of the phonatory, respiratory and protective functions of the larynx in their interdependent roles, the purpose of this investigation was the following:

1. To confirm the specificities of the phonatory function of the larynx following partial laryngectomy and reconstruction with fascia, and
2. to prove the hypothesis that the phonatory function of the larynx results from the interplay of the phonatory muscles and the vibrations of the mucosal membrane.

The function of the larynx was investigated in a total of 251 patients. This study included cases with vertical, combined or horizontal laryngectomy, and the control group. The laryngeal function had to be analyzed on the base of thirty-nine variables, in order to be able to investigate the complicated laryngeal functions following partial laryngectomy. The data were computerized at the University Computer Center in Zagreb. The examinees represented a nonhomogeneous group. Vertical and combined laryngectomies had in common laryngeal reconstruction with the fascia.

The following methods were used in the study of laryngeal function:
1. frontal tomography of the larynx during phonation and swallowing,
2. photofluorography of the act of swallowing,
3. spectral three dimensional acoustic analysis,
4. aerodynamic phonation tests, and
5. histology (with a special technique for demonstrating elastic fibers of the mucous membrane).

Several variations in phonation were observed in two groups of examinees (vertical and combined laryngectomy) and in the control group:
1. supraglottic phonation,
2. glottic phonation,
3. glottic phonation and supraglottic constriction, and
4. phonatory insufficiency.

The phenomenon of supraglottic horizontal vibrations was recorded in the group of examinees with supraglottic phonation. The voice produced by such vibrations was characterized in the sonographic analysis by complete periodicity, low frequency of the fundamental laryngeal tone and acoustic impulses of 0–8000 Hz. The majority of examinees with supraglottic phonation developed supraglottic constriction without vibration. Then, depending on the diameter of the supraglottic constriction, the sonogram recorded either a very high tone or only a noise.

Glottic phonation was very infrequent in patients with vertical and combined laryngectomy. The acoustic picture of the glottic phonation revealed only a few harmonics and formants, an absence of noise and an acoustic lack in the upper two-thirds of the sonogram. In the control group of examinees with glottic phonation and vibration of both vocal cords, a significantly higher number of harmonics, formants and acoustic impulses of 0–8000 Hz were recorded.

The glottic phonation and the simultaneous supraglottic constriction were, as a rule, associated with the appearance of the noise and the periodic distribution of acoustic energy in the lower portion of the sonogram. In cases of single vocal cord vibration, that periodic section of the diagram was significantly narrower than when both vocal cords vibrated. The frequency of the fundamental laryngeal tone was relatively high in all partial laryngectomees, but this did not statistically differ from the frequency of the fundamental laryngeal tone of the control group.

The dependence of noise on the presence of supraglottic constriction was clearly demonstrated with the acoustic voice analysis both before and after surgical removal of the supraglottic folds. The noise was not recorded in cases where the supraglottic folds vibrated horizontally during phonation.

The histologic analysis of individual parts of the laryngeal tissue and the correlation with the vibrating properties in each individual case showed the following: 1. vibrating supraglottic folds have a sufficient number of elastic fibers and thus they can vibrate under certain aerodynamic conditions (if the vocal cords do not vibrate); 2. non-vibrating supraglottic folds (those which do not vibrate in spite of glottic insufficiency) were histologically constructed of non-elastic fibers without glandular elements; and 3. there were no elastic fibers in the laryngeal mucous membrane where the fascia was incorporated and that part of the larynx did not participate in the vibrating process in any of the cases.

When evaluating and comparing our results with those obtained by other scientific investigations of this kind, the following conclusions emerged. Hyperkinesia which leads to supraglottic constriction plays an important role in the phonatory function following partial and vertical laryngectomy. Supraglottic constriction serves as a compensatory mechanism, since surgery and reconstruction have disturbed the natural function of the glottic area. In addition to preserving the vibratory mechanism in the glottic area, supraglottic constriction acts as a generator of noise which fundamentally disturbs the phonatory effect. In this way a de-differentiation of an otherwise highly differentiated phonatory function occurs, since this mechanism normally develops during deglutition.

Phonation results from the interaction of the phonatory motor activity and the mucosal vibratory process. The disturbance of the vibratory process changes the motor activity, or changes of the motor activity of the larynx can stimulate the vibrations of other structures instead of the vocal cords. Hoarseness is etiologically and acoustically a complex phenomenon which is not always due to a periodicity of the glottic area. On the contrary, the supraglottic constriction which generates supraglottic noise leads to severe hoarseness, with complete maintenance of the periodic function of the glottic area.

Oncological Results of Supraglottic Horizontal Partial Laryngectomy (Alonso Operation)

W. STEINER, Erlangen

Between 1976 and 1980, 45 patients were subjected to a supraglottic partial resection of the larynx. The post-operative histological classification revealed an early-stage cancer (pT_1) in only 8 patients. In contrast, 62% of the patients proved to have an advanced lesion ($pT_{3/4}$) (Table 1).

In 1976, the cervical lymph nodes were subjected to primary radical resection on one side, and, when indicated, a second operation on the contralateral side. From 1977 onwards, bilateral functional block dissection of the neck was usually performed. In 30% of the patients, metastases – bilateral in 5% – were verified histologically, all being located in the anterior triangle of the neck (Table 1). As expected, a comparison of the post-operative "T" and "N" stages shows that the probability of cervical metastases becomes greater with increasing tumour size (Table 1). On the basis of our experience to date, admittedly based on a limited number of cases, metastatic spread to the cervical lymph nodes is not to be expected in a supraglottic T_1 carcinoma, classified post-surgically.

Follow-up

By December 31, 1982, 27 (60%) of the 45 operated patients were still alive. Three patients had died of post-operative complications, and one patient each of cervical or cerebral metastases (Table 2).

An analysis of the three recurrent cases, all of whom died of their cancers, shows that only one patient had a residual tumour. An elderly, blind patient had presented with a supraglottic carcinoma ($pT_4N_1M_X$) extending into the piriform sinus. The site and size of the recurrent lesion, together with the time interval of 8 months strongly suggest that it was a residual, not a new cancer.

Table 1. Post-therapeutic TNM distribution (UICC classification, 1979) of 45 patients after surgical treatment of primary supraglottic cancer and the cervical lymph nodes

Supraglottic partial resection (Alonso) 1976–1980 (n = 45)
pTNM-distribution
pN_0: 70%/pN_+ bilateral 5%

pT \ pN	0	1	2	3
1	8	–	–	–
2	7	2	–	–
3	11	3	1	1
4	5	6	1	–

Table 2. Oncological results in 45 patients subjected to supraglottic partial resection and unilateral or bilateral neck dissection

Supraglottic partial resection (Alonso) 1976–1980 (n = 45)	
Follow up: (Dec. 31, 1982)	
Alive	27
Death	16
Due to postoperative complication	3
Tumour unrelated	7
Tumour related	
Local recurrence or second carcinoma in the oro- hypopharynx	3
Late neck metastasis	1
cerebral metastasis	1
second carcinoma oesophagus	1
Lost to follow-up	2

In the other two patients, the time interval of 18 months between the first operation and the appearance of the recurrent tumour, and the site of the lesion on the lateral wall of the sinus piriformis, at the junction of the oro- to hypopharynx suggests that the second lesion was a new carcinoma of the upper digestive tract.

The fact that, up to 31. 12. 83, no tumour had been observed in the residual larynx, and in particular in the glottic regions indicates that the critical period of two years for the appearance of recurrent disease had been exceeded in all patients, despite the fact that in the anterior commissure and in the region of the arytenoid cartilage, it had been possible to excise the tumour with a safety margin of only a few millimetres. This confirms the histological evidence for a lymphatic barrier between the supraglottic and glottic region in the anterior part of the larynx (Kirchner, page 209; Olofsson, page 211).

This fact, together with the clinical follow-up observations, justifies the use of horizontal partial resection even when the lesion extends to the glottis. It is my impression that too many laryngectomies are still being performed in patients in whom a partial resection would be oncologically justified.

It is, however, not merely the oncological results achieved with this technique that are so impressive; the complete functional rehabilitation of most of these patients is, in view of the alternative of mutilation by laryngectomy, a highly satisfactory result, both for the patients and the surgeon (compare also Serafini, page 223; Staffieri, page 228; Vega, page 226).

To date, it was possible to close the tracheostomy in all but one of our patients, in whom the hyoid bone also had to be removed. He required 6 months to learn to swallow again, while all other patients were decannulated, and learned to swallow food and drink within a couple of weeks.

In this connection, the author wishes to draw attention to a technical modification of the procedure. After tumour resection, no sutures were placed in the pharynx or arytenoid region, only the hyoid and thyroid cartilage were adapted by sutures in the usual manner.

This is possibly the explanation for the rapid restitution of the swallowing function, even in patients of advanced age (more than 80 years).

References

Alonso JM (1954) Cancer laryngeo. Paz Montalvo, Madrid
Denecke HJ (1980) Die oto-rhino-laryngologischen Operationen im Mund- und Halsbereicn, Bd. V/Teil 3. Springer, Berlin Heidelberg New York
Naumann HH (1972) Kopf- und Hals-Chirurgie, Bd. 1, Thieme, Stuttgart
Steiner W (1982) Chirurgie des Larynxkarzinoms. Munch Med Wochenschr 124:198

Oncological Results of Horizontal Partial Laryngectomy

J. Wilke, Erfurt

When we started to perform horizontal partial resections of the larynx immediately after its inauguration by Alonso in 1954 a voluntary anterior fistula was established by suturing the outer skin to the mucosa of the endolarynx. It was kept open for six months to allow check up. Today we follow Bainfai's recommendation of reconstruction of a substitute for the ary-epiglottic folds by mobilizing the mucosa of both the medial wall of the piriform sinus and of Morgagni's ventricle. The lateral thirds of the base of the tongue are sutured on both sides to the anterior mucosa of the piriform sinuses in order to provide a substitute for the ary-epiglottic fold.

A triangular mucosal flap is then directed downward to the defect of the thyroid cartilage, and is sutured to the mucosal wound above the anterior commissure. Finally, the lower border of the hyoglossus muscle is sutured to the mylohyoid muscle, and this one to the sternohyoid muscle. This type of surgery was carried out even in cases with tumour invasion of the lingual surface of the epiglottis or with penetration into the retrolingual area. For these cases post-operative irradiation was provided.

Some patients had difficulty in swallowing due to persistent edema of the arytenoids and the interarytenoid region. The tracheostomy had to remain in place for more than four weeks in some instances.

In principle the perivascular lymphatic sheaths were controlled bilaterally. N_1- and N_2-cases were treated by en bloc resection of the enlarged lymph nodes, while those cases with fixed lymph nodes (N_3 stages) were submitted to radical neck dissection.

Table 1. 3 years symptom-free survival after H.P.L. according to the T- and N-stages

T_1N_{0-2}	59/71	(83%)
T_1N_3	7/12	(58%)
$T_{3-4}N_{0-2}$	6/8	(75%)
$T_{3-4}N_3$	11/28	(39%)

Table 1 gives the oncological results of 119 horizontal partial laryngectomies (H.P.L.), performed between 1970 and 1979 in terms of 3 years survival. There were 83 (70%) T_1-tumours and 36 (30.6%) T_{3-4}-tumours. All patients with T_3- or T_4-tumours, due to infiltration of the base of the tongue, had post-operative radiotherapy.

The overall 3-years symptom-free survival for all patients, irrespective of the tumour stage and the modality of treatment was 69.75 percent.

References

Alonso JM (1954) Cancer laringeo. Paz Montalvo, Madrid
Banfai J (1965) Konservative horizontale Larynxexstirpation. Monatsschr Ohrenheilk 99:412
Naumann HH (1972) Kopf- und Halschirurgie Bd. 1 (Hals) Thieme, Stuttgart

Horizontal Supraglottic Laryngectomy with Total Glossectomy – Oncological and Functional Results

P. Kothary and R. Dev, Bombay

Introduction

Cancer of the base of the tongue is one of the most common malignancies of the oral, pharyngeal and laryngeal regions in males in western India. An average of 500 new cases of carcinoma of the tongue base is seen every year. By and large they fall into two main categories, i.e. 1. large exophytic growth at the primary site with minimal neck nodes and 2. small infiltrative growth at the primary site with large neck nodes.

All patients except the very advanced cases with fixed nodes are treated with radiation therapy as the primary mode of treatment. Surgery is offered as a salvage treatment for the failures. Those with residual or recurrent lesions of the vallecula, base of the tongue and/or lingual surface of the epiglottic are offered surgery, i.e. supraglottic laryngectomy with excision of the base of the tongue. Extended supraglottic laryngectomy with total glossectomy is offered to those with recurrent or residual lesions in the suprahyoid regions with minimal palpable neck nodes. The paper presents our work in this field over a period of 20 years.

Material

This is a report of 15 cases in which extended horizontal supraglottic laryngectomy with total glossectomy was performed between 1967 and 1980. These cases were selected from the patients attending the E.N.T.-clinics at the Departments of Surgery at the Sir H. N. Hospital and Tata Memorial Hospital. The cases selected for the operation had extensive cauliflower-like lesions localized to the vallecula, base of the tongue and lingual surface of the epiglottis, not involving the ary-epiglottic fold and/or lateral pharyngeal wall. They had no lymphadenopathy outside the suprahyoid triangle. All these patients had primary radiation therapy as the mode of the treatment.

Besides the extent of the growth other factors taken into consideration before the surgery were the general physical condition of the patient, presence of any systemic disease and the cardio-vascular and pulmonary status of the patients. Their respiratory reserve was normal and their motivation was more than average. All the patients were informed of the nature of the operation and the need for temporary tracheostomy and the use of nasogastric feeding tube.

There were ten males and five females in this series. Their age varied from 30 to 60 years. All of them had the primary disease as described, which was confirmed by direct laryngoscopy to note its extent and the non-involvement of the ary-epiglottic fold, false cords and the lateral pharyngeal wall, etc. These patients had swelling, pain and excessive salivation with varying degrees of dysphagia, bleeding and altered breathing. Five patients had enlarged palpable neck nodes in the suprahyoid region, but only two had histologically proved metastases. The mobility of both the vocal cords was normal and there was very little restriction of the mobility of the tongue. The floor of the mouth was free of the disease.

Our experience with radical total glossectomy for advanced cancers of the tongue with minimal neck nodes have convinced us of the utility of this procedure as a curative procedure without subsequent difficulty in swallowing and phonation. With this in mind the horizontal supraglottic laryngectomy was extended to include total glossectomy in the above group of patients.

Technique of Operation

1. An endotracheal tube was introduced through the initial tracheostomy opening under local anaesthesia.

2. A transverse incision was made at the level of the mid-thyroid region. The incision was deepened to the platysma and the flaps retracted to the level of the lower border of the mandible. Care was taken to preserve the mandibular branch of the facial nerve. The deep fascia was incised at the level of the hyoid and along the posterior belly of the digastric muscle, and the facial vein was clamped, cut and ligated. The submandibular salivary gland was retracted upwards, and the facial artery was identified, severed and ligated.

The standard horizontal supraglottic laryngectomy was performed and is now extended to include the body of the hyoid bone, upper one-fourth thyroid alae with the complete epiglottic/pre-epiglottic space and the complete tongue with all its musculature without excising the floor of the mouth, i.e. the mylohyoid musculature (Fig. 1).

Reconstruction of the excised thyro-hyoid membrane and of the area above the mylohyoid muscle was achieved by the use of a fascia lata graft from the patients lateral aspect of the thigh.

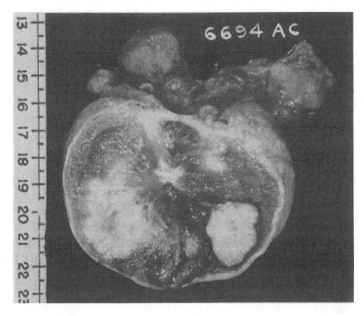

Fig. 1. Operated specimen

No prophylactic neck dissection was performed. The closure of the wound was achieved without any drainage as we feel that continuous intra-oral suction of the saliva and the use of probanthin is of great help in providing a dry oral cavity.

Post-Operative Management

Care of the air passage was achieved by use of cuffed and endotracheal tube and periodic deflation and inflation of the tube with proper use of suction of the oral cavity and the region of the surrounding tracheal area.

Intravenous glucose therapy was used for the first 24 hours, and the feeding via the nasogastric tube was kept for at least two weeks after surgery. This was removed only after the patient was able to breeth normally and speak adequately following surgery.

Post-Operative Mortality and Complications

There were no deaths in the above series and there was no breakdown of the wounds. Two patients had small fistulas which spontaneously closed after a period of two weeks by routine care.

Follow-up and Oncological Results

Of these 15 cases treated from 1967 to 1980, 8 are alive for more than 10 years, 3 were alive for more than 5 years and 2 had recurrent disease in the floor of the mouth requiring secondary surgery after 3 years. One had a recurrence at the level of the false cord anteriorly requiring total laryngectomy. And one was lost to our follow-up after three years.

Functional Results

The rehabilitation of these patients regarding deglutition and speech was highly successful and they were able to return back to their work. The dynamic aspect of swallowing was studied in five of these patients by cine-radiography (Fig. 2). The larynx being preserved in these cases, with restoration of the thyro-hyoid membrane by a fascia lata graft has helped to allow phonation following surgery. An attempt is made to describe the separate components of the continuous process of deglutition in the normal and altered conditions following extended horizontal supraglottic laryngectomy with total glossectomy.

Oral Phase

This is a voluntary phase and includes the propulsion of the bolus from the mouth through the isthmus of the fauces into the oropharynx. It is at this stage that the tongue plays a predominant part. Solid food is first chopped by chewing. This masticatory process may be voluntary or reflex and is not altered after a total glossectomy. Normally, fluid is drawn into the mouth by creating a sub-atmospheric pressure in the mouth by retraction of the tongue in contact with the palate. With the removal of the tongue and the infra-glossal musculature, it is not possible to produce a negative pressure within the mouth and hence the act of the sucking is not possible. Fluids have therefore to be poured into the mouth, and the normal labial and facial muscles facilitate this process.

In a normal person, the lubricated bolus of food is forced backwards by a piston like movement of the tongue resulting from elevation of the floor of the mouth by the mylo-hyoid complex of muscles. This is combined with a backward movement of the base of the tongue by the hyoglossus and styloglossus muscles. The anterior part of the tongue is also elevated and pressed against the hard palate. With the removal of the tongue this is not possible. To compensate for this, the patient is advised to take smaller amounts of food, so that the resulting bolus requires very little propulsive movement. He is also advised to place it near the region of the last molar teeth, to facilitate the decanting of the bolus by raising the head backward, a process which is not necessary in normal human beings. The palato-glossal contact being disturbed, the closure of the faucial opening is not possible, and the ingesta cannot be held in the mouth. Once the bolus touches the posterior pharyngeal wall, the entire pharyngeal musculature seems to rise to receive the bolus of food like a magnet attracting an iron piece, and the pharyngeal phase starts (Fig. 2).

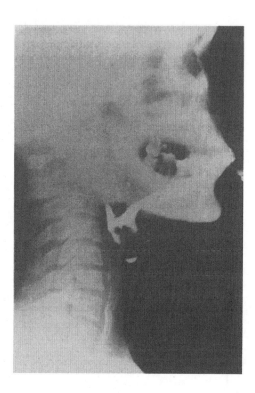

Fig. 2. Barium swallow film 6 weeks after surgery

Pharyngeal Phase

The reflex by which the pharynx rises to meet the descending bolus, is initiated by the receptors in the soft palate and the pharynx. In glossectomized cases, this action seems to be more pronounced and compensates a great deal of the lack of propulsive movements in the oral phase. This observation necessitates the preservation of the pharyngeal musculature in toto during extensive surgery of the tongue.

Normally the bolus is prevented from escaping into the nasopharynx by the apposition of the soft palate with Passavant's ridge on the posterior pharyngeal wall. The lateral and posterior pharyngeal walls also participate in this action. This mechanism is not disturbed after glossectomy.

More important is the prevention of the bolus from entering the endolarynx. This is achieved by the following factors:

1. During the second stage of swallowing, respiration is inhibited. This remains intact after glossectomy.

2. The larynx is suddenly and forcibly elevated into contact with the base of the tongue. The entrance to the larynx is thus drawn upwards under the shelter of the backward protruding base of the tongue, the powerful elevation being mainly effected by the stylohyoid, stylopharyngeus, digastric and mylohyoid muscles. Following this type of total glossectomy, this mechanism is almost totally lost. The larynx is a little elevated by the newly constructed floor of the mouth and by the contraction of the few muscles left behind (Mm. mylohyoideus, stylohyoideus, stylopharyngeus

and the posterior belly of the digastric). However, this elevation is not of much value as there is no protection available by the base of the tongue.

3. Closure of the laryngeal aditus: the aryepiglottic folds are approximated by the sphincteric action of the aryepiglottic and oblique arytenoid muscles. At a lower level, the thyro-arytenoid muscles approximate the false vocal cords or ventricular folds in a second line of defence. The Rima glottitis is closed by the lateral cricoarytenoid muscles adducting the vocal cords, and by the approximation of the arytenoid cartilages.

These protective mechanisms are most important following a total glossectomy with preservation of the larynx. The sensory component of the reflex is important. Following surgery the preservation of the superior laryngeal nerves and the pharyngeal branches of the vagus nerve have helped in a near normal sensory laryngeal component.

Esophageal Phase

The passage of a peristaltic wave down the pharyngeal constrictor muscles brings the bolus to the opening of the esophagus. There is a natural stop at the cricopharyngeus sphincter, and a possibility of laryngeal aspiration, especially with a shorter and shallower piriform fossa in a glossectomized patient. To obviate this, we advise the patients to initiate coughing towards the end of a swallow.

Discussion

Depending on the motivation, intelligence, and vigilance of the patient the ability to swallow was achieved within 2 to 6 weeks following surgery. Initial aspiration problems were reduced to a minimum by training the patients to cough out the residual fluid and saliva lying over the false cords. These patients were trained in this skill by one of the well trained motivated patients, and were advised to do this prior to sleep. The sensory denervation of the larynx was prevented by careful preservation of the superior laryngeal nerves during surgery. The compensatory mechanism of the false and true cords have helped in prevention of any aspiration problems. This was confirmed by cine-radiographic studies. One has to emphasize the importance of the recovery of strong pharyngeal movements and the powerful development of pharyngeal muscular action for the development of a near normal act of swallowing liquids and solids following glossectomy. Any further extension of surgery involving the pharyngeal musculature would necessitate the removal of the larynx. Hence defunctioning of even a small segment of the pharyngeal musculature of the middle constrictor by surgery or damage to the pharyngeal branch of the vagus nerve have to be avoided.

Rehabilitation of Phonation

The following hypotheses have emerged from our studies: 1. The restoration of the ability to swallow was a precondition of phonatory rehabilitation, and 2. there are

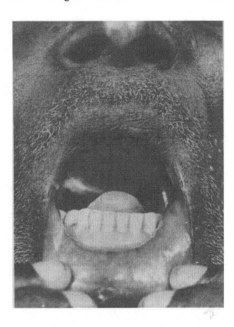

Fig. 3. Speech device used to improve the speech following surgery

phonatory components of the compensatory articulation patterns after glossectomy. They were developed by the glossectomy patients training mandibular, labial, buccal and palatal movements. These were examined by means of cinefluorography.

An artificial tongue made of silastic material was anchored on the lower teeth to serve as the anterior third of the tongue and another attached to the upper alveolus served as posterior one-third of the tongue (Fig. 3). To study the acoustic effect of this device certain experiments were carried out with selected vowels and consonants. Speech samples including the vowels 'I' 'U' were paired with consonants 'D' 'G' 'S' 'R' and 'Y'. The general result of the experiment indicates that this device is far behind in action and mobility compared to the natural tongue. Although the intelligibility test of the patient's speech showed improvement in 'G' 'R' and 'F' with the speech device.

For the total group of patients, the team concluded that 'Z' was produced by means of a bilabial tension obstruction with the lips in closer approximation than usual; 'n' was produced by momentary velar contraction followed by quick uvular relaxation with the lips almost approaching complete adduction. The 'g' was produced by pharyngeal constriction with a slight bulging of the retroglossal pharyngeal wall. Lower lip contact with upper alveolar ridge produced 'd'. Both 'l' and 'r' appeared to be produced by a combination of pharyngeal, uvular and buccal movements. For the 'l' a slight uvular vibration may provide the air stream division critical for this phoneme. An adequate frontal 'l' was developed recently by bowing the lips, causing them to adduct only in the center, with air stream outlet at each corner. The 'r' is normally achieved by tongue dividing the oral cavity into a large posterior and small anterior cavity, coupled by a narrow channel. The glossectomee compensates by retroflexing both lips, thrusting the mandible forward and elevating it so that the small anterior cavity is created within the lower retroflexion. The 'th' can be successfully made by anterior folding of the upper lip, which then is drawn up and back over the lower lip, with quick, sharp air explosion. Patients with total glossectomy consistently use an anterior mandibular thrust at varying excursions for the vowels.

More than 80% of the above 15 operated patients had intelligible speech for communication with the members of their family and with the people working with them in their various occupations.

References

Kothary PM, et al. (1973) Swallowing without tongue. Bombay Hospital Journal, Vol 15, 2:58–60
Kothary PM, et al. (1974) Radical total glossectomy. J Surg 61:109–212
Kothary PM (1975) Cancer of head and neck. Vol: Editor Chambers: 175–178. Excerpta Medica Series

Cineradiographic and Manometric Measurements of Deglutition Following Horizontal Partial Laryngectomy

E. Mozolewski, K. Jach, M. Sulikowski, and R. Wysocki, Szczecin

The pharyngeal phase of deglutition following regular and extended horizontal supraglottic laryngectomy was studied in 53 cases clinically, by cineradiography (frame by frame more than 300,000 single pictures) and by manometry (perfusion-manometry was applied in only 5 cases). In the present report only the most significant results were considered. The pharyngeal phase of deglutition was impaired considerably following resection of the supraglottic part of the larynx. Aspiration of food particles into the lower respiratory tract could be shown in 34% of cases. Two main forms of inadequate protection of the respiratory tract have been found, viz.: post- and intra-deglutition overflow. The time course of deglutition was approximately similar to the normal only in about 20%. In the remaining cases the time of deglutition was extended considerably up to as much as 10 sec. Beside anatomical changes of the residual larynx and the tongue base, the following factors influence the deglutition:
1. close topographic connection between the residual larynx and the tongue base
2. efficient glottis closure
3. extent of mobility of the residual larynx
4. extent of inferior and posterior mobility of the tongue
5. efficient peristalsis of pharyngeal muscles
6. proper coordination between propulsive power of the tongue and pharynx and relaxation of the pharyngeal sphincter.

Our methods of proceeding were based on the above investigations. They allowed a smooth deglutition more frequently compared to earlier surgical methods.

Two conclusions could be derived from our cineradiographic studies:
1. Deglutition following typical or extended supraglottic horizontal laryngectomy may show many undesirable disturbances, though usually of low intensity, due to the altered anatomy of the larynx, pharynx and tongue, their topographic relations and especially to the reduced mobility.
2. Our cineradiographic and manometric studies of the pathophysiology of deglutition have helped to understand the mechanisms of these disturbances and showed how to manage them.

E. Surgical Management of the Lymphatic System

Why Perform a Functional Neck Dissection?

C. Calearo, G. P. Teatini, and A Staffieri, Ferrara

Nomenclature

CND = Classic neck dissection, developed by G. Crile in 1906 (synonym: radical neck dissection).
FND = Functional neck dissection, developed by O. Suarez and popularized in the sixties by E. Bocca.

Advantages of FND (in Comparison with CND)

FND spares – whenever permitted by pathology – the sternomastoid muscle and the internal jugular vein. Therefore
a) a bilateral operation is feasible in the same session,
b) the carotid arteries remain covered by the sternomastoid muscle,
c) the cosmetic result is excellent.

Common Errors About FND

1. FND is but a conservative modification of CND. Consequently,
2. FND is less radical than CND. Consequently,
3. FND is indicated only as a prophylactic procedure (in N_0 cases).
All three statements are *wrong*.

1. The surgical principle of FND thoroughly differs from CND. In the latter, all muscular and vascular structures of the lateral neck compartments, with the single exception of the carotid arteries, are severed caudad, elevated from the underlying planes in a cranial direction and excised (as an alternative procedure one may commence cephalad and proceed towards the clavicle). The principle of FND consists of elevating the fascias from the underlying planes. Thus, the contents of the spaces enveloped by the fascias can be safely removed. As the sternomastoid muscle and the internal jugular vein lie outside these spaces, they may be dissected and preserved.
   Consequently,
2. with regard to the removal of lymph nodes FND is as radical as CND.
   Consequently,

3. FND can be also applied in cases of metastases, provided they have not broken through the lymph node capsule.

Outline of Surgical Technique

FND starts with the *incision of the external cervical fascia* (Fig. 1). Its elevation exposes the external aspect of the sternomastoid muscle, as well as the submandibular gland with the digastric and stylohyoid muscles running below (Fig. 2).

One important landmark is Erb's point indicating the exit of the spinal accessory nerve from the posterior margin of the sternomastoid muscle.

The First Space to be Dissected is the Lateral Cervical Triangle. Its top which abuts the mastoid process, is covered by the sternomastoid muscle, and is called the submuscular recess. To expose it, the medial margin of the sternomastoid muscle must be strongly retracted posteriorly (Fig. 3). When the dissection of the recess is accomplished, the specimen has to be slid under the sternomastoid muscle and conveyed into the lower part of the lateral space, corresponding to the posterior neck triangle (Fig. 4). This is dissected after the spinal accessory nerve has been isolated at its entrance into the trapezius muscle (Fig. 5).

Important Landmarks are:

in the submuscular recess
    the transverse process of the atlas, identified by palpation, corresponds to the internal jugular vein and (along the posterior border of the vein) to the spinal accessory nerve (blunt dissection is required here!);
    the ventral margin of the levator scapulae muscle corresponds to the posterior limit of the recess;
in the posterior neck triangle
    the anterior border of the trapezius muscle marks the posterior limit of the triangle;
    the phrenic nerve runs along the external aspect of the anterior scalenus muscle (caution during elevation of the fascia!).

The next step is the *dissection of the carotid sheath* (Fig. 6). The sheath must be completely dissected only in the layer which separates the lateral space from the paravisceral space, i.e. from the upper pole of the thyroid gland to the posterior belly of the digastric muscle. Below and above these limits, one confines oneself to elevating the fascia from the carotid arteries and the internal jugular vein. Within these limits, the vein is skeletonized along its whole circumference, and its tributary vessels are ligated and severed. The dorsal branches of the cervical plexus are also sectioned.

The last step is the *dissection of the paravisceral space,* from its caudal tip to its cranial border, i.e. to the arbitrary margin at the level of the posterior digastric muscle belly. The arteries feeding the viscera run on the floor of this space: they should remain untouched. The hypoglossal nerve is isolated from its surrounding venous plexus (Fig. 7).

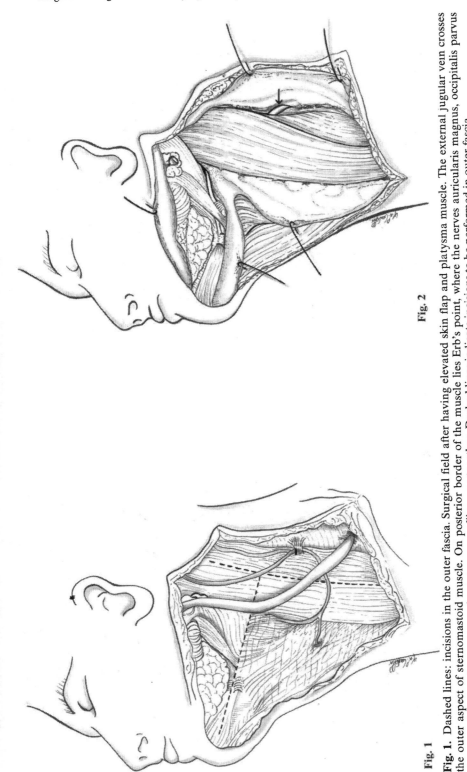

Fig. 1. Dashed lines: incisions in the outer fascia. Surgical field after having elevated skin flap and platysma muscle. The external jugular vein crosses the outer aspect of sternomastoid muscle. On posterior border of the muscle lies Erb's point, where the nerves auricularis magnus, occipitalis parvus sive mastoideus and transversus sive cutaneous colli merge together. Dashed lines indicate incisions to be performed in outer fascia

Fig. 2. Surgical field after elevation of the fascia. Arrow indicates Erb's point. External jugular vein has been ligated at the inferior parotis pole. The outer fascia has been incised, elevated from the underlying planes and retracted by means of hooks. Arrow indicates the spinal accessory nerve, which emerges from the posterior margin of the sternomastoid muscle within 2 cm above Erb's point

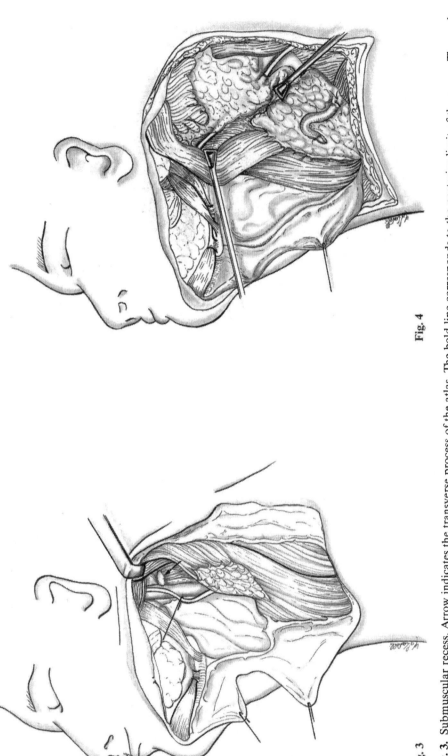

Fig. 3. Submuscular recess. Arrow indicates the transverse process of the atlas. The bold line corresponds to the posterior limit of the recess. The angle between digastric and sternomastoid muscles is widely opened by means of retractors. The transverse process of the atlas (*arrow*) is identified by palpation and uncovered, together with the internal jugular vein and the spinal accessory nerve which run before it. The submuscular recess can thus be thoroughly dissected up to the anterior border of the levator scapulae muscle (*bold line*) which markes the posterior limit of the space

Fig. 4. The specimen from the submuscular recess is slid under the sternomastoid muscle and pushed into the posterior neck triangle. After having elevated the fascias both from the upper aspect of the levator scapulae muscle and from the inner aspect of the sternomastoid muscle, the specimen from the submuscular recess is slid under the sternomastoid and conveyed into the posterior neck triangle

Surgical Management of the Lymphatic System

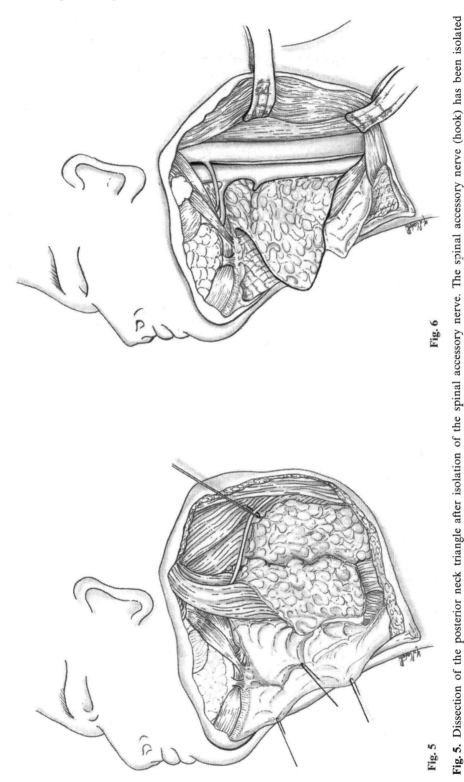

Fig. 5. Dissection of the posterior neck triangle after isolation of the spinal accessory nerve. The spinal accessory nerve (hook) has been isolated throughout its course in the posterior neck triangle. The specimen is slid under the nerve and the caudal portion of the triangle can now be dissected

Fig. 6. Surgical field before starting the dissection of the carotid sheath. Sternomastoid muscle is now retracted backward, while the specimen from the lateral space is strongly pulled in a medial direction. Sheath dissection commences with uncovering vagus nerve

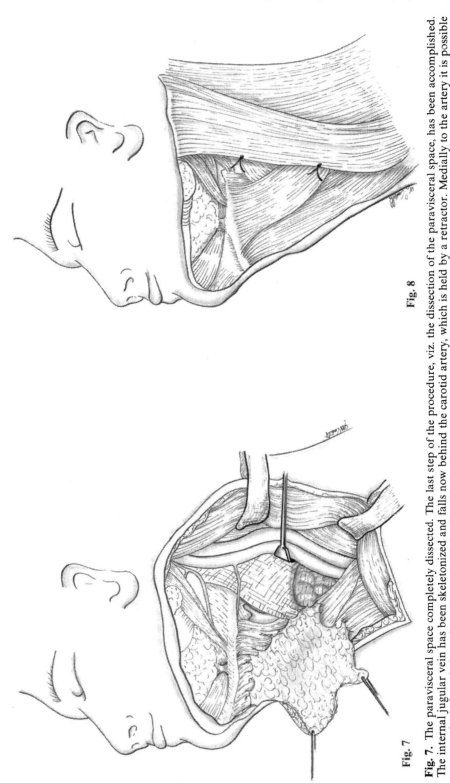

Fig. 7. The paravisceral space completely dissected. The last step of the procedure, viz. the dissection of the paravisceral space, has been accomplished. The internal jugular vein has been skeletonized and falls now behind the carotid artery, which is held by a retractor. Medially to the artery it is possible to appreciate, from below, the upper pole of the thyroid gland, the visceral sheath covering the inferior constrictor muscle with the superior thyroid artery running upon it and the hypoglossus nerve

Fig. 8. Covering of the vessels before wound closure. The sternomastoid muscle is sutured to the strap muscles in order to shelter the big neck vessels

Before closing the wound, the anterior edge of the sternomastoid muscle is sutured to the floor of the paravisceral space, in order to cover the carotid arteries (Fig. 8).

References

Bocca E (1966) Supraglottic laryngectomy and functional neck dissection. J Laryngol Otol 80:831–838

Calearo C, Teatini GP (1983) Functional neck dissection. Anatomical grounds, surgical technique, clinical observations. Ann Otol Rhinol Laryngol (to be published as a supplement)

Crile G (1906) Excision of cancer of the head and neck. JAMA 47:1780–1786

Suarez O (1963) El problema de las metastasis linfaticas y alejadas del cancer de laringe e hipofaringe. Rev Otorinolaringol Santiago 23:83–99

Surgical Treatment of the Cervical Lymph Node System in Laryngeal Carcinoma

W. STEINER, Erlangen

Over the last 20 years, different therapeutic concepts for the treatment of the cervical lymphatics have been employed at the Department of Oto-Rhino-Laryngology at Erlangen.

Roughly three periods can be distinguished:

Between 1962 and 1971, an explorative, usually bilateral dissection of the main cervical lymph nodes in the jugular chain was performed simultaneously with laryngectomy or partial resection of the larynx (LND) (Theissing, G., 1971). Whenever metastases were seen, radical, or, rarely, conservative neck dissection was performed.

Between 1972 and 1976 in accordance with a more stringent concept of radicality, as propagated by several authors in the United States, radical neck dissection (RND) was obligatory, either as a prophylactic measure in cases with advanced tumour stages with no palpable lymph nodes, or curatively in all cases with palpable lymph nodes.

The third period saw the introduction of functional neck dissection. The pathologic-anatomical basis for functional neck surgery worked out by Italian head and neck surgeons, the precise surgical anatomy introduced by Suarez, together with the oncological and functional results reported by the Italian working group (Bocca and Molinari, Milan; Calearo, Staffieri, A., and Teatini, Ferrara), encouraged us, from the beginning of 1977, largely to abandon radical neck dissection, in particular prophylactic radical neck dissection, in favour of a function-preserving procedure (FND).

This article first compares the results achieved with LND and RND in the two above-mentioned periods between 1962 and 1976. It then presents the preliminary results obtained with functional lymphatic neck surgery in laryngeal carcinoma over the period 1977–1981.

As a prerequisite for a comparison of the oncological results, the following features should be mentioned:

All the patients had laryngeal carcinomas treated predominantly by laryngectomy, or by vertical and horizontal partial laryngectomy.

In all the three groups, the histology and tumour stages were very similar; thus, in our comparative reassessment, these parameters need not be taken into further account. All detected lymph node metastases were stage N_1 or N_2, and were localized in the anterior triangle of the neck.

The differences, therefore, relate predominantly to the surgical procedure. In the following analysis of the data the post-therapeutic stage of lymph node invasion (pN) will be the basis for discussion.

The pretherapeutic lymph node stage (N, according to UICC) merely represents a palpatory finding, which is purely subjective. It forms the basis for the pretherapeutic decisions regarding prophylactic or curative therapy. Of greater relevance for the retrospective evaluation of cancer treatment statistics, however, is the true histological stage of the disease.

Patients with Partial or Total Laryngectomy Without Neck Metastases (pN₀)

First a comparison is made between patients with bilateral lymph node dissection of the carotid-jugular space (LND) (n = 111, 1962–1971) and those with radical neck dissection (RND) (n = 74, 1972–1976) (Table 1). After RND 40%, after LND 24% of the patients received radiotherapy to the neck.

Oncological Results. In the group of patients with pN₀ subjected to explorative bilateral lymph node dissection, the five-year survival rate is 51%, and 59% in the patients who received a prophylactic radical neck dissection. In both groups, the percentage of subsequent irradiation is about identical at 17.5% and 16%, respectively. Among the 57 patients with LND who survived for more than five years, a local tumour recurrence with late metastasis occurred in the neck of only one patient. The malignant secondary disease was successfully managed by combined surgery and radiotherapy. In a patient subjected to radical neck dissection, a late metastasis was observed on the contralateral, non-treated, side of the neck. This patient is the only one with malignant secondary disease out of the 44 patients in the group in whom a prophylactic radical neck dissection was performed, and he survived for more than five years.

In the patients who did not survive five years – 49% after bilateral LND, and 41% after RND – malignant secondary disease occurred in more than 50%. In Table 1, it must be pointed out that in one and the same patient several secondary diseases, for example a recurrent tumour, a late metastasis or, a distant metastasis, might have occurred.

Of the patients who died within five years, 77% of those subjected to RND had been given radiotherapy, compared with only 31% after LND. In the LND group

Table 1. Oncological course of laryngeal carcinoma in patients treated by lymph node dissection (carotid-jugular space) (LND) or radical neck dissection (RND), prophylactically (pN₀), between 1962 and 1976

Neck therapy surgery	(1962–1971) Lymphnode dissection (carotid-jugular space) bilateral (LND) (n = 111 pat.)	(1972–1976) Radical neck dissection (RND) unilateral (n = 74 pat.)
Postoperative radiotherapy	27 (24%)	30 (40%)
Survival		
> 5 years	57 (51%)	44 (59%)
Radiotherapy	10 (17.5%)	7 (16%)
Local recurrence or second primary	1	–
Late neck metastasis	1	1
Survival		
< 5 years	54 (49%)	30 (41%)
Radiotherapy	17 (31.5%)	23 (77%)
Local recurrence or second primary	7 (13%)	2 (7%)
Late neck metastasis	13 (24%)	7 (23%)
Stomal recurrence	8 (15%)	7 (23%)
Distant metastasis	4 (7%)	7 (23%)
Causes of death		
Tumour-related	25 (46%)	16 (53%)
Tumour-unrelated	11 (20%)	7 (23%)
Unknown	18 (34%)	7 (23%)

13% of the patients had local recurrent lesions or second primaries in the oropharynx and hypopharynx, compared with 7% in the RND group. Late metastases in the neck were observed about equally frequently (24% and 23%, respectively). In the RND group, stomal recurrences (23%), and distant metastases (23%) predominated vis-a-vis the LND group (15% and 7%, respectively).

Unequivocally tumour-related deaths occurred in 53% of the RND patients and 46% of the LND patients. In the latter group, the percentage of deaths for reasons unknown is, at 34%, markedly higher than in the RND group (23%). Roughly every fifth LND patient, and every fourth RND patient is known to have died from tumour-unrelated causes.

Patients with Partial or Total Laryngectomy with Neck Metastases (pN₁/₂)

Comparison between lymph node dissection of the carotid-jugular space (n = 27, 1962–1971) and radical neck dissection (n = 27, 1972–1976) (Table 2)

Of the 54 patients with histologically confirmed neck metastases after LND (27) or RND (27), about two-thirds were given post-operative radiotherapy.

Table 2. Oncological course of laryngeal carcinoma in patients treated curatively (pN$_{1/2}$) by lymph node dissection (carotid-jugular space) (LND) or radical neck dissection (RND)

Neck therapy surgery	(1962–1971) Lymph node dissection (carotid-jugular space) bilateral (LND) (n = 27 pat.)	(1972–1976) Radical neck dissection (RND) unilateral (n = 27 pat.)
Postoperative radiotherapy	19 (70%)	18 (66%)
Survival		
> 5 years	5 (18%)	11 (41%)
Radiotherapy	5 (100%)	7 (64%)
Late neck metastasis	–	1
Survival		
< 5 years	22 (82%)	16 (59%)
Radiotherapy	14 (64%)	11 (69%)
Local recurrence or second primary	6 (27%)	3 (19%)
Late neck metastasis	7 (32%)	7 (44%)
Stomal recurrence	8 (36%)	4 (25%)
Distant metastasis	1 (5%)	2 (12%)
Causes of death		
Tumour-related	17 (77%)	11 (69%)
Tumour-unrelated	1 (5%)	4 (25%)
Unknown	4 (18%)	1 (6%)

Oncological Results. The five-year survival rate of 41% in RND patients (n = 11) is much higher than the 18% of the LND group, all of the latter being subjected to post-operative radiotherapy (Table 2). In this group of patients, a late metastasis in the neck was found in only one patient.

Eighty-two percent of the LND group compared to 59% of the RND group died within 5 years. The difference of 23% is high; the percentage of patients subjected to post-operative radiotherapy is almost identical at 64% and 69%, respectively. Most patients (77% after LND and 69% after RND) unequivocally died of their cancer disease; in four of the LND group, the cause of death is unknown.

In these patients with (primary) neck metastases (pN$_{1/2}$), post-therapeutic malignant local and/or regional secondary disease, almost always fatal, is considerably more frequent than in patients with no (primary) metastasis (pN$_0$).

A comparison of the patients with primary neck metastasis (pN$_{1/2}$) who died within 5 years revealed that, for example, a local tumour recurrence, or a second carcinoma in the oro- and hypopharynx was observed somewhat more frequently after LND (27%) than after RND (19%). In contrast, ipsilateral and contralateral late metastases in the neck (44%) were more frequently observed after RND than after LND (32%). The stomal recurrences were more numerous after LND (36%) than after RND (25%). Distant metastases, however, were more frequently found in the radical neck dissection group (12%) than in the LND group (5%). Here, too, it must be remembered that in the 1970s, a more intense interdisciplinary search for distant metastases was undertaken.

In this group of 54 patients (pN$_{1/2}$), too, the figures quoted for malignant secondary diseases must not simply be added together, since some of the patients presented with "multiple disease", either simultaneously or consecutively.

Patients with Partial or Total Laryngectomy and Functional Neck Dissection (1977–1981)

81 patients with laryngeal carcinomas were subjected to 128 complete or regional functional neck procedures, unilateral or bilateral, depending upon stage and localization (1977–1981) (Table 3).

30 of the 128 surgical specimens (23%) proved to have one or more metastases (pN$_{1/2}$).

Complete Functional Neck Dissection (FND) (1977–1981)

In 32 patients (pN$_{0-2}$), 48 complete functional neck dissections (FND) were performed, a metastasis being confirmed histologically in 16 specimens (33% of the neck dissections) (Table 3).

Table 3. Oncological course of laryngeal carcinoma in patients treated by functional (regional) neck dissection, prophylactically (pN$_0$) or curatively (pN$_{1/2}$), between 1977 and 1981. For a detailed explanation of the multiple findings in patients with secondary malignant disease, and their relationship to death, see text

	Complete functional neck dissection (FND)	Regional functional neck dissection (rFND)	Exploration lymph-node dissection (carotid-jugular space) (LND)
Patients (n = 81)	32	33	16
Neck surgery (n = 128)	46	56	26
pN$_0$ (n = 98)	30	43	25
pN$_{1/2}$ (n = 30)	16 (35%)	13 (23%)	1
Postop. radiotherapy	14 (43%)	17 (52%)	11 (69%)
Alive (1. 1. 1983)	17 (53%)	25 (76%)	12 (75%)
Deaths	15	8	4
– tumour-unrelated	10	3	3
– tumour-related	4 (12.5%)	4 (12%)	1
unknown	1	1	–
Secondary malignant disease			
Local recurrence or second primary	1	4	2
Late neck metastasis			
pN$_0$	2$_c$	4$_i$	2
pN$_{1/2}$	1$_c$	–	–
Stomal recurrence pN$_0$	2	–	–
Distant metastasis	1	2	–

c = contralateral; i = ipsilateral

14 FND patients (43%) were subjected to post-operative radiotherapy on account of positive lymph nodes in the neck (pN$_+$).

Of the patients with pre-operatively negative palpatory findings (N$_0$), 15% had histologically verified metastases in the neck (pN$_+$) (false negatives).

Conversely, 67% with preoperatively palpable nodes (N$_{1/2}$) were shown to be false positives by frozen section histology, or definitive histological work up of the neck dissection specimens, that is no metastases were found.

All histologically detected metastases (pN$_{1/2}$) were localized exclusively in the anterior triangle of the neck.

Oncological Results – Follow up (Table 3). As on 31. 12. 1982, 53% of the patients were still alive. Of the 15 patients who had died by this date, however, only 4 (12.5% of the overall group), had succumbed to their cancer. Two patients later developed a contralateral metastasis, the functionally operated side of the neck having been free of metastases (pN$_0$). One of these two patients had, at the same time, a local recurrent lesion, or a second carcinoma; he subsequently died of his cancer.

In the group of 16 patients with metastases (pN$_+$) in the completely dissected neck, a secondary contralateral metastasis occurred in a single patient, who died of his tumour. Stomal recurrence developed in two patients submitted to prophylactic functional neck dissection (pN$_0$). One of these two patients proved to have metastases in the lungs; both died within one year after the appearance of the malignant secondary disease.

Regional Functional Neck Dissection (rFND) (1979–1981)

By rFND we mean dissection of the anterior triangle, that is the first step of the classical FND. It extends from the base of the skull to below the omohyoid muscle, laterally to beneath the sternocleidomastoid muscle, and down to the deep neck muscles; although the procedure spares the major vessels and nerves, it is oncologically radical.

Between 1979 and 1981, 56 regional functional neck dissections were performed in 33 laryngeal carcinoma patients subjected to partial or total laryngectomy. Metastases (pN$_{1/2}$) were found in 13 dissections (23%) (Table 3).

52% of the patients were submitted to post-operative radiotherapy, most (13) on account of positive lymph nodes in the neck (pN$_+$), the remainder (4) on account of the size of the tumour (pT$_4$).

Oncological Results – Follow up (Table 3). By 31. 12. 1982, 76% were still alive. Four patients (12%) had died of tumour-related causes.

In these, a post-treatment primary tumour recurrence of second primary developed in the oro- and hypopharynx, three of the four also developing a late metastasis on the operated metastasis-free side of the neck (pN$_0$). Cerebral metastases occurred in one patient. One patient with supraglottic cancer pT$_4$N$_0$ with ipsilateral late metastasis and pulmonary metastases, is still alive.

Explorative Lymph Node Dissection of the Jugular Chain (LND) (1980/1981)

The smallest group of patients (16) with the shortest follow-up period comprises patients in whom a, usually bilateral, prophylactic lymph node dissection (LND) (n = 26, 1980/1981) was performed (N_0). Only in one case was a micrometastasis found at definitive histological work-up in the anterior triangle of the neck, the frozen section diagnosis having been negative.

Post-operative radiotherapy was given in two-thirds of the cases (n = 11).

Oncological Results – Follow up (Table 3). On 31. 12. 1982, 75% of the patients were still alive, only one had died of tumour, after unsuccessful attempts at treating the primary tumour recurrence and ipsilateral late metastasis. At the primary exploration, no metastatic lymph nodes had been discovered (pN_0). A primary tumour recurrence in one other patient was successfully managed with combination treatment (surgery and radiotherapy).

Discussion

Results (pN_0 – Lymph Nodes Dissection of the Carotid-Jugular Space/Radical Neck Dissection)

A comparison of the oncological course of patients treated by partial or total laryngectomy, in whom no metastases (pN_0) were found histologically, shows no appreciable difference in the five year survival rate between LND (n = 111) and RND (n = 74).

The fact that in the LND group, a recurrent lesion or a second primary occurred almost twice as often, might be due to the fact that only 31% of the patients with LND were given post-operative radiotherapy as compared with 77% after RND. The percentage of late metastases (n = 7/23%) in the 30 RND (pN_0) patients who died within 5 years, is surprisingly high. Two patients developed a local recurrence or a second primary that might have been the source of the late metastases.

However, among these seven patients six presented with a contralateral metastasis, one with bilateral metastases. In this group of patients unilateral RND, tailored to the extent of the primary tumour, was performed; since no metastases were found (pN_0), a contralateral neck dissection was not performed.

Four patients received subsequent radiotherapy to the primary tumour site and both sides of the neck. Here, a serious drawback of RND manifests itself: since only one side can/may be operated on primarily, possible contralateral, clinically occult, metastases cannot be detected or treated. On average, patients with contralateral metastases survived for 34 months.

The prognosis for patients with ipsilateral or bilateral late metastasis, and in particular, with stomal recurrence, is appreciably poorer. All the seven patients who developed a stomal recurrence after RND (pN_0) – most of them with $T_{3/4}$ tumours of the supraglottic region – died of their cancer within an average of 14 months. Almost every second patient who died succumbed to his tumour.

Overall, among the patients who died within five years, death was tumour-related in 53% after RND, and 46% after LND, the percentage of deaths from unknown causes being 34% in the LND group, as compared with 23% in the RND group.

Results (pN$_{1/2}$ – Lymph Nodes Dissection of the Carotid-Jugular Space/Radical Neck Dissection)

As expected, in patients with histologically verified neck metastases, survival rates for the two groups LND/RND were poorer (by 30% and 20%, respectively) than in the patients with no metastases (pN$_0$).

The survival rate for patients with manifest metastases in the neck (pN$_{1/2}$) is, as expected, appreciably higher in the RND patients than in the LND patients. Despite the relatively small number of cases (27 patients in each group) it may be concluded that, if metastases are already present in the neck, an LND alone is not adequate.

Two-thirds of the patients who died within five years succumbed to their cancer irrespective of whether they had been treated by LND (77%) or RND (69%).

Understandably, late neck metastases were observed more frequently after neck dissection with confirmed metastases (pN$_{1/2}$, 44%), than with freedom from metastasis (pN$_0$, 23%).

An interesting observation, however, was that in the RND group (pN$_{1/2}$), late metastases occurred ipsilaterally in 5, and bilaterally in 2 patients; four of these seven patients were subsequently given radiotherapy. After RND, a late metastasis occurred about 10% more often than after LND, although somewhat fewer local tumour recurrences were observed after RND. Stomal recurrences occurred more frequently after LND. Taken together, late neck metastasis and stomal recurrence in patients who died of tumour within five years occurred with about equal frequency after LND and RND.

The logical consequence to be drawn from the oncological results achieved with extremely conservative or radical neck surgery in prophylactic and curative intent, was to search for a compromise. Here, an orientation to the long-term results achieved by Italian head and neck surgeons with functional neck dissection suggested itself, for they were able to show that the survival rates were roughly identical for both radical and functional neck dissection (Molinari et al. 1980).

Although the observation period does not extend to five years for all the patients most of them have been followed up for at least three years, so that, in view of the fact that the frequently fatal malignant secondary disease (i.e. local recurrence, a second primary, late metastasis in the neck or stoma usually occurs within the first two years after primary treatment, it is indeed possible to make a statement.

Three-year survival means that the majority of the patients have already passed beyond the oncologically critical phase. This is of particular importance when our concern is to justify the modified surgical dissection of the neck, which cannot be held responsible for a primary tumour recurrence which, perhaps, again metastasizes to the ipsilateral or contralateral side.

The relative paucity of metastases, their predilection site at the angle between the facial and jugular veins, the reliability of the intraoperative frozen-section evaluation, and the favourable post-therapeutic oncological course, even in the presence of metastases, achieved by functional neck dissection, represent the basis and the justification of a more conservative, regional, functional surgical removal of the lymphatics.

Depending upon the size and localization of the primary tumour, and also on the pre-operative and intra-operative clinical and histological lymph node findings

($N_{0/1}$), the decision is taken during surgery as to whether the patient should receive a radical or complete functional neck dissection.

An analysis of the oncological courses of 81 patients make it clear that stomal recurrence after functional neck surgery is far less frequent that after LND or RND. With only a few exceptions, a late metastasis occurred either ipsilaterally in consequence of a primary tumour recurrence or a second primary, or contralaterally on the non-treated side. In no way does this militate against the (regionally restricted) functional surgical treatment concept. So far, fewer patients have died of their cancer. Almost all the FND procedures were carried out by the author himself, while the standard RND procedures were performed by a number of surgeons, not all of whom were equally experienced.

Conclusions

Prophylactic RND (N_0) is overtreatment, irrespective of the stage of the laryngeal carcinoma, and should be just as emphatically rejected as the practice of performing no dissection when a supraglottic $T_{3/4}$ or T_2 lesions presents, since in about 15% of these latter cases, clinically occult metastases ($N_0 \rightarrow pN_+$ – "false negatives") can be expected. Late metastases frequently prove fatal.

In advanced laryngeal carcinoma with bilateral spread, or predominantly supraglottic localization, *unilateral RND* is not a suitable form of treatment (even when no metastases are found), since, at the *primary* operation, the contralateral side, which may already have clinically occult metastases, cannot be included in the therapeutic concept. Provided that freedom from metastatic disease (pN_0) has been confirmed histologically, LND is adequate therapy. The most important topographic region (with respect to the probability of metastasis) is explored.

Preoperatively non-palpable lymph nodes can be removed at surgery and subjected to histological examination. In pN_0 patients, the five-year survival rate after LND is almost as good as after RND.

The *histological frozen-section examination* of the soft tissue containing the lymph nodes, obtained from the jugular chain (in LND) or from the entire anterior triangle (in rFND), is a reliable diagnostic technique, for which the false negative rate is 3%.

With this examination, as a rule, only micrometastases might possibly escape detection, that is, are recognized only in the definitive histological work-up – so that if a rFND has been performed there is no risk for the patient, since in such cases regional dissection is adequate therapy. In the rare cases of a primarily negative frozen-section examination, but positive definitive histology after LND, a regional FND can be performed subsequently, or radiotherapy can be given.

The relatively high rate of false positive lymph node findings in more than two-thirds of patients (preoperative or intraoperative palpable lymph nodes – intraoperative or postoperative histologically confirmed metastases, emphasizes the expediency of always carrying out intraoperative frozen-section examinations. The demonstration of enlarged lymph nodes in the jugular space, should no longer justify a radical, or even a complete functional, dissection of the neck.

In the presence of metastases (pN_+) in the anterior triangle, LND is not adequate as the sole treatment of the cervical lymphatics.

Although in these cases appreciably better survival rates were obtained with RND than with LND, nevertheless, rFND or, if required, complete FND – usually performed bilaterally in a single session – provides identical oncological safety. Additionally, functionally important organ structures can thus be preserved.

The systematic functional dissection of the anterior triangle using the rFND procedure, makes possible the early detection of metastases on both sides at the same time, more reliably than LND alone. In the case of solitary metastases of less than 2 cm in diameter, it represents adequate neck treatment.

Depending upon the size and number of the metastases verified by frozen-section examination, this intervention can be extended at any time, and a complete FND performed.

The oncological results obtained since 1977 with functional neck surgery form the basis for our present diagnostic/therapeutic concept (Fig. 1). In the case of tumour stage T_1 and T_2 carcinomas of the glottis, as also T_1 tumours of the supraglottis and negative palpatory findings (N_0), neither surgical nor radiotherapeutic prophylactic neck therapy is performed.

In contrast, in the case of fixed neck metastases (N_3) a classical radical neck dissection with subsequent radiotherapy is always carried out irrespective of the primary tumour stage.

If in a supraglottic T_2 tumour or a $T_{3/4}$ laryngeal carcinoma, a vertical or horizontal partial resection or laryngectomy is performed, in the absence of pre-therapeutic negative palpatory findings (N_0), the anterior triangle of the neck on either side is explored.

Exception: In the case of strictly unilateral tumours originating in the glottis which are treated by means of a vertical partial resection, e.g. hemilaryngectomy, merely a homolateral exploration is performed. If no suspicious lymph nodes are found at surgery, we limit our procedure to this prophylactic, diagnostic intervention.

In the absence of palpatory findings (N_0), but in the presence of suspicious lymph nodes detected during the exploration (N_0 pre-operative → N_1 intra-operative) a regional function neck dissection is carried out. The same applies in the presence of a suspicious pre-therapeutic palpatory finding (mobile lymph nodes $N_{1/2b}$).

Here, the anterior triangle of the neck, that is, the region most likely to be invaded by metastasis in advanced laryngeal carcinoma, is dissected. The entire preparation is then subjected to a frozen-section examination.

The further surgical procedure is decided, in the first instance, by the histological frozen-section diagnosis ($pN_{0/+}$). Also determinative for the therapeutic procedure are the size, localization and number of metastases. In the absence of metastases (pN_0), or if only a small solitary metastasis is detected, the regional neck dissection forms the complete treatment of the neck.

In the presence of a large solitary metastasis (diameter in excess of 2 cm), or multiple metastases, the functional neck dissection is usually completed by subjecting also the posterior (lateral) triangle of the neck and the supraclavicular fossa to a surgical functional dissection. If the definitive histological work-up of the neck dissection specimen reveals positive lymph nodes in the lateral triangle of the neck

Surgical Management of the Lymphatic System

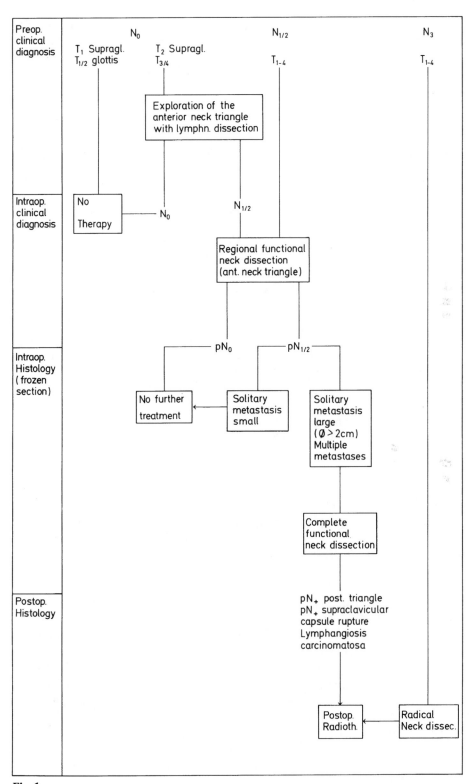

Fig. 1

and/or in the supraclavicular fossa, too, and/or if a capsule rupture is detected histologically, and/or a lymphangiosis carcinomatosa presents, postoperative radiotherapy is given.

The region of the primary tumour is subjected to radiotherapy in partial resection or laryngectomy only if the tumour has not been (or might not have been) removed completely.

References

Bocca E (1972) Chirurgie der Halslymphknoten. In: Naumann HH (Hrsg) Kopf- und Hals-Chirurgie, Bd. 1. Thieme, Stuttgart
Bocca E (1976) Critical analysis of the techniques and value of neck dissection. Nuovo Arch Ital Otol 4:151
Calearo C, Teatini GP (1976) Lo svuotamento funzionale laterocervicale. II – Tecnica chirurgica. Nuovo Arch Ital Otol 4:177
Molinari R, Chiesa F, Cantu G, Grandi C (1980) Retrospective comparison of conservative and radical neck dissection in laryngeal cancer. Ann Otol Rhinol Larnygol 89:578
Staffieri A (1976) Lo svuotamento funzionale laterocervicale. III – Resoconto statistico. Nuovo Arch Ital Otal 4:302
Steiner W (1978) Erfahrungen mit der funktionellen Neck dissection. 1. Erlanger Operationskurs für Kopf- und Halschirurgie, Erlangen, 14.–17.06.1978
Steiner W (1982) Die funktionelle Neck dissection beim Larynxkarzinom – Ergebnisse und Indikationen. Symposion über experimentelle Tumorforschung in der Hals-Nasen-Ohren-Heilkunde, Düsseldorf, 25.–27.02.1982
Suarez O (1963) El problema de las metastases linfaticas y alejados del cancer de largine e hipofaringe. Rev Otorrinolaringol (Santiago/Chile) 23:83
Teatini GP, Zampano G (1976) Lo svuotamento funzionale laterocervicale. I – Basi anatomiche. Nuovo Arch Ital Otol 4:159
Theissing G (1971) Kurze HNO-Operationslehre. Bd. 1. Thieme, Stuttgart

Surgical Management of the Lymphatic System with Regard to Supraglottic Resections of the Larynx

H. BRYAN NEEL III, Rochester (Minnesota)

Neck metastases account for most surgical and radiation failures in patients with supraglottic carcinoma. Therefore, management of the cervical nodes often determines the eventual outcome of the disease. My associates and I (Coates et al. 1976; DeSanto et al. 1977) advocate neck dissection for virtually all patients except those with small epiglottic (T_{1a}) tumors; for these patients, a wait-and-watch policy is followed. The low morbidity and mortality (1.6%) after the operation and the long-term outcome of the patients at the Mayo Clinic justify this approach. Furthermore, neck dissection facilitates the execution of the supraglottic operation and gives the surgeon surgical staging information. The close cooperation and assistance of a surgical pathologist skilled and efficient in fresh-frozen section diagnosis of nodal cancer are required. In our practice, the neck dissection is carried out on one side of the neck in a noncontiguous operation. The nodes are sectioned and studied by the pathologist while the primary tumor is being excised.

When the nodes in the neck dissection specimen are negative, no further surgery in the opposite side of the neck is required. If positive nodes are identified, we usually dissect the other side in the form of a functional dissection, sparing the accessory nerve and sometimes the internal jugular vein and the sternocleidomastoid muscle.

The Patient with Clinically Apparent Nodes

When cervical adenopathy is palpable and significant, a complete (radical) neck dissection is done. When the clinically apparent positive nodes involve both sides of the neck, bilateral complete (radical) neck dissections are carried out at the same operation in most cases. In the rare situation in which nodes are palpable on the side opposite the primary lesion (clinically significant nodes contralateral to the primary tumor), bilateral simultaneous neck dissections are usually carried out. A radical neck dissection is done on the side bearing clinically palpable nodes, and a modified dissection is done on the opposite side; at least the spinal accessory nerve is spared.

The Patient Without Clinically Apparent Nodes

If the primary tumor is located on one side of the supraglottic region, a neck dissection, usually with sparing of the spinal accessory nerve, is carried out on that side. As noted above, this facilitates the execution of the supraglottic operation. If no nodes are palpable and the supraglottic lesion is midline, either side of the neck may be dissected, once again with sparing of the spinal accessory nerve. If the surgical pathologist finds histologically positive nodes in the neck dissection specimen while the surgeon is performing the supraglottic laryngectomy, a modified neck dissection that preserves the accessory nerve and often the internal jugular vein and sternocleidomastoid muscle is usually carried out on the opposite side, provided that the patient's health is favorable.

In many institutions, the indications for an elective neck dissection are not clearly delineated, and the decision to do an elective neck dissection is based on whether the information derived from the neck dissection and the extra security given to the patient can be clearly weighed against the extra time and the morbidity of the neck dissection (Coates et al. 1976; DeSanto et al. 1977; DeSanto et al. 1982). In our practice, the accessory nerve is routinely preserved in the elective operation. In a recent review, DeSanto et al. (1977) found that among all the patients who had surgery, the incidence of surgical deaths was low (1.6%). Each death occurred after irradiation failure.

In a review by Coates et al. (1976) of our patients, 2 of 71 patients with clinically negative cervical nodes had histologically positive nodes. Conversely, in the same study, neck metastases later developed in 12 of 39 patients (31%) who had had *no* neck dissections, and they were subsequently treated by neck dissection. (The other 27 patients remained free of neck metastases, and all 27 survived for 5 years or longer.) This result evokes the issue of microsopic foci of metastatic disease not detected by the pathologist by use of frozen section techniques. If the nodes in these clinically negative necks were subjected to permanent serial sections, a much higher incidence of microscopic foci would be found. This figure would be somewhere around 30%, because in patients not treated by initial neck dissection as the definitive operation, the incidence of subsequent neck metastases is about 30%, the generally cited incidence of occult metastases in supraglottic carcinoma. A wait-and-watch policy does not appear to reduce long-term survival, but this approach demands close follow-up and certainly subjects the patients to the danger of delayed treatment of larger nodes and a poorer chance of survival.

No ideal program of management of the neck in patients with supraglottic carcinoma exists. The controversy of the role of elective bilateral and functional neck dissections as part of the treatment for supraglottic carcinoma will continue. The principles cited above are applied in the context of our practice and other factors, such as the patient's age, general health, and pulmonary function and a variety of other subtle factors.

References

Coates HL, DeSanto LW, Devine KD, Elveback LR (1976) Carcinoma of the supraglottic larynx: A review of 221 cases. Arch Otolaryngol 102:686–689

DeSanto LW, Holt JJ, Beahrs OH, O'Fallon WM (1982) Neck dissection: Is it worthwhile? Laryngoscope 92:502–509

DeSanto LW, Lillie JC, Devine KD (June 1977) Cancers of the larynx: Supraglottic cancer. Surg Clin North Am 57:505–514

F. Radiotherapy and Chemotherapy

Sequential Chemotherapy and Radiotherapy in Advanced Head and Neck Cancer

P. M. STELL, Liverpool, J. E. DALBY, Merseyside, P. STRICKLAND, Middlesex,
J. G. FRASER, London, P. J. BRADLEY, Liverpool, and L. M. FLOOD, London

Summary and Conclusion

Eighty six previously untreated patients with advanced squamous cell carcinoma of the head and neck were entered into a prospective randomized controlled trial to evaluate whether the addition of a kinetically based chemotherapy regimen before and after radiotherapy would improve survival compared to radiotherapy alone. Survival at thirty months showed there was no evidence that the addition of chemotherapy to radiotherapy improved survival and that the chance of getting a significant result in favour of adjuvant chemotherapy was remote.

Introduction

The survival of patients with head and neck cancer treated by radiotherapy and/or surgery has not greatly improved during the last decade. It is hoped that the addition of chemotherapy to local treatment will improve survival (Green 1978; Wittes 1979/80).

A non-randomized study of synchronous chemotherapy with radiotherapy showed a two-fold improvement in survival compared with historical controls treated by radiotherapy alone (O'Connor et al. 1979; O'Connor 1980).

At present a kinetically based chemotherapeutic regimen (Price and Hill 1977) is claimed to have the highest tumour response of the regimens available, with minimum toxic effect (Hill and Price 1980). This regimen, when given before radiotherapy, has been reported in uncontrolled trials to improve survival (Price and Hill 1980; Sergant and Deutsch 1981).

A randomized controlled prospective trial to evaluate whether the addition of the kinetic chemotherapy regimen, designed by Price & Hill (Price and Hill 1977; Norton and Simon 1977) before and after radiotherapy improved survival compared to radiotherapy alone.

Material

All patients with previously untreated Stage III or Stage IV squamous carcinoma of the head and neck were considered for entry.

After histological confirmation of the disease and classification according to the UICC scheme (1978), the patients were seen jointly by a surgeon and a radiotherapist. If the patient had an advanced tumour fulfilling the criteria shown in Table 1, he was entered into the trial. Patients were excluded from entry for the following reasons: pregnancy, unavailability for follow up, poor general condition, second simultaneous malignancy, or age over 80 years. The patient was assigned randomly to two groups only one of which was to receive chemotherapy. Thirty six men with a median age of 63 years (range 39–75 years) and 11 women with a median age of 59 years (range 50–68 years) were randomized to be treated by chemotherapy and radiotherapy. Twenty eight men with a median age of 58 years (range 43–79 years) and 11 women with a median age of 63 years (range 41–74 years) were randomized to be treated by radiotherapy alone.

The site distribution is shown in Table 2. Because of the small number of patients with carcinoma of the oral cavity, oropharynx, nasopharynx and pyriform fossa these sites are grouped together and collectively referred to in this paper as "buccopharynx" (Table 2).

Each patient before, during and after chemotherapy, had regular monitoring of their peripheral blood count, absolute platelet count, liver function studies, and urinary creatinine clearance. Administration of chemotherapy was delayed if the haematological and biochemical results were unsatisfactory (Rowland 1981).

Table 1. Conditions of entry

All patients must have squamous cell carcinoma at the following sites:

Oral cavity	
Oropharynx	
Pyriform fossa	T_3N_x or T_4N_x
Larynx	
Nasopharynx	T_xN_x
T_x = any T	N_x = any N
All patients M_0	

Table 2. Material

	Chemotherapy & radiotherapy group	Radiotherapy group
Larynx	25	23
Oral cavity	5	4
Oropharynx	7	5
Nasopharynx	4	3
Pyriform fossa	6	4

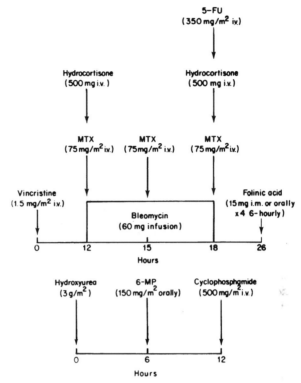

Fig. 1. Schedule I (*top*). Schedule II (*bottom*)

Method

All patients randomized to receive chemotherapy were given two regimens of cytotoxic drugs as shown in Figure 1. Schedule I was given on day 1 and schedule II on day 14. Radiotherapy began about day 28.

Patients who were randomized to be treated by radiotherapy alone began treatment on day 1, and received no cytotoxic drugs at any stage of treatment. Mega voltage radiation was given to all patients and a dose of 4000–6000 cGy was delivered in a three–six week period.

Patients who received chemotherapy before radiotherapy were to receive further chemotherapy on completion of radiotherapy, alternating between schedule I and schedule II at 21 day intervals, commencing about day 56, for a total of 12 courses over 36 weeks.

Results

Toxicity

Four patients, all in the "buccopharynx" group, ceased chemotherapy because of toxicity; one patient died from septicaemia following pancytopenia, one developed pulmonary fibrosis, one autonomic neuropathy and one alopecia.

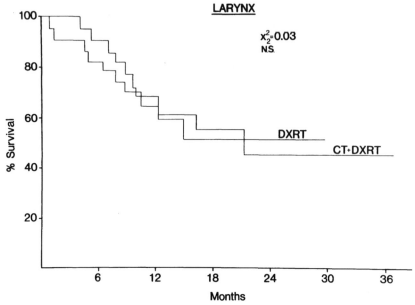

Fig. 2. Actuarial survival curve for laryngeal carcinoma

Follow-up Chemotherapy

Chemotherapy was stopped temporarily in four instances: three because of depression of bone marrow and one because of reduced renal function. Twenty two patients withdrew from further chemotherapy because of tumour growth in spite of chemotherapy after radiotherapy. Only six of the 47 patients in the chemotherapy group completed all 12 courses of chemotherapy after radiotherapy. Four patients all with laryngeal carcinoma are currently still receiving therapy.

Salvage Surgery

Seventeen patients had salvage surgery: ten had a laryngectomy, three a pharyngolaryngectomy, two a pelvimandibulectomy, one exploration of the postnasal space, and one had bilateral radical neck dissection. Four patients in the chemotherapy group, and four of six patients treated by radiotherapy who underwent a laryngectomy, are still alive. Three of the seven patients in the "buccopharyngeal" group who underwent salvage surgery are still alive. All three were treated by radiotherapy alone.

Survival

For the larynx the survival was virtually identical in both groups: 46% at 30 months for the chemotherapy + radiotherapy group and 52% for the radiotherapy alone group. (Fig. 2).

The patients with a tumour of the buccopharynx who received chemotherapy did particularly badly: all patients died within 24 months (Fig. 3).

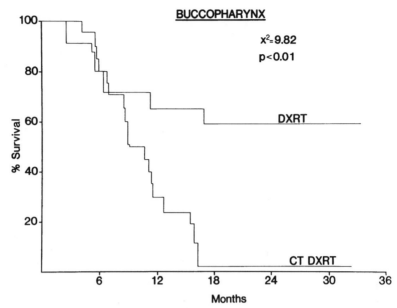

Fig. 3. Actuarial survival curve for buccopharyngeal carcinoma

Acknowledgement. The authors are grateful to the North West Cancer Research Fund for technical assistance.

References

Green M (1978) Chemotherapy of head and neck cancer. Head Neck Surg 1:75–86
Hill BT, Price LA (1980) The changing role of chemotherapy in the treatment of head and neck cancer. Cancer Topics 2:5–7
Norton L, Simon R (1977) Tumour size, sensitivity to therapy and design of treatment schedules. Cancer Treat Rep 61 (7):1307–1316
O'Connor AD et al. (1979) Advanced head and neck cancer treated by combined radiotherapy and VBM cytotoxic regimens – four year results. Clin Otolaryngol 4:329–337
O'Connor AD (1980) Head and neck cancer: 5 year experience with VBM and radiotherapy. Cancer Topics 2:8–9
Price LA, Hill BT (1977) A kinetically based logical approach to the chemotherapy of head and neck cancer. Clin Otolaryngol 2:339–345
Price LA, Hill BT (1980) Safe and effective combination chemotherapy for squamous cell carcinoma of the head and neck. J Laryngol Otol 94:89–90
Rowland CG (1981) Safer cancer chemotherapy, In: Price LA, Hill BT, Chilchik MW (eds) Bailliere Tindall, London, p 53–57
Sergant R, Deutsch G (1981) A preliminary report on the combination of initial chemotherapy and radiotherapy for advanced head and neck cancer. J Laryngol Otol 95:69–74
UICC (1978) TNM classification of malignant tumour. In: Harmer MH (ed) 3rd Edition, Geneva
Wittes RE (1979/80) Head and neck cancer: Chemotherapy. Bristol-Meyers Co.

Combined Radiation Therapy and Surgery for Limited Carcinoma of the Larynx

R. SAUER, Erlangen

The treatment of laryngeal carcinoma is considered to be one of the most productive fields of cancer management in terms of cure. A variety of therapeutic procedures is available which can achieve tumor control. These include total laryngectomy, conservation surgery, laser excision, radiation therapy, cryotherapy and others. Therefore, the choice of initial treatment has to take all clinical features of each individual patient into consideration. Moreover, surgeons and radiotherapists should know the strengths and weaknesses of their disciplines and the limitations of their specialty. It is the complementary and cooperative efforts of this team that ensure the welfare of patients with malignant disease: the extent of surgery may be reduced by supplementary radiotherapy; the local control of radiotherapy may be increased by salvage surgery.

At present, every effort is made to preserve the voice in the management of early laryngeal cancer. The following methods are available:
1. the modern techniques of radiotherapy (beam quality, field size, total dose, fractionation, etc. are of interest)
2. the different methods of limited surgery.

Each of these modalities has its own merits, indications and limits. Radiation alone for mobile vocal cord cancers ($T_{1/2}$ lesions) controls 80–90% of tumors (Goffinet et al. 1973; Harwood et al. 1981; Marks et al. 1973; Wang 1974) and 80–85% of failures can be salvaged by limited surgery (Biller et al. 1975; Norris and Peale 1966). In small exophytic supraglottic cancers, local control of the primary tumor by irradiation is excellent (Fletcher 1980; Ghossein et al. 1974). Radiation therapy must be considered as the best tissue and organ sparing procedure currently available. On the other hand, for certain early lesions limited surgery can be carried out expediently and effectively without significant functional and cosmetic mutilation and is, therefore, preferred.

Limited Surgery After Definitive Radiotherapy, Radiotherapy After Limited Surgery?

There are two important questions in the management of early laryngeal carcinoma:
Is limited surgery with preservation of voice still possible after curative radiotherapy?
How is postoperative radiotherapy tolerated after partial resection of the larynx?
These questions can be answered on the basis of the experience gained with complications associated with curative radiotherapy of the larynx. Here we might mention edema, necrosis and chondritis. The extent of radiation complications depends on quality of irradiation beam, total dose, duration of treatment, fraction size, and individual risks.

Type of Ionizing Radiation

Ionizing radiation is that radiation which, during absorption, causes the emission of orbital electrons. Such ionizing radiation may be electromagnetic or particulate. Electromagnetic radiation is divided into roentgen and gamma radiation. Examples of particulate radiations are the subatomic particles, electrons, protons, neutrons, negative pimesons etc.

In the therapy of larynx carcinoma it is important to employ high energy electromagnetic irradiation (megavoltage therapy). In contrast, X-rays with orthovolt-technique or particulate radiations such as electrons and neutrons are dangerous and should not be used. These radiation qualities are absorbed by bone and cartilage at higher rates than by soft tissue. As a result, dosage peaks increase the risk of bone necrosis and chondritis.

Total Dose and Fractionation

Radiobiologically, it is known that an approximately exponential relationship exists between the radiation dose administered to a cell population and the surviving fractions of these cells. Relatively low doses will inactivate a vast number of cells in a tumor. This is in agreement with the clinical observation that small microscopic aggregates of tumor cells, which cannot be palpated on physical examination inspite of previous histopathological verification, can be controlled by doses of 4500–5000 rads/5 weeks in more than 90% of cases (Fletcher 1972). However, for a larger tu-

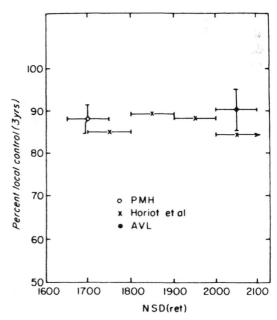

Fig. 1. Local control (percent), T_1 glottic cancer vs nominal standard dose. The dose cure curve is flat over the dose range 1650–2050 ret (from Harwood and Tierie, 1979)

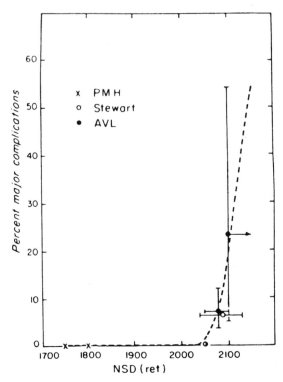

Fig. 2. Dose complication curve for the larynx. Once the dose of 2050 ret is exceeded the risk of complications rises rapidly (from Harwood and Tierie, 1979)

mor, i.e., T_1/T_2 larynx carcinoma higher doses such as 6000–7000 rads/7 weeks are required. The fractionation is 4–5 times a week.

The risk of serious complications due to radiotherapy increases with the total dose. Harwood and Tierie examined the results of treatment and the complications from two cancer centers. The Netherland's Cancer Institute, Antoni Van Leeuwenhoek Ziekenhuis (AVL), Amsterdam, Holland, and the Ontario Cancer Institute, Princess Margret Hospital (PMH), Toronto, Canada. Similar techniques were used at each center for the treatment of early glottic cancer; the dosage used at the former center (AVL) was in the upper range of that generally used, and the dosage of the latter (PMH) at the lower end of this range. For purposes of comparison the variables of dose, time, and number of fractions were reduced to a single number using the Ellis formula (3). It was concluded that the dose cure curve for early glottic cancer (T_{1a} and T_{1b}) is flat over the dose range 1650–2050 ret (5500 rads/6 weeks to 7500 rads/7–8 weeks). The dose usually used is 6000–6500 rads/6–7 weeks. Once the dose of 2050 ret is exceeded the risk of subsequent major chronic complications rises quite rapidly: larynx and/or cord necrosis, edema and/or laryngeal stenosis requiring tracheostomy (Figs. 1 and 2).

In the curative treatment of patients with early laryngeal cancer by radiotherapy, a decision must be made about the optimal dose on the basis of the benefits and risk of treatment.

Table 1. Relationship between fraction size, dose, duration of treatment and radiation complications for vocal cord cancer

Fraction size in rads	Total dose in rads	Duration in weeks	Dose in ret	Edema or necrosis
250	5000	4	1700	5/68 (9%)
240	6000	5	2000	
214	6000	5½	1800	3/330 (1%)
212	7000	6½	2000	

Fletcher, G.H. et al., Laryngoscope 85: 987–1003, 1975

Fraction Size

By reducing fraction size and increasing duration and total dose, Fletcher et al. (1975) were able to maintain a biologically equivalent dose and reduce the incidence of radiation complications (Table 1). Using the Ellis formula (3) and the same biologically equivalent dose of 1700–2000 ret, the risk of serious complications decreased from 9% to 1%.

Field Size

It is known that local control increases when the irradiation field measures at least 5×5 cm. On the other hand, the complication rate rises when the field size exceeds 50 cm^2. Today, early laryngeal carcinomas are treated with a field size of about 6×6 cm. In this way, complications can largely be avoided.

Individual Risks

Diabetes and other metabolic diseases, and hypertension exert a major effect of increasing the complication rate of treatment. This contribution of individual factors is striking at high dose levels. The observation that the severity of the acute reaction enables one to predict the subsequent risk of developing a major complication is inconsistent in the various series (Harwood and Tierie 1979).

In summarizing the facts mentioned above, the answers to the former questions are:

Even after curative radiotherapy, partial resection of a larynx free from complications remains possible without significantly increasing post-operative morbidity. The prerequisite is that a dose of 6000–7000 rads/6–7 weeks has not been exceeded, and that at least 6 weeks have elapsed since radiotherapy. This has been our experience at Erlangen.

A larynx already damaged by surgery is less resistent than the intact organ. The risk of radiation-induced complication rises. It has been, however, shown that a dosage of about 6000–6500 rads/6–7 weeks can be applied postoperatively after every type of partial larynx resection. Irradiation is usually carried out approximately 4–6 weeks after surgery or still later when the wound is healed. Here in Erlangen, we have given postoperative irradiation of about 6000–6500 rads over 6½–7 weeks following laryngeal partial resections, without any complications.

Management of Metastatic Nodes

The management of metastatic nodes in the neck from a primary tumour arising in the head and neck region depends upon the size, number of nodes, and the cell type and location of the primary lesion. Radiotherapy is highly curative for small, metastatic nodes. For metastatic nodes of laryngeal carcinomas, a combination of radiation therapy and surgery is the treatment of choice.

Frequency of lymph node metastases differs from tumors originating from different regions of the larynx due to variation in density of lymphatic vessels within the larynx according to region and site. Glottic cancers have the lowest incidence of lymph node metastases while supraglottic tumors have the highest. McGavran et al. found a significant increase of the incidence of lymphatic metastases for a number of primary tumor characteristics, including size greater than 2 cm, poor cellular differentiation, infiltrating peripheral growth patterns, and nerve sheath invasion. Unfortunately, most of these primary tumor characteristics cannot be determined before surgery and therefore are of little value in identifying those patients most likely to harbor clinically inapparent microscopic lymphatic metastases. Lacking the ability to predict subclinical lymphatic metastases, the clinican resorts to elective neck dissection or irradiation of regional lymphatics.

In the case of glottic cancers adjuvant radiation is not given before or after surgery for small lesions. Patients selected for postoperative irradiation include:
  those who require emergency tracheostomy since the incidence of subsequent recurrence in the tracheostoma is significant (Keim et al. 1965)
  those whose primary tumor has spread extensively within the paraglottic space.
  those with documented or significant potential for lymphatic metastases.
In the case of supraglottic cancers the rate of lymphatic metastases is approximately 25% for central and 50% for marginal lesions (Marks et al. 1979). If lymph nodes are palpable we favour integrated surgical removal of the primary tumor and regional lymphatics with adjuvant radiotherapy to the tumor region and the lymphatics after surgery. If palpable nodes are not present, we favour elective treatment by ipsilateral neck dissection or radiation to both necks. In the presence of histopathologically proven lymphatic metastases we apply postoperative radiotherapy in all cases.

Barkley et al. (1972) and Fletcher (1980) have shown that 5000 rads/5 weeks control aproximately 90% of subclinical microscopic lymph node metastases and

Table 2. Recurrences in the radically dissected neck

Memorial Hospital (Strong 1969)	M.D. Anderson Hospital (Barkley et al. 1972)
All sites	Oropharynx, supraglottic larynx, pyriform sinus, $N_1 - N_3$
RND alone 28.7%	RND alone 25.6%
Preop. Irradiation (2000 rads: 5 × 400) 17.6%	Pre- or postop. irradiation (at least 5000 rads) 7.6%

From Fletcher 1980

Table 3. Disease control – immediate postoperative irradiation versus irradiation for gross recurrence

	Immediate postop. irradiation	Irradiation for gross recurrences
Pts. treated	19	147
Pts. free of tumor	8	16
Percent	42% p 0.001	11%

Fletcher 1980

that postoperative radiation to the neck, pharynx and tracheostomy effectively reduces local recurrence at these sites.

Table 2 shows that after neck dissection, with positive specimens of different origins, recurrences occur in 26–29% (Strong 1969; Barkley et al. 1972). 2000 rads (500 rads × 4) cause only a modest diminuition of recurrences in the radically dissected neck. In contrast, the incidence of failures in the radically dissected neck with 5000 rads given either pre- or postoperatively is drastically reduced.

Table 3 is a tabulation of patients remaining free of cancer according to whether they had immediate irradiation for lack of surgical clearance or delayed irradiation for proven recurrence. The group of patients with elective postoperative irradiation have a statistically significant higher NED-rate. Treatment should not await recurrence in patients with a high risk of failure after a surgical procedure. Such patients should be given postoperative irradiation as soon as the wound heals (Fletcher 1980).

Summary

The major goals in the treatment of cancer of the larynx are to control the tumor and regional nodes and to preserve voice whenever possible. Local and regional tumor control is best accomplished by surgery or radiation, alone or in combination. Limited conservation surgery can be carried out, without significantly increasing postoperative morbidity, after definitive radiotherapy. Postoperative radiotherapy can be applied after every type of partial resection of the larynx. The prerequisite is that a dose of 6000–6500 rads/6–7 weeks has not been exceeded, that high-voltage therapy is employed and that account is taken of such individual risks as metabolic diseases and hypertension. Postoperative radiation to the neck, pharynx, and tracheostomy effectively reduces local recurrence at these sites.

References

Barkley HT, Fletcher GH et al. (1972) Management of cervical lymph node metastases in squamous cell carcinoma of the tonsillar fossa, base of tongue, supraglottic larynx and hypopharynx. Am J Surg 124:462–467

Biller HF, Barnhill FR et al. (1975) Hemilaryngectomy following radiation failure for carcinoma of the vocal cords. Laryngoscope 85:1318–1326
Ellis F (1968) Relationship of biological effect of dose-time-fraction factors in radiotherapy. In: Ebert M, Howard A (eds) Current Topics in Radiation Research, Amsterdam, North Holland, pp 357–397
Fletcher GH (1972) Elective irradiation of subclinical disease in cancers of the head and neck. Cancer 29:1450–1454
Fletcher GH (1980) Textbook of Radiotherapy, 3rd edition, Lea and Febiger, Philadelphia
Fletcher GH, Lindberg RD et al. (1975) Reasons for irradiation failure in squamous cell carcinoma of the larynx. Laryngoscope 85:987–1003
Ghossein A, Batini JP et al. (1974) Local control and site of failure in radically irradiated supraglottic cancer. Radiology 112:187–192
Goffinet DR, Eltringham JR et al. (1973) Carcinoma of the larynx: Results of radiation therapy in 213 patients. Am J Roentgenol 117:553–564
Harwood AR, Beale FA et al. (1981) T_2 glottic cancer: An analysis of dose-time-volume factors. Int J Radiat Oncol Biol Phys 7:1501–1505
Harwood AR, Tierie A (1979) Radiotherapy of early Glottic Cancer-II. Int J Radiat Oncology Biol Phys 5:477–482
Keim WF, Shapir MJ et al. (1965) Study of postlaryngectomy stomal recurrence. Arch Otolaryngol 81:183–186
Marks JE, Freeman RB et al. (1979) Carcinoma of the supraglottic larynx. Am J Roentgenol 132:255–260
Marks JE, Lowry LD et al. (1973) Glottic cancer: An analysis of recurrence as related to dose time and fractionation. Am J Roentgenol 117:540–547
McGavran MH, Bauer WC et al. (1961) The incidence of cervical lymph node metastases from epidermoid carcinoma of the larynx. Cancer 14:55–66
Norris CM, Peale AR (1966) Partial laryngectomy for irradiation failure. Arch Otolaryngol 84:558–562
Strong EW (1969) Preoperative radiation and radical neck dissection. Surg Clin North Am 49:271–275
Wang CC (1974) Treatment of glottic carcinoma by megavoltage radiation therapy and results. Am J Roentgenol 120:157–163

Vertical and Horizontal Partial Resections of the Larynx After Radiotherapy

J. CZIGNER, Budapest

Specific problems exist when partial laryngectomy is considered the treatment of choice after radiotherapy: 1. the therapeutic benefit of preoperative radiation in the surgical therapy of laryngeal carcinoma; 2. the management of persistent or recurrent laryngeal carcinoma after full-dose radiation therapy when a partial operation with all its advantages would suffice clinically; 3. the influence of radiation on postoperative complications.

In the treatment of glottic cancer primary curative radiotherapy, with salvage surgery reserved for radiation failures, has an important advantage (Harwood et al. 1980; Németh 1981). However, reported failure rates averaged 15% in T_1 and 32% in T_2 glottic lesions (Nichols et al. 1980). The residual or recurrent tumor can be removed by a conservation surgery procedure in well selected instances of glottic tumors (Norris and Peale 1966; Burns et al. 1979; Nichols et al. 1980).

In the management of supraglottic carcinomas, surgery not only has a cure rate significantly superior to telecobalt therapy but supraglottic horizontal laryngectomy is also able to preserve laryngeal functions (Sellars et al. 1981).

Marks, Ogura et al. (1979) stated that patients with carcinoma of the supraglottic larynx, who have been treated by preoperative low dose radiation, have a relatively favourable prognosis with conservation surgery. However, it is difficult to assess the real merits of this preoperative low dose radiotherapy when their 45% five years survival rate (140 patients were treated surgically after radiotherapy) is compared to the 58% five years survival rate of our 136 patients who underwent conservation supraglottic surgery alone.

Cachin's (1974) opinion seems to be well established that preoperative radiation before supraglottic horizontal laryngectomy does not improve survival rates.

A challenging problem is the surgical management of those tumors which persist or recur after full dose radiotherapy. The complication rates of this salvage surgery particularly after supraglottic horizontal laryngectomy are unacceptably high. Stell (1974) stressed that a patient who once had radiotherapy for supraglottic carcinoma cannot then have a supraglottic laryngectomy.

Burns et al. (1979) reported two of six successful patients undergoing horizontal partial laryngectomy after radiation, and no substantial postoperative complications were encountered. Nevertheless, few successful cases have been reported in the literature until now.

Patient Presentation

The age, sex and staging of our 24 patients in this study group are displayed in table 1. Details of the 16 vertical partial resections for radiation failure of early glottic carcinomas and 8 supraglottic horizontal laryngectomies performed after radiation therapy were available for analysis. Table 2 shows initial surgical treatment, subsequent total laryngectomy and the cause and number of deaths.

In the glottic group, one patient developed local recurrence 5 months after frontolateral resection. He was salvaged by total laryngectomy and paratracheal block dissection with histologically positive lymph nodes. He now is disease free after 39 months. One 70 years old patient with unfavourable pulmonary function died in the postoperative period of aspiration pneumonia. One patient died because of cervical

Table 1. Tumor stages of 24 patients with cancer of the larynx submitted to partial laryngectomy after preoperative radiation (19 males, 5 females, 37–81 years of age)

Glottic		Supraglottic	
T_{1a}	5	T_{1a}	2
T_{1b}	9	T_{1b}	6
T_2	2		

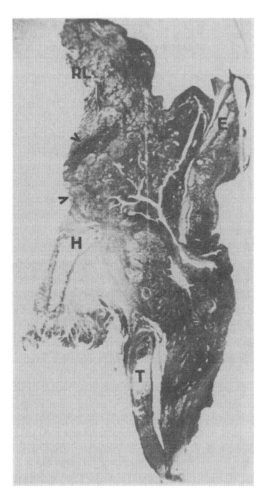

Fig. 1. Recurrent T_{1b} supraglottic carcinoma 8 months after a full dose telecobalt radiation, with deep invasion of the base of the tongue (*arrows*). Sagittal section of a specimen after supraglottic laryngectomy with resection of the base of tongue (RL). *E*, epiglottic cartilage; *H*, hyoid bone; *T*, thyroid cartilage

Table 2. Methods of conservation surgery of the larynx after radiotherapy (n=24) and subsequent fate

	Surgery		Death		
	Initial partial surgery	Subsequent total laryngectomy	Post-oper.	Tumor	Other
Cordectomy by EMS+C[a]	3				1
Cordectomy by thyrotomy	2				1
Frontolateral resection	6	1			
Vertical hemilaryngectomy	5		1	1	
Supraglottic laryngectomy	8	1	1	2	

[a] Endolaryngeal microsurgery + cauterisation

metastases with a tumor-free larynx, and 2 patients died of other diseases. Prolonged wound healing was noted in most patients. The following other complications were observed: 8 laryngocutaneous fistulas with perichondritis in 5 patients, 2 postoperative hemorrhages, 7 persistent oedema and/or granulation, but none of them remained dependent on a tracheostomy.

In the supraglottic group, 4 of the 8 patients had received preoperative radiation of 3000–4000 rads in other centres. All 4 are alive and well after supraglottic horizontal laryngectomy. Two of them had pharyngocutaneous fistulas for some weeks postoperatively, and two recovered without complications. 4 other patients had radiation failures after 6000–6500 cGy telecobalt therapy. They were operated on by supraglottic laryngectomy. One of them who was understaged by the preoperative examination (Fig. 1) died of major postoperative complications of complete wound break down and unsuccessful re-operation. The other 3 patients healed without postoperative complications but all 3 later developed lymph node metastases. Two of them underwent neck dissection but died because of neck recurrences and distant metastases. The third patient was salvaged by total laryngectomy and neck dissection.

Complete horizontal wound break down occurred in this salvage group in one of the 4 patients while it was observed only in 3 of our 217 patients who underwent supraglottic conservation surgery without radiotherapy.

Conclusions

The superficial spread of a tumor after failed radiotherapy may be observed but it is always difficult to define its deep extension. It seems particularly difficult to evaluate the size and extent of recurrent tumors when recurrence develops after a long tumor-free interval and when recurrent supraglottic tumor extends into the base of tongue (Fig. 1). Decreased vocal cord mobility is one important indication of deep tumor spread, and those patients who show fixed vocal cords should be treated by total laryngectomy.

Laryngeal conservation surgery for radiation failures is indicated as follows:
1. Cordectomy should be considered for T_{1a} glottic carcinoma when a complete course of radiotherapy has failed and the tumor can be recognized and operated upon at the earliest possible date;
2. Frontolateral partial resection and vertical hemilaryngectomy may be successful methods for T_{1b} glottic lesions after radiation failure with some increased postoperative complication;
3. Supraglottic horizontal laryngectomy as salvage surgery after full dose radiotherapy should be taken into consideration with inevitably unsatisfactory results.

The benefit of preoperative radiotherapy for supraglottic carcinoma remains controversial. The majority of our patients was treated by conservation surgery alone which achieved favourable rates of survival and voice preservation. These suggested that *primary treatment of supraglottic laryngeal carcinoma should be supraglottic partial laryngectomy.*

References

Burns H, Bryce DP, Nostrand AWP van (1979) Conservation surgery in laryngeal cancer and its role following failed radiotherapy. Arch Otolaryngol 105:234–239

Cachin Y (1974) Limitations of horizontal partial laryngectomy. Can J Otolaryngol CCLC Workshop 6:385–388

Harwood AR, Hawkins NV et al (1980) Radiotherapy of early glottic cancer. Laryngoscope 90:465–470

Marks JE, Freeman RB, Lee F, Ogura JH (1979) Carcinoma of the supraglottic larynx. AJR 132:255–260

Nemeth G (1981) In: Skolyszewski J, Reinfuss M (eds) The results of radiotherapy of cancer of the larynx in six european countries. Radiobiol Radiother (Berl) 22:32–43

Nichols RD, Stine PH, Greenawald KJ (1980) Partial laryngectomy after radiation failure. Laryngoscope 90:571–575

Norris CM, Peale AR (1966) Partial laryngectomy for irradiation failure. Arch Otolaryngol 84:558–562

Sellars SL, Mills EED, Seid AB (1981) Combined preoperative telecobalt therapy and supraglottic laryngectomy. J Laryngol Otol 95:305–310

Stell PM (1974) Discussion of roles and limitations of conservation surgical therapy for laryngeal carcinoma. Can J Otolaryngol CCLC Workshop 6:397–398

Radiotherapy and Partial Laryngectomy

H. J. Denecke, Heidelberg

According to the experience of the author for more than 25 years partial laryngectomy may be performed even after application of radiotherapy in doses up to about 60 gy (6000 rad) or after application of radonseeds. The postoperative course, however, may be delayed inspite of reconstructive measures with pedicle flaps. After application of two series of radiotherapy with total doses of up to 90 or 120 gy (9000 to 12000 rad) the laryngeal cartilages are damaged to such a degree that partial laryngectomy with reconstruction is no more possible. Total laryngectomy has to be performed in most cases. Only in very few of such cases was the author able to preserve the larynx and to rehabilitate respiration, phonation and deglutition by reconstructive measures, so that the patient could be decannulated and continue his professional life.

If in partial laryngectomy with reconstruction one of the three functions of the larynx – translaryngeal respiration, phonation and deglutition – cannot be restored because of the severe damage to the tissue from preoperative radiotherapy, then translaryngeal respiration is sacrified before the other two functions. In these cases the glottis should be reconstructed relatively narrow and the patient should wear a speaking cannula.

After high dose irradiation of the larynx the tissues develop prolonged edema especially after surgical interventions. Transposition of pedicle flaps into the irradiated region is, therefore, of particular importance. The flaps function as draining tissues: After time intervals of three to four months the lymphatic drainage recovers, the edema decreases, and the previously fixed arytenoid cartilages resume their function.

The transposition of large skin flaps such as the pectoralis major or deltopectoral flaps into the laryngeal area is difficult because of the continuous movements of the laryngeal region by the respiratory activities, by swallowing, and coughing. Special techniques of plastic reconstructive rehabilitation are, therefore, necessary together with great experience and patience.

Radiotherapy and Partial Supraglottic Resection

C. CALEARO and A. STAFFIERI, Ferrara

The following is a reassessment of the University of Ferrara E.N.T. Clinic Surgical Team's experience with radiotherapy in association with conservative supraglottic surgery.

Although this association causes no problems with regard to total laryngectomy it may become problematic in conservative surgery. It may have a negative influence on the functional abilities, while, from a cancerological point of view, its effect may be positive. Therefore, the usefulness of a preoperative irradiation of the larynx is doubtful and has been strongly contested.

It is our personal opinion that this combination of radiotherapy and surgery is useless for those indications of conservative surgery which can be managed by surgery alone. In fact, additional irradiation may even cause severe inconveniences.

However, there is one consistent exception: vestibular T_4 tumors with extension beyond the larynx. It is our experience that programmed and timed combination with radiotherapy preceeding horizontal supraglottic laryngectomy, can successfully be applied to these cases.

Although these tumors can also be treated by supraglottic surgery alone, dangers linked to location and extension are present as well as those dangers related to tumor spread and histology. These cases favour neither radiotherapy nor surgery alone and it, therefore, seems rational that both together would help to improve the prognosis. However, this improved prognosis is established at the cost of some inevitable inconveniences.

Our experience consists of 16 supraglottic tumors with glosso-epiglottic and/or pharyngo-epiglottic extension during the period from 1971 to 1978. All were preoperatively treated by high energy radiation. In all cases a total of 40–60 gy was administered, generally in doses of approximately 10 gy a week divided into 5 fractions of 2 gy each. The supraglottic laryngectomy, enlarged at the base of the tongue and/or at the lateral pharyngeal wall, was performed 30–60 days after termination of radiotherapy.

The results can be summarized as follows:

1. The surgical procedure and its post-operative sequelae were not appreciably deteriorated by unacceptable complications. Table 1 shows the duration of time

Table 1. 16 enlarged supraglottic laryngectomies with pre-operative radiotherapy

Closure of tracheostoma after	18–210 days
Removal of nasogastric tube after	14– 45 days

Table 2. Enlarged supraglottic laryngectomies

Survival rates	3 years	4 years	5 years
Radiotherapy + surgery (16 cases)	87.5%	83.4%	75.0%
Surgery alone (8 cases)	75.0%	57.2%	57.2%
Surgery + radiotherapy (6 cases)	66.6%	50.0%	33.3%

necessary for closing the tracheostoma (18–210 days) and for the removal of the nasogastric tube (14–45 days). The functional results were completely satisfactory. The recovery of deglutition and respiratory function took more time, but still within acceptable limits. While no cases of fistula were observed among our cases, Cachin observed 5 in a group of 32 horizontal supraglottic laryngectomies pre-treated by radiotherapy.

2. Table 2 separately demonstrates the oncological results with survival rates for surgery in combination with radiotherapy for 3, 4 and 5 years (87% at 3 years, 75% at 5 years). These results are compared to surgery alone and with postoperative radiotherapy.

In conclusion two data should be underlined: the survival rate at 5 years was 75% in cases which underwent surgery in combination with radiotherapy in comparison to 57% in those subjects who underwent surgery alone.

Aspects of Adjuvant Chemotherapy in Combination with Horizontal Partial Laryngectomy

J. THEISSING, Nuremberg

Discussion of the use of adjuvant pre-operative chemotherapy before horizontal partial resection of the larynx has to address the fundamental question whether chemotherapy in combination with a transverse resection in laryngeal squamous cell cancer is justified at all.

Because of the considerable risks and stress on the patient inherent in this treatment, chemotherapy is not indicated for tumors strictly confined to the supraglottic portion of the endolarynx and which do not involve the lingual area of the epiglottis.

In the present state of knowledge, the chance of remission of tumors, which can easily be removed by horizontal transverse resection, cannot be significantly improved by pre-operative chemotherapy. However, with tumors that have slightly crossed the borders of the false vocal cord down towards the vocal cord and are thus no longer accessible for a transverse resection, it appears tempting to achieve tumor remission by pre-operative chemotherapy, which would then still permit the minor, less mutilating operation of a transverse resection. It has to be considered, on the other hand, that macroscopical remission does not exclude persistance of microscopical tumor growth. For this reason resection after preceding chemotherapy has to be so extensive as to cover the entire region primarily involved.

Chemotherapy appears useful when a tumor has extended to the lingual surface of the epiglottis, the vallecula or the retrolingual region. Also regression starting from a vallecular tumor with transgression through the epiglottis into the endolaryngeal region makes a pre-operative chemotherapy worth consideration. But also in this case, it is by no means justified to reduce the extent of a later resection after tumor remission by chemotherapy. The expectations associated with adjuvant pre-operative chemotherapy rather aim at a decrease of the local recurrence rate, and at the prevention of metastatic spread of extensive tumors, as well as at the mobilization of fixed regional metastases.

To what extent these hopes are finally realized cannot be estimated at this time because of our too short and too limited experience with combined chemo-surgical therapy.

Preliminary Results

In our first attempts some remarkable remissions could be observed in squamous cell carcinomas of the hypopharynx and larynx after a combination therapy of Methotrexate (40 mg/m^2 on the 1st and 15th day), Bleomycin (10 mg on the 1st, 8th and 15th day), Cisplatin (50 mg/m^2 on the 4th day), in due case with an additional dose of Vincristin (2 mg on the 1st, 8th and 15th day).

After adjuvant chemotherapy resection specimens of tumors of the upper larynx region with extension into the vallecula were examined by serial sections. They showed no residual tumor in some cases, in one case there was merely circumscribed superficial growth of cancer. Also considerable remissions of lymph nodes were noticeable. However, the response to chemotherapy varies considerably. For the individual case it cannot be predicted whether the tumor will react with complete remission, partial remission or none. If there is no definite initial but only delayed remission chemotherapy will probably not cause persistant remission.

When selecting the patients, apart from the extent of their tumor, attention must be paid to their general condition and age. Patients of higher age (beyond 65 years) should not be submitted to combination therapy because of the increased risk of complications. Also for the young patients, the risks and side effects of mucosal lesions, loss of hair, blood dyscrasias are so significant that in each individual case critical considerations should be applied.

Surgical aspects, such as difficult dissection or healing complications are of no significance when weighing the pros and cons. Increased healing complications are generally not to be expected after chemotherapy. But it appears advisable to allow a time lapse of 14 days between the end of chemotherapy and the surgical intervention.

Postsurgical radiotherapy was applied as a rule. The single doses of irradiation had to be smaller, however, because of increased reactive mucosal edema and frequent moniliasis, and increased radiosensitivity of the external skin. These reactions were ascribed to the previous chemotherapy. To what extent late effects on the haematopoietic system can occur, as are known in Hodgkin's disease, cannot be predicted at present.

In conclusion it has to be questioned whether adjuvant pre-operative chemotherapy prior to a horizontal resection and/or a combination with additional follow-up radiotherapy provides definite improvements of the results. The initial and significant tumor remissions however, seem to justify their application in the treatment of supraglottic carcinoma of the larynx.

G. Postoperative Course After Vertical and Horizontal Partial Laryngectomy

I. Complications After Partial Resections of the Larynx

Postoperative Care After Partial Resections of the Larynx

P. Federspil, Homburg/Saar

The postoperative care after laryngeal surgery depends on the preceding procedure. It therefore seems relevant to differentiate between patients with or without tracheostomy and a feeding tube.

A *tracheostomy is performed* in subtotal reconstructive laryngectomies, supraglottic partial laryngectomies, hemilaryngectomies and in most extended frontolateral laryngectomies. The incidence of tracheostomy will be higher in departments without an intensive care unit where emergency intubation could be performed around the clock.

Personal care of the patient by the surgeon during the early postoperative period is essential. Clear instructions for the emergency case have to be issued to the doctors and nurses in charge. The administration of corticosteroids or enzymes such as Varidase, Alphachymotrase, or Traumanase before intubation or tracheostomy should be scheduled for possible acute laryngeal edema with acute respiratory disorders. Although prophylactic tracheostomy in a patient with a partial resection of the larynx will protect him against acute respiratory deficiency, this patient deserves full postoperative attention. Problems may arise from displacement of the tube. If the patient can breath without a big problem through his larynx in case the displaced cannula is removed, the reintroduction of the cannula is not an emergency. However, if the patient suffocates if the cannula is not reintroduced at once or if the Mikulicz larynx tamponade is not removed immediately, the medical staff must know that the Mikulicz tamponade may be removed instantly without problems in case the reintroduction of the cannula is difficult.

Patients Without a Tracheostomy Tube and a Feeding Tube

After cordectomy, and sometimes after frontolateral partial laryngectomy patients do not need a tracheostomy or a feeding tube. These patients are preferably accommodated in the semiprone position in a quiet room. This position avoids irritating cough and facilitates coughing and respiration. Only week cough supressant drugs are given on demand. Depending on the preceding anesthesia the patient is allowed to get out of bed at the day of the operation. From the first postoperative day physiotherapy should be applied. A *sufficient air humidity* should be provided. A nebulizer or humidifier should be available. The patient should have the opportunity to rinse his mouth with ice-water and to aspirate his saliva by a suction tube, if he has difficulties with swallowing. He is not allowed to speak for four to eight days.

On the first postoperative days the patient receives a semi-solid diet which should contain sufficient calories as well as sufficient fluid. In cases with serious difficulties of swallowing or frequent deglutition parenteral nutrition or food via a naso-pharyngeal feeding tube is recommended for some days.

The *per- and postoperative antibiotic therapy* takes into account the essential organisms such as staphylococcus aureus or pseudomonas aeruginosa, and also the streptococci and anaerobic bacteria and consists in a combined use of penicillinase-resistant penicilline or a betalactamase inhibitor and pseudomonas-penicillin as for example azlocillin, piperacillin or ticarcillin. The new cephalosporin cefsulodin, which is active against pseudomonas and staphylococci, may be used alone or combined with these penicillins or cefuroxime, cefamandole, cefotaxime, cefoperazone or cefmenoxime. With patients suffering from penicillin allergy one should consider moreover fosfomycin, which is very efficient against all staphylococci and pseudomonas and, of course, fosfomycin or the aminoglycosides, for example in combination with clindamycin and metronidazole. It is important to realize the deficiencies of the antibiotics used and to remedy them, if possible, immediately. We have never encountered complications under postoperative antibiotic therapy. Perioperative antibiotic prophylaxis seems too short, but studies with the newer antibiotics are not available. In case of complications, one should think of the synergistic effect between penicillin and aminoglycoside antibiotics and treat according to the antibiogram.

The *first change of dressing* should take place *on the 3rd day* and the removal of the sutures on the 5th/7th day. Particularly during the *first 24 hours* it is necessary for the patient on the *ENT intensive care unit* to have a recovery room nurse watching him closely for respiration (obstruction of the tube, displacement of the tube into the pretracheal space), pulse and blood pressure as well as an appearance of emphysema, postoperative bleeding or a possible pneumothorax.

Patients with a Tracheostomy and Feeding Tube

In these particular cases, in addition to the already mentioned recommendations (see p. 291), we stress the importance of sterile suction of the tracheal secretion and sufficient fluid intake (in tracheotomized patients about one liter in addition to the standard regimen).

Sufficient fluid intake, ultrasound atomizer and early application of a protection of the tracheostomy helps to avoid the development of crusts. The tracheostomy protection may consist of a compress which helps to filter, moisten and warm the inspired air. If necessary Tacholiquin can be applied as aerosol or for example Bisolvon intravenously.

To avoid tracheal stenosis after a correctly performed tracheostomy the cuff must be deflated as soon as the patient is awake or, after horizontal laryngectomy, at least after 24 hours. Every two or three hours the cuff should be deflated for some minutes with the sucker available. The inner tube is removed and checked every four to six hours and cleaned if necessary while the outer tube remains in situ. For hygienic reasons it seems important not to suck the tube and the mouth of the patient with the same catheter. Suction should be continued for short intervals at any one time and steps taken to aspirate from both bronchi. This is best achieved by using a catheter with a slightly angled tip which can be directed to each bronchus. The patient will be taught to cough out, and thus suction will mostly be limited to the tube.

The *first change of the tube* should be carried out on the 2nd or 3rd postoperative day together with the removal of the iodoform tamponade. On this occasion one should consider the use of a second tube of different length in order to avoid tracheal lesions. The Mikulicz tamponade can be removed on the 2nd or 3rd day. The tube is then plugged to accustom the patient to the normal airway. The decannulation will be performed the next day.

In frontolateral laryngectomy a *naso-oesophageal feeding* tube is only introduced if important parts of the arytenoid cartilage are removed. In supraglottic partial resections or subtotal laryngectomies a feeding tube is always placed by the anaesthetist after the induction of anaesthesia and intubation. Even in the above mentioned extended frontolateral laryngectomy the naso-oesophageal tube can be removed at least after one week. In supraglottic partial resection when both laryngeal nerves could be preserved or in subtotal laryngectomy with epiglottoplasty, cricohyoidoepiglottopexy or cricohyoidopexy an attempt to swallow milk can be made on the 10th or 14th day. We have to warn of a too early removal of the feeding tube in elderly patients with potential renal functional disturbances. Utmost care should be taken that the tube is fixed at different positions of the nose every day or at least every second day in order to avoid ulcers.

Swellings of the larynx which persist over 14 days or that appear after a fortnight are to be treated by enzymes such as Alphachymotrase, Varidase, Alphintern or also antiphlogistics as Tanderil, Voltaren, Felden or by a steroid. The dose of steroid should not be too great and it should not be given over too long a period because of the risk of diminishing the immune response and inducing ulceration of the stomach. Endoscopic removal of edema is very rarely indicated. The Redon or Penrose drainage can be removed after two or three days.

Finally, all these posttherapeutic rules should also imply the mental well-being of the patient. A daily visit by the surgeon is, therefore, essential. After the operation the patient is informed of the "good course" of the surgical procedure. This is repeated to him on the following days. Moreover the results of postoperative histopathologic data are given to him if they are good. Bad news will be retained in general for some days or longer if the patient does not require an immediate second operation.

Early and Late Complications After Laryngofissure or Vertical Partial Laryngectomy

H. Bryan Neel III, Rochester (Minnesota)

Of the 182 patients with early squamous cell cancer of the true vocal cord treated from 1962 to 1974 at the Mayo Clinic, 47 (26%) had complications during the operation, during the postoperative hospitalization, or later (Table 1) (Neel et al. 1980). All complications – major and minor – were noted and reported. For most, hos-

Table 1. Complications in 47 (26%) of 182 patients undergoing laryngofissure or partial vertical laryngectomy for laryngeal cancer

Complication	No.[a]
During operation	
Cardiac arrest	1
During hospitalization	
Atelectasis	6
Pneumonia	6
Subcutaneous emphysema	4
Bleeding	3
Wound	7
Hematoma	1
Infection	3
Perichondritis	2
Breakdown	1
Recannulation	2
After hospitalization	
Granulation, larynx	20
Poor voice	6
Cyst	3
Sequestrum	2
Laryngeal stenosis	2
Large web	1

[a] Some patients had more than one complication

pitalization was not prolonged; indeed, the median duration of hospitalization was the same in the group with postoperative complications as in the group without postoperative complications. There were no deaths attributable to complications.

During Operation

There was one cardiac arrest. The operation was completed satisfactorily, and the patient made a total recovery.

After Operation

Complications consisted of atelectasis, pneumonia, subcutaneous emphysema of the neck and face, bleeding from the tracheotomy site or within the larynx, wound problems, and airway obstruction requiring replacement of the tracheotomy tube.

Late

Laryngoscopy and removal of granulation, usually 3 to 4 months after surgical treatment, to evaluate for recurrent or residual tumor were accomplished in 20 patients.

None had recurrent cancer. Six patients complained of having a poor, breathy voice. Laryngeal retention cysts formed in the ipsilateral false cord in three patients. Delayed wound healing and extrusion of cartilaginous sequestrum occurred in two patients. Two patients had laryngeal stenosis, and one patient had an obstructing web.

Hospitalization

The median duration of hospitalization was 6 days in the group with and the group without postoperative complications. The duration of hospitalization for patients with postoperative complications, however, was 4 to 30 days and exceeded 8 days in 24%. For patients without postoperative complications, the duration was 3 to 16 days and exceeded 8 days in 9%.

The survival data and these data substantiate our belief that the laryngofissure and partial vertical laryngectomy operations, and their minor variations, are an expeditious and highly successful means of eradicating glottic cancers.

Reference

Neel HB III, Devine KD, DeSanto LW (1980) Laryngofissure and cordectomy for early cordal carcinoma: Outcome in 182 patients. Otolaryngol Head Neck Surg 88:79–84

Early and Late Complications After Partial Resections of the Larynx

M. F. VEGA, Madrid

The operative care extends from the preparation of the patient for sugery, until his discharge from the hospital.

Preoperative Care

From the moment of his arrival at the hospital, and before any decision is taken, the patient must undergo a series of examinations to study his general health. Preoperative care also should include informing the patient about the operation to be performed, personal hygiene and care related to the operation itself, to the postoperative period, and the preparation of the room (cleaning, airing, disinfection, humidification, etc.). Small details are essential for a good postoperative recovery.

Per-operative Care

Redon drainage in the supraclavicular area.
Uniform cervical and supraclavicular gauze dressing.
A naso-gastric tube for enteral feeding after the first 24 hours.
A cuffed tracheostomy tube for 48 hours, beginning deflation after 14 hours.
Serum therapy for 24 hours and antibiotic therapy (celasporine) by I.V. while serum is administered intramuscularly till the 8th day.

Postoperative Care

Change of the cuffed tube for a metal tube after 48 hours.
Plugging the tube after the 4th day thus permitting natural phonation and breathing.
Keeping the initial dressing and drainage until the 7th day if nothing unusual happens.
Removing the cannula when feeding is satisfactory, which normally occurs over a period of between 15 and 45 days.
Beginning the reeducation of swallowing from the 10th day. Food that passes to the bronchial tree will be easily expelled by coughing, and does not produce atelectasia by bronchial obstruction. We use boiled potatoes at the beginning of the reeducation of swallowing.
The naso-gastric tube is usually removed between 5 and 10 days.

Postoperative Complications

In the following table we can see the type and frequency of complications we have had in our patients (Table 1).

Table 1. Complications in 240 cases of horizontal partial laryngectomy

	Cases
Local infection	44
Aspiration pneumonia	12
Laryngostomas	5
Base of the tongue haemorrhage	4
Cervical haemorrhage	3
Septicemia	4
Gastric haemorrhage	3
Hepatitis	2
Cardial infarction	4
Postoperative death	12

Local Infection

The impairment of general condition, fever, amount and characteristics of the secretions, and a bad smell leads us to suspect the existence of local infection and requires immediate removal of the dressing. If we find that the skin appears oedematous, with a little necrosis on the edge of the tracheostoma, but adheres to the lower planes without purulent discharge this usually indicates minor necrosis at the level of the glottic stump. Cleaning and disinfection of the wound, antibiotic therapy, and antiseptic gargling usually leads to rapid cure, and the normal postoperative period is not delayed. In other cases we have found a sero-haematoma due to the obstruction of the drain caused by an infection of the haematoma. It is essential to empty the haematoma or empyema immediately and to prescribe antibiotics according to the antibiogram. This complication occurred in 18% of our patients.

Aspiration Pneumonia

This complication was particularly frequent in extended supraglottic laryngectomy with resection of the base of the tongue or of the arytenoids. The entry of saliva into the bronchial tree is a typical problem in the early postoperative period. This situation is managed by the use of a cuffed tracheostomy tube. The problems which arise 10 or 12 days after surgery, at the time of reeducation for swallowing, are obvious and are seen in almost all patients. For this reason we emphasize the need for the patient to be in good respiratory condition, in order to expel by coughing the food which might otherwise enter the bronchial system. It is also important that during the process of reeducation the patients receive only oral food that would dissolve after entering the bronchial tree and would not produce obstruction. We use boiled potatoes. Usually the patient will soon learn to swallow solids, but liquids continue to be a problem for some for at least one month.

Extensive Necrosis

This is the most severe local complication and usually appears on the 7th day. The general condition worsens, the temperature rises and a bad odour appears. These are the danger signals. These complications are common and appear later (after 12–14 days) in radiated or diabetic patients. The development of this necrosis is severe and can lead to death by haemorrhage in the base of the tongue, massive bleeding from the carotid artery or by septicemia. If the breakdown is not fatal the recovery is encouraged by tracheostomy and subsequent reconstructive surgery.

Postoperative Death

This may be due to local or general complications. The causes of mortality in our series are listed in Table 2.

The total percentage of complications has been 33.5%, causing death in 5% of the cases. The most frequent complication was local infection in 18% of the cases, managed without sequelae. We had 5% of severe swallowing problems with repeated aspiration pneumonia. The most severe complication was extensive necrosis in 6.5% of the cases, and also 4% of general complications.

Table 2. Causes of postoperative mortality

		Cases
Local	Haemorrhage from base of the tongue	4
	Septicemias	4
General	Cardial infarction	2
	Gastric haemorrhage	2

Most of the complications occurred in postirradiation surgery and in extended laryngectomies, but the number of complications seems to have diminished in recent years, probably due to the better preparation of the patients, and a better care of the patients in the postoperative period.

Early and Late Complications After Supraglottic Partial Resection of the Larynx

J. Czigner, Budapest

There is no doubt that patients who have had a successful supraglottic partial laryngectomy are in a more acceptable state than total laryngectomees. On the other hand, these procedures bring about some undesired consequences although not all of these have to be considered as real complications. Transitory mucosal edema of the residual larynx and various difficulties of swallowing occur in all patients for some days. They resolve spontaneously, but patients must have an effective cough as well as adequate pulmonary function. By the end of the second or third postoperative week, the airway becomes adequate and both the tracheostomy tube and the nasogastric tube can be removed. Oral feeding is attained in most of the patients (Calearo and Teatini 1972).

The peri-operative complications are similar to those experienced with total laryngectomy but two complications are specific to conservation supraglottic surgery: Laryngeal incompetence/spillover/ and swallowing difficulties (Sellars et al. 1981). The development of a cutaneous fistula is very rare after an ordinary partial supraglottic laryngectomy (Bocca et al. 1968; Som 1974). Preoperative radiotherapy has an unfavorable influence on postoperative complications. Marks et al. (1979) reported 16% major and 26% minor complications in their patients after low dose preoperative radiation and conservation supraglottic surgery. Sellars et al. (1981) reported that the postoperative complication rate and the duration of hospitalization was related significantly to the extent of surgery.

Patient Presentation

226 cases of conservation supraglottic surgery were analysed related to early and late postoperative complications. Swallowing difficulty was an inevitable conse-

quence of this surgery in the early postoperative period. It remained difficult for some patients to swallow fluids after removing the feeding tube and occasionally it became necessary to reinsert a tube to correct the fluid intake. The nasogastric tube was removed between three and sixty-seven days (on average: 19 days). The tracheostomy tube could be removed between the 6th and 68th postoperative day (on average: 23 days).

Early Major Complications: 14 (6%)

1. Peri-operative mortality within 60 days was seven of 226 cases (3%). Deaths were due to aspiration pneumonia with lung abscess in one, wound break down in one, myocardial infarction in two, pulmonary embolism in one and external carotid rupture in two patients.

2. Complete horizontal wound break down (Fig. 1) occurred in 4 patients (1.8%), one of which resulted in death after salvage surgery and unsuccessful re-operation. The other 3 were reconstructed successfully with a second operation and all 3 required minor endolaryngeal surgical excision of the oedematous mucous membrane, later.

3. Rupture of the external carotid branch appeared in three patients (1.3%) due to wound infection, two of which were lethal.

Early Minor Complications: 42 (19%)

Aspiration with or without pneumonia was the most common early complication (14%) with spontaneous recovery in most of the patients, but permanent laryngeal incompetence remained in 3%. Other complications were the following: Wound in-

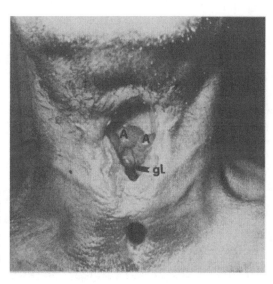

Fig. 1. Postoperative complete horizontal wound break down after supraglottic horizontal laryngectomy in a restful state before reoperation. *"AA"*, oedematous mucous membrane of the arytenoids; *gl,* glottic level *(arrow)*

fection (9%), pharyngocutaneous fistula (3%) with perichondritis in three patients, prolonged oedema and/or granulation (13%) and prolonged de-cannulation time (7.5%).

Late Postoperative Complications: 14 (6%)

1. Permanent laryngeal incompetence (Fig. 2) remained in 7 patients (3%). In the beginning 2 of them were corrected by paraffin, and later one patient by teflon injection to improve the glottic closure. All these three and one other had been operated on by extended supraglottic surgery with the excision of one vocal cord and arytenoid. They required a plastic tube to drink fluids. One patient got a lung abscess and underwent thoracic surgery, but refused any other corrective surgery and died within two years. The remaining 2 patients achieved glottic closure by thyrotomy, suturing together of the anterior 2/3 of the vocal cords, and a permanent tracheostomy but some aspiration of fluids remained in both.

2. Postoperative stenosis: 11 of the 17 patients who had prolonged de-cannulation time developed moderate stenosis above the glottic level, and a massive stenotic scar developed in the other 6 patients.

Endolaryngeal excision and coagulation was employed in all stenotic cases and resulted in the restoration of the air-passage in 9 patients. Endolaryngeal microsurgery combined with Kleinsasser's anterior commissure plasty was used in two patients, but only one was effective. Four patients were operated on by thyrotomy and excision of the scar and insertion of a plastic tube for three or four months. Two of them were successful.

Five patients of the stenotic group needed a permanent tracheostomy, but two of them died later because of recurrent tumor.

3. Late perichondritis with partial sequestration of thyroid cartilage occurred in one patient in the fourth postoperative year. He was treated conservatively.

Our experience shows that swallowing difficulties occur more frequently after extended supraglottic surgery; there was no clear clinical evidence that the extent of

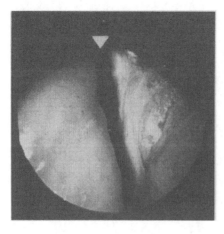

Fig. 2. Laryngeal incompetence at the true cord level. Arrow shows the spacing anterior commissure. Laryngomicroscopic view after extended supraglottic subtotal laryngectomy. The reconstructed pseudocord is on the left side

surgery increased the early postoperative complications; the careful surgical technique of the reconstruction is the most important factor in the prevention of the late postoperative complications of laryngeal incompetence and stenosis.

References

Bocca E, Pignataro O, Mosciaro O (1968) Supraglottic surgery of the larynx. Ann Otol Rhinol Laryngol 77: 1005–1026
Calearo C, Teatini P (1972) Unsere Erfahrung mit der supraglottischen Teilresektion des Kehlkopfes. HNO 20: 11–15
Marks JE, Freeman RB, Lee F, Ogura JH (1979) Carcinoma of the supraglottic larynx. AJR 132: 255–260
Sellars SL, Mills EED, Seid AB (1981) Combined preoperative telecobalt therapy and supraglottic laryngectomy. J Laryngol Otol 95: 305–310
Som ML (1974) Discussion of roles and limitations of conservation surgical therapy for laryngeal carcinoma. Canad J Otolaryng CCLC Workshop 6: 403–411

Functional Complications After Supraglottic Laryngectomy

P. M. STELL, R. P. MORTON, and S. D. SINGH, Liverpool

Introduction

Supraglottic laryngectomy for carcinoma of the supraglottic larynx has been in use for about 70 years (Trotter 1913; Orton 1938) but was popularised by Alonso in 1947.

Ogura (1958) later described extended forms of this procedure in which part of the base of the tongue, one arytenoid or one vocal cord could be removed (Ogura et al. 1961). If the base of the tongue was removed (up to the foramen caecum) the defect was closed in the usual way by approximation of the base of the tongue to the remnant of the thyroid cartilage. If one arytenoid was removed the remaining part of the now immobile glottis on this side was fixed in the midline by a suture posteriorly. Finally, if the true cord was removed a neoglottis could be created from a sliver of cartilage.

Descriptions of the technique, and results of surgery abound in the recent literature (e.g. Bocca et al. 1968; Shumrick 1969; Som 1970; Piquet et al. 1972; Coates et al. 1976). Attention has generally focused on the place of radiotherapy in combination with supraglottic laryngectomy, on the actual extent of resection, and in the use of elective neck dissection in association with the surgery. Alonso (1966) warned of the danger of aspiration pneumonia (1966) after extended supraglottic resection, and this was reinforced by clinical reviews in which adverse pulmonary changes after supraglottic laryngectomy were reported (Staple et al. 1967; Staple and Ogura 1966; Litton and Leonard 1969). Radiographic studies (Staple and Ogura 1966) showed that aspiration occurred more readily with thin liquids than with food of thick consistency. Not surprisingly, the greater the aspiration the higher the incidence of pulmonary complications (Staple et al. 1967).

A review of several papers in which pulmonary complications are mentioned shows that a total of 96 from 592 patients (16%) either died from pulmonary disease or developed pneumonia after supraglottic laryngectomy.

Very little detailed information is available concerning the relationship between the surgery performed and the pulmonary complications that follow. Both Sessions et al. (1975) and Litton and Leonard (1969) concluded that cricopharyngeal myotomy helped prevent aspiration. The other factor that has been reported to be associated with a higher risk of pulmonary complications is the "extended" supraglottic laryngectomy (Sessions et al. 1975; Staple and Ogura 1966; Litton and Leonard 1969).

The present paper is devoted to a study of the pulmonary complications of supraglottic laryngectomy related to the extent of the operation.

Material

This paper is based on a personal series of 85 patients undergoing supraglottic laryngectomy between January 1965 and January 1982.

Of the 85 patients, 41 had had a classical supraglottic laryngectomy with preservation of both arytenoid eminences, both vocal cords and all of the base of the tongue, 9 had resection of part of the base of the tongue, 25 of one arytenoid, and 10 resection of one vocal cord with replacement of the cord by a mucosal or cartilaginous flap.

All patients had cricopharyngeal myotomy done at the time of surgery.

Method

The patients have been followed up for a median period of 50 weeks (range 0–750). The following evidence of deficient function of the larynx was looked for: failure to resume swallowing by mouth within three months of operation, progression of chronic bronchitis, later appearance of chest infection, and death due to chest infection. The ability to rehabilitate was measured by the number of days spent in hospital (of those patients who left hospital alive).

Results

Swallowing

The number of patients who did not resume swallowing by mouth is shown in Table 1. Inability to resume swallowing was confined, with one exception, to patients undergoing supraglottic laryngectomy extended to removal of one arytenoid or one

Table 1. Inability to swallow

	Standard operation	Extended operation		
		Base of tongue	Arytenoid	True cord
Normal swallowing not returned within 3 months	1/41	0/9	2/25	2/10

Table 2. Number of days spent in hospital

	Standard operation	Extended operation		
		Base of tongue	Arytenoid	True cord
Mean	37.0	28.8	49.4	64.5
(S.E.)	2.9	7.3	9.4	21.2

Table 3. Death from chest infection

	Standard operation	Extended operation		
		Base of tongue	Arytenoid	True cord
In hospital	0/41	0/9	1/25	2/10
Later	1/41	0/9	3/25	1/10

vocal cord. 4/35 (11%) of patients undergoing extended supraglottic laryngectomy were unable to swallow satisfactorily.

Only one patient was unable to swallow after simple supraglottic laryngectomy: he had been irradiated previously and should have had a total laryngectomy but refused.

Days in Hospital

The number of days spent in hospital (of those patients who left hospital) is shown in Table 2.

Length of stay in hospital of patients undergoing resection of the arytenoid or true cord was prolonged.

Death from Chest Infection

The number of deaths in hospital and after leaving hospital due to chest infection and/or aspiration is shown in Table 3.

7 patients out of 35 (20.0%) undergoing extended supraglottic laryngectomy (removal of arytenoid or true cord) died before leaving hospital, or later, of the effects of aspiration. Only one of 50 undergoing supraglottic laryngectomy, with or without resection of part of the base of the tongue, died. These differences were significant (Fisher-Irwin exact test $p=0.007$).

Table 4. Later chest infection

	Standard operation	Extended operation		
		Base of tongue	Arytenoid	True cord
Later infection	4/41	2/9	9/25[a]	6/10
Progression of radiological changes of bronchitis	2/41	0/9	1/25	1/10
Total	6/41	2/9	10/25	7/10

[a] 2 patients required injection of teflon and 1 total laryngectomy to control this

Progression of Bronchitis and Later Chest Infection

In addition to the patients who died in hospital of chest infection, some later developed chest infection, and some who already had chronic bronchitis suffered progression of the disease (Table 4).

Once again the patients undergoing extended supraglottic laryngectomy came off badly, and the differences were again statistically significant ($\chi^2_3 = 13.80$, $p < 0.01$).

Several patients required later surgery to protect the airway — this included injection of Teflon into a cord rendered immobile by removal of one arytenoid, and total laryngectomy.

Acknowledgements. The authors are grateful to the North West Cancer Research Foundation for technical support, and to Mrs Morton who did the typing.

References

Alonso JM (1947) Conservative surgery of the cancer of the larynx. Trans Am Otolaryngol 51:633–642
Bocca E, Pignataro O, Mosciaro O (1968) Supraglottic surgery of the larynx. Ann Otol Rhinol Laryngol 77:1005
Coates HL, De Santo LW, Devine KD (1976) Carcinoma of the supraglottic larynx. Arch Otolaryngol 102:686
Litton WB, Leonard JR (1969) Aspiration after partial laryngectomy: cineradiographic studies. Laryngoscope 79:887–908
Ogura JH (1958) Supraglottic subtotal laryngectomy and radical neck dissection for carcinoma of the epiglottis. Laryngoscope 68:939–1903
Ogura JH, Saltzstein SL, Spjut HJ (1961) Experiences with conservation surgery in laryngeal and pharyngeal carcinoma. Laryngoscope 71:258–276
Orton HB (1938) Cancer of the laryngopharynx. Arch Otolaryngol 28:344–354
Piquet JJ, Desaulty A, Decroix G (1972) La laryngectomie horizontale sus-glottique dans le traitement des cancers sus-glottiques et de la margelle laryngee. Ann Otolaryngol Chir Cervicofasc 89:35–48
Sessions DG, Ogura JH, Civalsky RH (1975) Late glottic insufficiency. Laryngoscope 85:950–959
Shumrick DA (1969) Supraglottic laryngectomy. Arch Otolaryngol 89:91–97
Som ML (1970) Conservation surgery for carcinoma of the supraglottis. J Laryngol Otol 84:655–678

Staple TW, Ogura JH (1966) Cineradiography of the swallowing mechanism following supraglottic sublateral laryngectomy. Radiology 87:226–230

Staple TW, Ragsdale EF, Ogura JH (1967) The chest roentgenogram following supraglottic laryngectomy. Am J Roentgenol 100:583–587

Trotter W (1913) The principles and techniques of the operative treatment of malignant disease of the mouth and pharynx. Lancet 1:1147–1152

Late Complications and Recurrences After Partial Resections of the Larynx

Z. KRAJINA, Zagreb

Introduction

On the basis of preceding studies of the particular behaviour of laryngeal carcinomas we have extended the classical indications for partial laryngectomy: fixation of one vocal cord no longer was a contraindication if the tumor had not invaded the laryngeal skeleton. The most important principle is a wide excision of the tumor with a healthy margin what must be proven by frozen section. The size of the excisional defect has no upper limit, as it can easily be closed by a rotation flap of sterno-hyoid fascia. Three quarters of the uninvolved, mobile vocal cord should be preserved as a minimum. Our ten years' experience with this technique was published 1979 in the Journal of Laryngology.

This paper will deal with the late complications observed in those patients which had undergone extended partial laryngectomy between 1969 and 1978.

Material and Method

During ten years between 1969 and 1978 211 partial laryngectomies were performed: 110 vertical and frontolateral, 51 supraglottic, 47 combined resections, and 3 subtotal laryngectomies. Preoperative radiotherapy, with doses of 20–30 gy, was applied to patients with poorly differentiated tumors invading the superior or inferior hypopharynx. Postoperative radiotherapy of up to 60 gy was provided for the cases who had preoperative irradiation or for those cases whose borders of resection were dubious histologically. All cervical lymph nodes were examined intraoperatively: This was carried out on both sides in horizontal laryngectomy.

Results

As late complications we have defined all changes which appeared as anatomical abnormalities in the neck or in distant organs after time intervals of six months up to ten years. The data are figured out in the Tables 1–5.

Table 1. Partial laryngectomies 1969–1978 (211 cases)

	Total	Alive	Dead	Lost
Horizontal laryngectomies	51	40	9	2
Vertical and frontolateral laryngectomies	110	90	11	9
Combined laryngectomies	47	40	4	3
Subtotal laryngectomies	3	2	1	0
	211 (100%)	172 (81%)	25 (12%)	14 (7%)

Table 2. Recurrences after vertical and frontolateral partial laryngectomy (n = 120)

	Without radiotherapy (n = 64)				With radiotherapy (n = 56)			
	Total	Alive	Dead	Lost	Total	Alive	Dead	Lost
Leucoplacia	2	2	0	0	3	3	0	0
Recurrence of tumor	3	2	1	0	5	2	2	1
Recurrence of neck metastases with or without local recurrence of tumor	5	2	2	1	9	5	2	2

Table 3. Complications after vertical and frontolateral partial laryngectomy (n = 120)

	Without radiotherapy (n = 64)	With radiotherapy (n = 56)
Stenosis of larynx	2	1
Synechias of larynx	4	0
Hypertrophy of larynx	5	1
Insufficiency of glottis	1	1
Obliteration of sinus piriformis with dysphagia	0	1

Table 4. Recurrences and survival rates after horizontal partial laryngectomy and radiotherapy (n = 51)

	Total	Alive	Dead	Lost
Occurence of bilateral neck metastases	6	1	5	0
Occurence of unilateral neck metastases after 1–3 years	3	3	0	0
Occurence of pulmonary carcinoma after 4–6 years	3	0	3	0
Local recurrence of tumor (after 11 years)	1	1	0	0

Table 5. Complications after horizontal partial laryngectomy and radiotherapy (n = 51)

Stenosis of larynx	2
Edema of larynx	2
Synechia of anterior commissure	1

Discussion

Patients undergoing vertical and frontolateral laryngectomy were divided into two groups: those who were treated only by surgery, and those who had a combined treatment of surgery with radiotherapy. In both groups the development of leukoplakia or recurrent tumor was observed on the operated or on the contralateral side. The occult or multicentric growth of carcinoma in the environment of a visible focus offers severe difficulties. According to our experience no vertical or frontolateral resections are indicated in diffuse laryngeal edema. Stout, and Miller and Fisher have published cases with glottic carcinoma who showed a carcinoma in situ on the contralateral side. Miller and Fisher emphasized that in ten of their cases recurrences were observed even after postoperative irradiation.

We have not observed bilateral neck metastases in our material. Unilateral lymph node metastases were observed in 14 cases (13%) of both our groups after one to three years postoperatively.

This happened in combination with a recurrent laryngeal carcinoma in five cases. Radical neck dissection was the salvage therapy in seven patients. We conclude that additional radiotherapy is no protection against secondary metastatic growth in the regional lymph nodes. Minor complications such as hypertrophy of the contralateral cord or synechia were not relevant. Laryngeal stenoses were rare but occurred in both groups. There were two cases of glottic incompetence which induced aspiration during the intake of liquids.

Five of our 47 cases (11%) with combined partial laryngectomies developed stenoses of the larynx irrespective of the application of irradiation. In three of these cases the stenosis could be removed by minor interventions such as microlaryngoscopy or laser therapy. In this group (combined partial resections) no bilateral metastases, but only unilateral recurrence of neck metastases were observed, sometimes after irradiation, neck dissection or adjuvant chemotherapy. Three patients developed insufficient glottic closure, but none suffered from swallowing difficulties.

In two of three cases with subtotal laryngectomy the malignant process was eradicated, and decannulation was possible in one of them.

In conclusion, the evaluation of the postoperative course of 211 patients with partial laryngectomy showed a cure rate of 81%: 172 patients were free of disease after the observation time mentioned above.

References

Krajina Z, Kosoković F, Večerina S (1979) Laryngeal reconstruction with sternohyoid fascia in partial laryngectomy. J Laryngol Otol 93:1181

Miller AH, Fisher HR (1953) Carcinoma-in-situ of the larynx. Ann Otol Rhinol Laryngol 62:358

Stout AP (1953) Intramucosal Epithelioma of the Larynx. Am J Roentgenol 69:1

II. Early Detection and Management of Recurrences

Follow-up Examination After Partial Laryngectomy. Early Detection of Recurrences

W. STEINER, Erlangen

The pre-therapeutic and post-therapeutic diagnostic work-up is the domain of endoscopy, cytology and biopsy. Other methods such as xerography, X-ray tomography, computed tomography, ultrasound and biochemical investigations of the blood, cannot provide appropriate early evidence of residual or recurrent cancer. The preconditions for the early detection of recurrent tumour in the larynx were better than in any other organ system, since recurrent lesions or second primaries were usually confined to the surface of the mucosa, and were relatively easily identified by endoscopy.

More difficult is the early detection of residual or recurrent disease in scar tissue or beneath the skin graft used to close a defect.

In follow-up examinations, the entire mucosa of the endolarynx must be inspected, using the 90° angled telescope and the flexible endoscope aided by cotton wool carriers or the suction tube. It is not always feasible to perform microlaryngoscopy under anaesthesia in the presence of surgery-related anomalies of the larynx that make inspection difficult.

The use of a cotton wool carrier has proved of value, for example, both for rendering visible the mucosa covered by a prolapsed arytenoid cartilage, and also for obtaining cytological swabs. Between 1973 and 1978, 100 postpartial resection patients were examined by magnifying endoscopy and swab cytology. In three cases cytology revealed recurrent disease, although endoscopy failed to show anything suspicious. A problem is the assessment of cytological swabs in a larynx previously subjected to radiotherapy for carcinoma; here, in particular, with findings classed as Papanicolaou IV, misinterpretations are possible. Any proliferation must be investigated irrespective of its clinical appearance. The histological investigation of the material resected with the aid of the endoscope provides information on whether the lesion really is a locally circumscribed process that can be appropriately treated with preservation of function, or whether the macroscopically recognizable circumscribed lesion represents the "tip of an iceberg" and the surgical scar conceals an extensive submucosal residual or recurrent tumour.

Thoroughgoing, regular, long-term follow-up continued beyond 5 years makes it possible to detect new lesions in good time to permit mucosa-sparing surgery that is also capable of preserving functionally important structures. Thus, for example, patients who developed a second primary up to 33 years after partial resection, have been spared a mutilating laryngectomy.

The appearance of an endolaryngeal recurrent tumour in partially resected or irradiated patients, by no means always requires radical, often mutilating, surgery. The recurrent lesion or second carcinoma can be successfully treated surgically or, if detected early, even using the microlaryngoscopic technique, depending upon its (histological) spread. We consider the cytological swab to be an important additional diagnostic measure. In particular in cases with prior surgery requiring defect closure, or prior radiotherapy, resulting in a situation that is difficult to assess, the swab, carried out under magnifying endoscopic control after spray anesthesia, can provide valuable information on a concealed tumour. However, it can never replace the endoscopic removal of accessible proliferations with histological work-up.

For the prevention of recurrent disease or a second primary, a systematic "clean up" of the upper airways aimed at achieving complete healing of the mucous membranes, together with the elimination of inhaled agents in particular the carcinogens contained in cigarette smoke, is necessary.

References

Jaumann MP, Steiner W, Münch E, Pesch H-J (1981) Endoskopische Krebsnachsorge im oberen Aero-Digestiv-Trakt. Arch Otorhinolaryngol (NY) 231:656

Steiner W (1979) Vergleichende Beurteilung endoskopischer Diagnostik- und Therapieverfahren beim Kehlkopfkrebs und seinen Vorstadien. Habilitationsschrift, Erlangen

Early Detection of Recurrent Tumours After Previous Treatment of Laryngeal Carcinomas

J. Olofsson, Linköping

Prerequisites for early detection of recurrent or new tumours after previous treatment of laryngeal carcinomas are:
a) A well organized follow-up system at oncologic centres with necessary expertise available,
b) regular laryngoscopies – with a microlaryngoscopy a few months after treatment,
c) the follow-up should be based on the histopathological findings,
d) impaired mobility of the vocal cord after previous endoscopic surgery or radiotherapy means recurrent tumour until the opposite is proven,
e) to exclude residual or recurrent carcinoma in a persistent postradiologic oedema,
f) that the increased risk for multiple primaries is taken into account, but also that,
g) preventive measures should be undertaken.

Oncologic Centres

Patients with head and neck cancers in general should be treated at oncologic centres with adequate equipment and necessary expertise available. This means patient materials large enough to provide possibilities for systematized studies to evaluate the treatment results. The computer is more and more becoming an integrated part of the routine work at oncologic centres for an easy patient follow-up and for continuous statistical work. The computer analysis may also reveal the patients at high risk. The follow-up in Scandinavian oncologic centres are mainly performed in joint ENT-radiotherapy clinics. Under all circumstances the patients are best followed by specialists, who are able to take care of the patients with recurrent disease.

A correct assessment and classification of the tumour is the base for the treatment planning and is best performed by direct laryngoscopy using the operating microscope − microlaryngoscopy − which also allows excellent opportunities for photographic documentation. This examination may be complemented by photographic documentation using the telescope. A good photographic documentation of the tumour and a detailed radiographic mapping increases the chance to detect a recurrent tumour. A post-therapeutic radiograph is a valuable reference too. The latter examination should be performed when the oedema has settled and can preferably be done at the same time as the first control microlaryngoscopy. The value of such a reference radiogram is especially valid if the Toronto "radiate and see" policy for T_3 and T_4 carcinomas is adopted (Harwood 1982).

Examination of the Larynx

Microlaryngoscopy should be performed about 3 months after completion of the radiotherapy or after partial laryngectomy for a laryngeal carcinoma. At this time most of the postradiologic or postoperative oedema has settled. Smear cytology can be a diagnostic aid but is less sensitive after previous radiotherapy (Lundgren et al. 1981). Biopsies should be taken from all clinically suspect areas but one should be careful after previous radiotherapy not being to aggressive and thereby introducing an infection with the risk of subsequent chondritis.

In most series with head and neck cancer 90% of the recurrences occur within the first two years. The checkings must therefore be more frequent during this period of time. As a rule the patients can be examined every second month during the first year after therapy and every third month for the following two years and every fourth month up to 5 years. After this, examination every sixth month will be enough. After the initial microlaryngoscopic examination the following examinations can be performed as mirror laryngoscopies or using a telescope, which also allows photographic documentation. The mirror laryngoscopy can for glottic carcinomas be supplemented by the use of the operating microscope which gives an excellent assessment of the vocal cord mucosa. Stroboscopic examination may further increase the chance for early detection of recurrent glottic carcinoma.

If the larynx is difficult to inspect due to e.g. an overhanging epiglottis the fiberscope provides an excellent possibility for a close and easy inspection of the laryngeal surface of the epiglottis, the ventricles, vocal cords, anterior commissure and subglottis. A special laryngofiberscope may be used or a regular bronchofiberscope, which has a greater versatility. The fiberscopic examination is easily performed as an outpatient procedure.

Histopathology

The intervals between the laryngoscopies certainly depend on the location and extent of the tumour. The histopathological examination of the biopsy specimen and the surgical specimen should be taken into account. Jakobsson (1973) showed that the use of a morphologic malignancy grading system proved to give additional information about the prognosis. For glottic carcinomas nuclear polymorphism, mode of invasion and total malignancy points were factors of importance in the prediction of the 5 year results. DNA measurements may give additional information (Hellquist 1981). When dealing with severe dysplasia and carcinoma in situ it is the well differentiated and diffuse lesions that seems to give most problems with recurrences and development of invasive carcinoma (Hellquist et al. 1982). Patients with carcinoma developing in a chronic laryngitis have an increased risk for further carcinomas in a diffusely changed mucosa after partial surgery or radiotherapy. They often get a longstanding oedema, and a red swollen, slightly granulated mucosa is common after radiotherapy. The chronic laryngitis is not a histopathologic premalignant condition *per se* but may act as a "promoting factor" for cancer development (Glanz and Kleinsasser 1976).

The surgical specimen should be carefully examined. The margins of resection need special attention. However, histologically positive resection margins do not necessarily mean recurrent disease. In a series of 39 patients with cancer involvement of a margin in the hemilaryngectomy specimen 7 (18%) later developed a biopsy proven local recurrence. Four out of 72 patients (6%) with no tumor at the resection margin developed a recurrence (Bauer et al. 1975). Under all circumstances the histopathology gives us an idea where to look for a recurrent tumour.

Impaired Vocal Cord Mobility

Impaired mobility or fixation of the vocal cord appearing after previous minor endoscopic surgery or radiotherapy indicates recurrent disease until the contrary is proven. Repeated radiological examination – soft tissue plain films and computed tomograms – should be taken. At this situation a reference, immediate posttherapeutic, radiologic examination may be of great value. Microlaryngoscopy should be performed and multiple biopsies taken if there is no visible tumour. Especially after radiotherapy but also after partial surgery there is a risk for a recurrent entirely submucosally growing tumour. After partial surgery the natural barriers within the larynx are removed and the tumours may spread outside the larynx into the soft tissues.

Postirradiation Problems

Postirradiation oedema may complicate the laryngoscopic examination. A red, swollen epiglottis and arytenoids may hide the vocal cords for an indirect inspection. In some centres a short-term steroid therapy is employed in these cases at least before the first post-therapeutic inspection (Wey 1979). If the oedema does not settle, or if it settles down and later flares up, this may indicate an underlying chondritis and result in chondronecrosis of the larynx. Early cases may respond to medical treatment, but a laryngectomy is required as soon a chondronecrosis has developed according to Stell and Morrison (1973). Ward et al. (1975) presented a material where persistent oedema 6 months or more after completion of the radiotherapy indicated residual carcinoma in 23 out of 43 cases (53%) and only 6 out of these 23 (26%) were salvaged by total laryngectomy, indicating the difficulties involved to diagnose the residual or recurrent tumour in these cases. DeSanto and his colleagues (1976) recognized the irradiation failures too late to be able to utilize conservation surgery.

Irradiation induced carcinoma is not common but has to be taken into account (Baker and Weissman 1971; Glanz 1976; Aanesen and Olofsson 1979). These tumours are often diagnosed decades after the irradiation therapy, which implies that patients who have undergone irradiation treatment have to be followed for lifetime.

Multiple Primaries

A number of reports stress the importance to detect synchronous or metachronous second and third primaries in patients with head and neck carcinomas. Wagenfeld et al. (1980, 1981) found a high incidence of second primary respiratory tract neoplasms in patients with laryngeal carcinoma. 6.5% of patients with a glottic carcinoma and 12.3% with a supraglottic carcinoma had a second primary within the respiratory tract and more than half of these tumours were located in the lungs. Multiple primaries with dissimilar histology may occur within the larynx (Ferlito 1980). Prospective panendoscopic examinations have been performed in patients with mucosal neoplasms in the upper aero-digestive tract and have disclosed a high percentage of synchronous multiple primary carcinomas (McGuirt et al. 1982). The value of such "screening" examinations has to be further assessed but certainly introduce interesting aspects in the treatment of patients with aero-digestive tract carcinomas.

Preventive Measures

The patients who continue to smoke are at a higher risk than those who quit smoking (Rudin and Sandberg 1972). The same may be true for excessive consumption of alcohol. The doctors play an important role in preventive oncological medicine. The doctor treating a patient for a laryngeal malignancy should use all efforts to try to get his patient to quit smoking. The advices are certainly more efficient if the doctor is a non-smoker or has quit smoking himself.

References

Aanesen JP, Olofsson J (1979) Irradiation-induced tumours of the head and neck. Acta Otolaryngol [Suppl] (Stockh) 360:178–181

Baker DC, Weissman B (1971) Postirradiation carcinoma of the larynx. Ann Otol Rhinol Laryngol 80:634–637

Bauer WC, Lesinski SG, Ogura JH (1975) The significance of positive margins in hemilaryngectomy specimens. Laryngoscope 85:1–13

DeSanto LW, Lillie JC, Devine KD (1976) Surgical salvage after radiation for laryngeal cancer. Laryngoscope 86:649–657

Ferlito A (1980) Double primary synchronous and metachronous cancer of the larynx and hypopharynx with dissimilar histology. Five case reports and review of the literature. Arch Otorhinolaryngol (NY) 229:107–119

Glanz H (1976) Late recurrence or radiation induced cancer of the larynx. Clin Otolaryngol 1:123–129

Glanz H, Kleinsasser O (1976) Chronische Laryngitis und Carcinom. Arch Otorhinolaryngol (NY) 212:57–75

Harwood AR (1982) Cancer of the larynx – the Toronto experience. J Otolaryngol [Suppl] 11:1–21

Hellquist H (1981) Dysplasia of the vocal cords. Linköping University Medical Dissertations, No 105. Linköping

Hellquist H, Lundgren J, Olofsson J (1982) Hyperplasia, keratosis, dysplasia and carcinoma in situ of the vocal cords – a follow-up study. Clin Otolaryngol 7:11–27

Jakobsson P (1973) Glottic carcinoma of the larynx. Factors influencing prognosis following radiotherapy. Thesis, Stockholm

Lundgren J, Olofsson J, Hellquist HB, Strandh J (1981) Exfoliative cytology in laryngology. Comparison of cytologic and histologic diagnoses in 350 microlaryngoscopic examinations – a prospective study. Cancer 47:1336–1343

McGuirt WF, Matthews B, Koufman JA (1982) Multiple simultaneous tumors in patients with head and neck cancer. A prospective, sequential panendoscopic study. Cancer 50:1195–1199

Rudin R, Sandberg N (1972) Ökad recidivfrekvens hos rökare med larynxcancer. Medicinsk riksstämma p 372

Stell PM, Morrison MD (1973) Radiation necrosis of the larynx. Etiology and management. Arch Otolaryngol 98:111–113

Wagenfeld DJH, Harwood AR, Bryce DP, van Nostrand AWP, de Boer G (1980) Second primary respiratory tract malignancies in glottic carcinoma. Cancer 46:1883–1886

Wagenfeld DJH, Harwood AR, Bryce DP, van Nostrand AWP, de Boer G (1981) Second primary respiratory tract malignant neoplasms in supraglottic carcinoma. Arch Otolaryngol 107:135–137

Ward PH, Calcaterra TC, Kagan AR (1975) The enigma of post-radiation edema and recurrent or residual carcinoma of the larynx. Laryngoscope 85:522–529

Wey W (1979) Suspicion of persistent or recurrent carcinoma of the larynx after radiation therapy. ORL 41:301–311

Early Detection and Management of Recurrences After Vertical Partial Laryngectomy

H. BRYAN NEEL III, Rochester (Minnesota)

Postoperatively, patients are examined every 2 to 4 months, usually over a period of 12 to 18 months. The larynx is examined with use of mirrors and, occasionally, fiberoptic instruments in the office. The neck should always be palpated carefully, although the likelihood of metastasis from early cordal cancers is small.

Seven (4%) of the 182 patients with early cordal cancers had recurrences: three in the larynx only, one in the larynx and neck, and three in the neck only (Neel et al. 1980). Of the four patients with laryngeal recurrences, two were alive and well at long-term follow-up; both had laryngectomies, one of which was preceded by irradiation. One patient died as a consequence of distant metastases after a laryngectomy preceded by irradiation, and one died of regional and distant cancer after irradiation, thyroidectomy, and excision of tumor from the tracheoesophageal tissues.

Recurrence of tumor after laryngofissure and cordectomy or partial vertical laryngectomy is uncommon if one does not attempt to overstep the indications for the operation. Because irradiation is unlikely to eradicate a recurrence after removal of cartilage in a partial vertical laryngectomy, my associates and I prefer to do a total laryngectomy, usually with a complete neck dissection on the side of the major recurrence. The spinal accessory nerve is spared if there is no obvious metastatic tumor in the neck.

Three of the 182 patients had metastases to the neck, although the larynx was free of cancer. Metastasis from an early cordal cancer is quite rare and occurs in less than 1 to 2% of patients. One patient with ipsilateral neck metastasis and one patient with contralateral neck metastasis were successfully treated by radical neck dissections. A third patient, who had metastasis to the neck and axillary nodes treated by irradiation, died as a consequence of distant metastases. Prophylactic neck dissections are unnecessary, and a complete (radical) neck dissection is carried out in the rare patient in whom metastatic disease develops.

Reference

Neel HB III, Devine KD, DeSanto LW (1980) Laryngofissure and cordectomy for early cordal carcinoma: Outcome in 182 patients. Otolaryngol Head Neck Surg 88: 79–84

Early Detection and Management of Recurrences After Vertical Partial Laryngectomy

Y. Guerrier, Montpellier

The follow-up of patients submitted to vertical partial laryngectomy must be very close. According to the precise indications for this type of surgery the postoperative follow up should be carried out by the team which performed the operation and which is familiar with the size and localization of the primary tumour and with the clinical details. The prediction of a recurrence relies on the intraoperative observations, on the histological examination with classification and grading of the tumour, especially on the scrupulous examination of the excisional borders. Also the volume of the tumour is meaningful. The individual hygiene, e.g. continued smoking or abstinence is important. Collecting all this information we can separate a group of high risk patients which should be followed up with particular attention.

Material and Methods

This paper is based on the evaluation of the charts of 292 patients undergoing vertical partial laryngectomy between January 1, 1970 and December 31, 1981. During this period 774 total laryngectomies were performed.

Detection of Recurrences

Follow-up examinations have the following schedule: during the first six months the patients are seen every month, during the next year every third month, then every sixth month over two years, and finally once a year.

Some patients are difficult to inspect by indirect laryngoscopy because of increased reflex activity. One should not hesitate to provide direct laryngoscopy for this group. This technique should also be applied in all cases that have been dubious by indirect inspection. Some patients offer definite problems either due to difficult laryngoscopy or by bad discipline in keeping to their follow up schedule, may be because they are anxious of the examination. All these belong to a high risk group of recurrences.

After vertical partial laryngectomy the anterior commissure remains a site of incertainty because this region offers particular problems during the follow-up period:

1. Scar formation in the anterior commissure may be the result of tissue repair but may be suspicious of tumour recurrence if red granulations are visible. The ordinary scar has a white to gray colour.

2. Unilateral immobility of the glottis is frequent in cases of tumour proliferation in the paraglottic space. This is the case after the operation of Leroux-Robert and even after St. Clair-Thompson's operation. A vocal cord which becomes fixed after an initial period of free mobility is always suspicious and must be submitted to

direct laryngoscopy using an angle optic. This optic tool has considerably increased the reliability of postoperative follow-up.

3. The late development of a cutaneous fistula is an undoubted sign of tumour recurrence. Cytologic examination of a smear from the fistula will verify the nature of this lesion.

4. Since we know that the lymphatic drainage from the glottis has a dorso-ventral direction we generally have to assume a recurrent tumour growth in the anterior commissure.

In this connection we must remember the necessity of removing all lymphatic tissue in front of the crico-thyroid region with exposure of the anterior angle of the thyroid cartilage, of the conus elasticus, and the anterior face of the cricoid cartilage. This strategy holds for all kinds of vertical partial laryngectomies.

The excised specimens must always be sent for histological examination. Involvement of the delphian node, situated on the conus elasticus, is always a bad prognostic sign. In this, fortunately rare, occasion we plan postoperative irradiation of the central neck region and the superior mediastinum. The delphian node drains to the mediastinal lymph nodes without regional interruption in cervical lymph nodes.

Local Recurrences

Among 102 cases of T_1 tumours treated by cordectomy, there were 8 local recurrences. All of them were late: six were observed after three years, two after eight years. This fact may emphasize the importance of prolonged aftercare even in small glottic cancers. There was one recurrence in a series of 12 T_{1b} cases submitted to bilateral cordectomy. Three local recurrences were observed in 21 cases of hemiglottectomy performed for involvement of the vocal process of the arytenoid without extension to the anterior commissure.

There were also three recurrences in 17 hemilaryngectomies by Hautant's method carried out in glottic cancer with tumour growth directed to the central area of the subglottis.

Severe problems are offered by the T_2 tumours crossing the anterior commissure and invading the opposite vocal cord. They were treated by fronto-lateral laryngectomy. Not included were those carcinomas arising in the anterior commissure, inspite of preserved mobility of the glottis.

In a series of 140 frontolateral laryngectomies we found
18 local recurrences
3 regional lymph node metastases, and
3 local recurrences with regional lymphatic spread.
That is 21 local recurrences in 140 frontolateral laryngectomies (17.1%). A critical reevaluation of these cases showed, that in 16 patients the tumour mass was comparatively large, and the cord mobility was difficult to judge. In 12 of these 21 cases the histologic examination of the specimen had been favourable.

We changed our strategy two years ago: in cases like the above described we now prefer a subtotal laryngectomy with crico-hyoidopexy.

Certainly, in all the 21 cases of recurrences total laryngectomy or vertical partial laryngectomy had been considered. It has to be emphasized, however, that between the radical and mutilating procedure of total laryngectomy there exists a type of subtotal reconstructive surgery which also offers functional rehabilitation.

Treatment of Local Recurrences

If the local recurrence of carcinoma is associated with regional lymphatic spread we perform total laryngectomy with monobloc neck dissection.

If there exists only a local recurrent growth of tumour therapy depends on the size of the recurrence:

1. Small lesions are irradiated administering 45 gy from small fields. During the last decade we have not used fronto-lateral laryngectomy after unsuccessful cordectomy.

2. In cases of medium size recurrence subtotal, reconstructive laryngectomy is carried out.

3. For the large recurrent carcinoma of the larynx with fixation of the glottis an enlarged total operation is used. This is called laryngectomy-en-bloc. Its principle consists of the ablation of all the adjacent prelaryngeal scar tissue in connection with the larynx. Its technique is described in the following paragraph.

Technique of Laryngectomy-en-bloc

The main feature of this operation is the combined removal of the larynx and the hyoid bone in connection with the prelaryngeal structures including the skin. Irre-

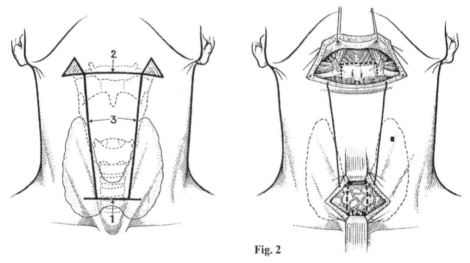

Fig. 1. En-bloc laryngectomy. Skin incisions (see text)

Fig. 2. En-bloc laryngectomy. *Above:* Dissection of the suprahyoid muscles and resection of the hyoid bone. *Below:* Resection of the thyroid isthmus for inferior tracheostomy

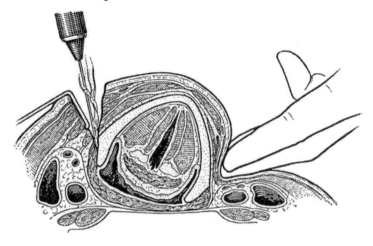

Fig. 3. En-bloc laryngectomy. The surgeon's left hand rotates the larynx in order to expose the dorsal edge of the contralateral thyroid cartilage. The electric knife sections the inferior constrictor muscles of the pharynx

spective of the actual scar formation this technique is optimal for safe removal of the possibly involved prelaryngeal zone of danger.

The skin incisions are demonstrated in Fig. 1. The basal horizontal incision has a length of 4 centimetres (*1*). The superior horizontal incision has a length of 8 centimetres (*2*). The supraphyoid muscles are severed and the dissection will reach the bottom of the valleculae. Hemostasis of the lingual veins and section of the hyoid body follow (Fig. 2).

Two vertical incisions 3 cm above and 2 cm below from the median plane (*3*) connect the horizontal incisions. Using scissors the subhyoid muscles are dissected, and the larynx is mobilized to its posterior edge on both sides. The constrictor muscles are freed from the thyroid cartilage (Fig. 4). The thyroid gland is dissected

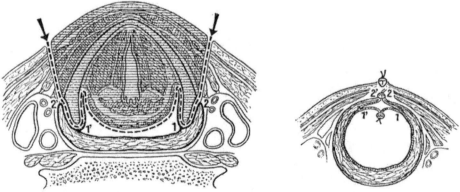

Fig. 4   Fig. 5

Fig. 4. En-bloc laryngectomy. Wound closure in three planes. The sutures 1 and 2 may be achieved by chromic cat gut or using atraumatic needles

Fig. 5. En-bloc laryngectomy. Skin closure by single sutures

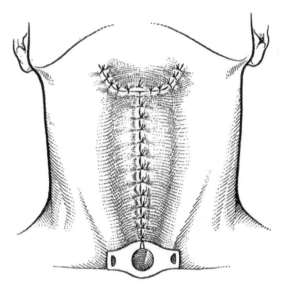

Fig. 6. En-bloc laryngectomy. Schematic drawing of the bloc excision. Note the exposure of the thyroid cartilage following the oblique line

and its isthmus divided. After ligation of the superior thyroid vessels a typical laryngectomy is performed with a small pharyngeal opening. The posterior extent of the laryngeal carcinoma is checked. This pharyngostoma is then closed in the typical manner (Figs. 4 and 5). The skin wound can be closed after triangular skin excision (Fig. 1), and "per primam" wound healing is established in most cases. This technique has proven useful in reconstructive surgery after radiotherapy. The extension of the en-bloc laryngectomy in the horizontal plane is illustrated by Fig. 6.

Treatment of Recurrences After Supraglottic Horizontal Laryngectomy (S.H.L.)

M. F. Vega, Madrid

The possibility of recurrence requires strict posttherapeutic follow up of all patients. In our practice the patient is checked monthly for the first year, every three months in the second and third years and every six months in the fourth and fifth year, and annually from the sixth year on. Nevertheless, the number of not followed up patients is very important as we can see when we study the results. Also the stage the patient reaches with a recurrence is discouraging and in most cases valuable treatment will be impossible.

Early Detection and Management of Recurrences   321

Table 1. Incidence of recurrence in a series of 240 horizontal partial laryngectomies

Localization of recurrence	Number of cases	%
Local	26	10.8
Regional	30	12.5
Distant	3	1.25
Total recurrences	59	24.6

Table 2. Incidence of local recurrences with regard to the type of surgery

Technique	Cases	%
S.H.L. extended to the base of the tongue	6/24	(25.0)
S.H.L. extended to a piriform sinus and hypopharynx	3/8	(37.5)
S.H.L. extended to a vocal cord	3/17	(17.5)
S.H.L. extended to an arytenoid	2/34	(6.0)
S.H.L. simple	12/149	(8.0)
Horizonto-vertical L.	0/8	(0.0)

Table 3. Therapy of 26 local recurrences after S.H.L.

Treatment	Cases
Total laryngectomies	5
T-Co-T	9
Chemotherapy	2
Without treatment	10

Local Recurrences

26 patients had local recurrence (Table 1). The incidence of these failures according to the technique is given in Table 2.

The treatment of local recurrences varied with their stage. The different kinds of their treatment are listed in Table 3. Of the 26 cases, only three patients remained free of recurrence, two of them treated by a total laryngectomy, and one by telecobalt therapy (T-Co-T).

Regional Recurrences

3 patients had regional recurrence. The following classification is based on the previous treatment:

In necks not treated	4/23 (17.5%)
In necks treated with T-Co-T	9/53 (17.0%)
In necks treated with neck dissection	17/164 (10.0%)

In the necks previously treated the recurrence was:
  Homolateral   9 cases
  Contralateral   8 cases
Of the 9 homolateral cases, 6 were after radical neck dissection (N_3); 2 cases after functional neck dissection (N_{1b}); and one after functional neck dissection (N_0).

Of the 30 cases, 10 are alive without showing any sign of recurrence. All were treated by neck dissection complemented with T-Co-T in four cases. The necks of 3 of the cases had not been treated previously. Six of the cases had been treated previously. Six of the cases had contralateral nodes at the previous neck dissection and only one case after a previous functional neck dissection.

Distant Metastasis

Only three patients had lung metastases from which they died, but at the moment of death the larynx and neck were free of tumor.

The analysis of the data reveals the following: The percentage of local recurrences after horizontal supraglottic laryngectomy is low (10.75%), but the percentage of patients curable by a total laryngectomy or radiotherapy is also very low (11.5%). The highest percentage of cure is to be found in the operations extended to the base of the tongue and the piriform sinus (37.5%). When the tumor involves the cord the recurrence rate is higher when treated by three-quarter laryngectomy (17.5%) than when treated by a horizontal-vertical laryngectomy.

Involvement of the arytenoids, with preserved mobility does not mean a worse prognosis. In recurrences after simple supraglottic laryngectomy the highest percentage is to be found in the techniques "a minimum".

The percentage of node recurrences in patients treated by simple supraglottic laryngectomy or complemented with irradiation, but without surgery for the nodes is 17%. On the other hand, in the supraglottic laryngectomy associated with neck dissection, in N+ as in N–, the rate is 10%. Of the 13 cases of nodal recurrence in patients previously treated by simple laryngectomy or with complementary irradiation, only three recovered, a total failure rate of 13%. On the other hand, of the 17 nodal recurrences of patients treated by neck dissection with or without complementary irradiation, 7 cases recovered, a global failure of 6%.

H. Final Synopsis of Conservating Surgery for Carcinoma of the Larynx

Resumé of the Course on Conservation Surgery for Carcinoma of the Larynx, Erlangen 1982

G. P. TEATINI, Ferrara

The organizing committee had intended that the last round table should be a kind of resumé of the whole course, shedding light on the points which both gained unanimous consensus and gave rise to controversy. To this purpose, an unusually high number of panelists were coopted and the chairman was asked to touch as many topics as the allotted time permitted. The chairman and the co-chairman had prepared a list of 8 questions, but only the following 5 could be discussed.

The first question, which was put especially to the pathologists, was:

1. "Do you consider that conservative surgery of laryngeal tumours builds upon clear pathological grounds, or is it mainly a heuristic procedure, viz. based on favourable clinical results?"

The surgical excision of a cancer is still guided by the well-established principle of the safety distance. In other words, during removal, a coat of healthy tissue must surround the tumour in order to be sure that no remnants have been left behind. The breadth of such a coat varies from tumour to tumour and from organ to organ.

Neoplasms of the same histological type, such as squamous cell carcinomas, which represent the object of this surgery in the great majority of instances, may require different safety distances according to their different kinds of proliferation. A deep infiltrating cancer, for example, often has an indented growth front which obliges one to place the excision line farther off. In the larynx the tumour expansion may be hindered in some places by the presence of anatomical barriers, like cartilage, muscles or ligaments. In such cases the safety distances may be legitimately reduced, providing that the barrier itself has not been invaded.

Therefore, conservative surgery of laryngeal tumours seems to be fully justified from the point of view of the pathologists. Of course, a partial resection demands accurate histological controls of the specimen margins. In this context two requirements were emphasized: the need for a strict cooperation between surgeon and pathologist and for more indepth investigations into the modalities of tumour expansion.

2. "Which are the main prerequisites for the success of conservative procedures from a surgeon's point of view?"

A proper selection of patients was unanimously considered the most important element. The indications and contraindications of each procedure are very specific. One must know them perfectly and apply them rigidly to each single case. When this does not take place, i.e. indications are broadened or modified to fit the individual case, a disaster can be expected. The motto "life is more important than voice" should always be present in the surgeon's mind.

Modern technology has provided us with multifarious tools that, in most patients, permit an extremely precise preoperative assessment. And yet the surgeon must be ready to change his programme according to the peroperative findings, whether endoscopical or pathological (frozen sections).

Other elements which pave the way for the success of conservative procedures are:

thorough mastery of the techniques which are, in general, more difficult than radical surgery;
careful respect for the limits of each procedure, avoiding personal modifications and interpretations not supported by long clinical experience;
facility for meticulous patient follow-up, which must be carried out by a very skillful person at regular time intervals, thus supplying long-term feedback as to results.

One main difficulty is the exact choice of the first procedure which always conditions the whole course of the disease. In many cases radiotherapy may be a valuable alternative to surgery. The dilemma between treatments cannot be solved on the basis of firm guidelines, since it depends on personal convictions and previous experience.

Finally, two requirements were stressed:
the incidence of conservative surgery could be significantly raised if laryngeal cancer were diagnosed earlier. This might occur by improving both our technical tools and patients' health education;
investigations into new surgical procedures must be pursued with special emphasis not only on pathology but also on physiology, especially of deglutition and phonation.

3. "Two statements about functional surgery of laryngeal cancer are often considered as rules: according to the first, advanced age should be a contraindication. Do you agree?"

Such a rule can be disregarded, especially if one takes into account not the chronological but the biological age. Nevertheless, those procedures, such as horizontal supraglottic laryngectomy, which involve major rehabilitation effort require some caution in very old patients.

4. "The second statement says: a failure of conservative surgery should never be treated by a second conservative procedure, but rather by radical surgery. Do you agree?"

This was probably the question which brought forth the greatest diversity in opinions. Starting from the unconditional "yes" of Alonso and Calearo, who consider radiotherapy the only viable alternative to total laryngectomy after a failure, we pass through many nuances to less categorical answers. In selected cases, providing the extent of the growth can be accurately assessed (which may be difficult in a previously operated larynx), the majority of the panelists seemed not to exclude – and

Steiner definitely approved – the possibility of a second conservative approach, especially when one is not dealing with a residual or recurring, but rather with a new primary tumour.

The distinction between these two conditions is rarely easy. When the growth is to be found within or quite close to the region of surgery and is surrounded by scar tissue, it is likely that this is a recurrence or a residual tumour; in all other cases it can be considered as a second primary cancer.

5. "The treatment of neck is an important stage in the treatment of most laryngeal cancers. Do you employ
a) classical (radical) or functional,
b) elective (prophylactic) or curative neck dissection?"

In regard to the first subquestion, the choice between the two procedures depends on the surgeon's conviction and skill, since both are equally indicated in N_0 and N_1 cases. Functional neck dissection is technically more difficult, but in experienced hands it may be preferred in the aforesaid instances, given the advantages it secures. On the whole, functional neck dissection seems to have gained popularity in recent years.

When the tumour has broken the lymphnode capsule, a classical neck dissection must be carried out. However, the prognosis is then extremely poor: Calearo reported only a 10% 6-year-survival in supraglottic T_{2-3} N_3, treated with horizontal supraglottic laryngectomy and neck dissection in association with radiotherapy.

The second subquestion, regarding elective versus curative neck dissection, is much more controversial. By rights it was remarked that when a problem has been debated for more than 40 years without having found an appropriate solution, it is highly probable that there is no solution.

To briefly review the answers, Alonso, Kirchner, Neel and Piquet were explicit about their use of elective surgery in all cases with a high tendency to metastatization, viz. supraglottic tumours. Olofsson favours prophylactic irradiation. The chairman reported that in the Ferrara Clinic, where elective neck dissection was previously the rule, a trial was started in 1981, based upon a randomization of N_0 patients, half of whom are prophylactically operated, while the remainder is being clinically controlled and submitted to curative surgery whenever necessary. The behaviour of Erlangen Clinic was detailed by Steiner: in supraglottic T_1 and in glottic T_{1-4}, in the absence of palpable lymphnodes, a simple peroperative inspection of the jugular chain is performed. In all other cases, with the obvious exception of N_3, an elective functional neck dissection is executed, but it is limited to the anterior neck triangle. Only when routine peroperative histology reveals a tumour, is the dissection extended to the posterior neck triangle and the supraclavicular fossa.

Most panelists employ postoperative irradiation in the case of N_+. Preoperative irradiation in the presence of fixed lymphnodes was advocated by Neel.

At the close, the chairman remarked that the whole course, as well as this round table, had clearly demonstrated that functional surgery has today gained full citizenship among the methods for curing laryngeal cancers. A few decades ago, absolute radicality was imperative, with the single exception of laryngofissure cordectomy. Then some pioneers broke these fetters and several procedures started being applied. At least one of these, horizontal supraglottic laryngectomy, has enjoyed worldwide acceptance.

However, a further step has begun. Other pioneers (among them mainly the Erlangen team) have shown that an endoscopical treatment is feasible in selected patients and that this approach is also valuable as palliation. Even those who are not ready to follow this new trend should look charitably upon the efforts of these people who are striving to improve the quality of life of patients suffering from laryngeal cancer.

L. Michaels

Pathology of the Larynx

1984. 222 figures. Approx. 385 pages
ISBN 3-540-13237-6

Contents:
- The Normal Larynx
- Non-Neoplastic Lesions
- Squamous Cell Neoplasms
- Non-Epidermoid Neoplasms
- Subject Index

From the Preface:

"The purpose of this work is to review the current knowledge of laryngeal pathology...

The role of histopathological investigations in the care of patients with diseases of the larynx is given special consideration. Radiological study of the larynx has become more refined in recent years with the introduction of computerised tomography. Microlaryngoscopy with biopsy of the interior of the larynx is now a frequent procedure in the diagnosis of laryngeal disease. In the effort to interpret the findings from these methods, the need for a monograph outlining the pathological basis of laryngeal disorders has arisen..."

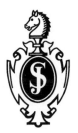

Springer-Verlag
Berlin
Heidelberg
New York
Tokyo

The Management of Head and Neck Cancer

With Contributions by L.W. Brady, S.K. Choksi, L.W. Davis, J.B. Drane, J.E. Hamner III., D.P. Shedd

Editor: **J.E. Hamner III**

1984. Approx. 250 figures. Approx. 320 pages. ISBN 3-540-13279-1

Contents:
- Introduction
- Etiology and Epidemiology
- Detection
- Diagnosis
- Pretreatment Evaluation
- Treatment
- Follow-Up
- Rehabilitation
- Series of Case Examples
- Subject Index

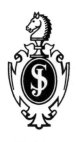

Springer-Verlag
Berlin
Heidelberg
New York
Tokyo

Printed by Publishers' Graphics LLC USA
MO20120905-307